Diary of a Detour

WRITING MATTERS!
A series edited by Lauren Berlant, Saidiya Hartman,
Erica Rand, and Kathleen Stewart

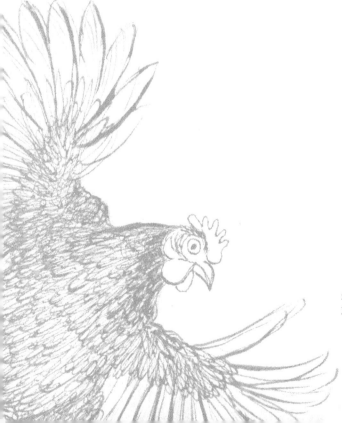

DUKE UNIVERSITY PRESS
Durham and London   2020

Diary of
a Detour

Lesley Stern

With illustrations by Amy Adler

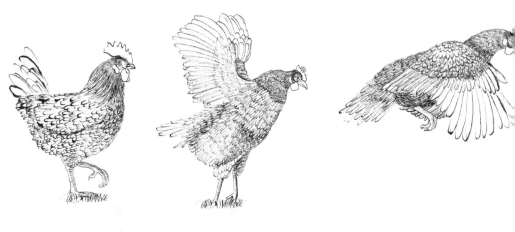

Designed by Courtney Leigh Richardson
Typeset in Whitman by Copperline Book Services

Library of Congress Cataloging-in-Publication Data
Names: Stern, Lesley, author. | Adler, Amy, illustrator.
Title: Diary of a detour / Lesley Stern ; with illustrations by Amy Adler.
Other titles: Writing matters! (Duke University Press)
Description: Durham : Duke University Press, 2020. | Series:
Writing matters! | Includes bibliographical references.
Identifiers: LCCN 2019054737 (print)
LCCN 2019054738 (ebook)
ISBN 9781478008811 (hardcover)
ISBN 9781478009672 (paperback)
ISBN 9781478012290 (ebook)
Subjects: LCSH: Stern, Lesley. | Chronic lymphocytic leukemia—Patients—
Biography. | Authors, Australian—20th century—Biography. | Chronic
lymphocytic leukemia—Treatment. | Cancer—Psychological aspects.
Classification: LCC PR9619.3.S796 Z46 2020 (print) |
LCC PR9619.3.S796 (ebook) | DDC 828/.9303 [B]—dc23
LC record available at https://lccn.loc.gov/2019054737
LC ebook record available at https://lccn.loc.gov/2019054738

COVER ART: Chickens for Lesley © Amy Adler 2019.
Courtesy of the artist.

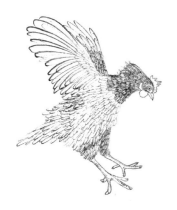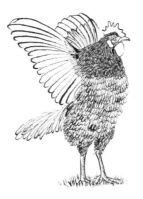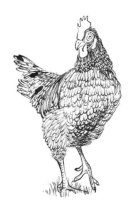

IN MEMORY OF THOSE, *dear to me, who died during the writing of this book. With some I traveled fleetingly, others have shared many journeys and detours, all have made my life, and* Diary, *richer.*

Miriam Hansen	*Paul Willemen*	*Ryoko Amani Geoken*
Milane Christiansen	*Jack Counihan*	*Bengitj Ngurruwuthun*
Christine Alavi	*Fran Ruda*	*Peter Casey*
Viv Kondos	*Sylvia Lawson*	*Scott Nygren*
Martin Harrison	*David Antin*	*Elvis, the King of the Cats*

Contents

Acknowledgments

Jeffrey Minson: For everything, always.

Genevieve Lloyd came up with the perfect title, for which I am very grateful, as well as for the many long walks and talks about writing and politics and other things.

For many years Amy Adler and I talked, as we perused the antics of the chickens, about her doing drawings for the book. In the end she acted swiftly and generously, when she should have been on holiday relaxing. Her drawings are perfect. Thank you, Amy.

This book took shape over many years, and many people have read and contributed comments and ideas that have shaped the final version. It began life as a blog, and many unnamed friends contributed; I appreciate every comment. In particular I would like to acknowledge the generous engagement and writing friendship of John Frow, Leslie Dick, Eleanor Bluestein, Tracy Cox-Stanton, Eileen Myles, and Amelie Hastie. Others read carefully and commented astutely and helpfully on parts of the book: Jane Goodall, Katrin Pesch, Anne Freadman, Patricia Montoya, Lesley Ruda, Erica David, and the four anonymous readers of the manuscript for Duke University Press. For help with the science-related aspects of this book I am indebted to Chandra Mukerjee, Donna Haraway, and Curt Wittenberg. In particular, Curt, a molecular geneticist and cheese-making and fermentation co-conspirator, read a lot and was both critically helpful and always encouraging. Needless to say, they are not responsible for any relapses from the truth.

I was fortunate, during the writing of some of this book, to belong to a wide-ranging, floating, group of writers interested in writing as a process of both worlding and negotiating the parameters between fiction and criticism: Katie Stewart,

Allen Shelton, Lauren Berlant, Anna Tsing, Donna Haraway, Susan Harding, Stephen Muecke. From each and every one of them I have learned so much.

Without the encouragement and support of friends who helped in a variety of ways—from flying across the world to making meals to driving me to the hospital, sitting with me during chemo, suggesting crucial things to read, pruning and weeding my garden, bringing pictures and other gifts to brighten dark days—this book would never have materialized. My thanks to all of them, but above all to Helen Barnes and Lesley Ruda.

I have been incredibly lucky to have the incomparable Dr. Thomas Kipps, at UCSD Health, as my CLL oncologist. Without him I doubt I would have had the energy to write this book. I cannot thank him enough and, also, his team: Drs. Michael Choi and Januario Castro and Research Nurse Sheila Hoff, an extraordinarily informative and supportive resource. Dr. Marlene Millen, my primary care physician, is one of a kind, always there, an inspiration and constant support. The infusion team at Hillcrest UCSD Hospital are simply great; what better tribute can I offer than to say I look forward to seeing them every month: Amelita Angkianco, Desirée–the Queen–Valdez, Marcie Diamond, Bill Sleeman, Risé Thompson.

Thanks to my colleagues and students at the Universities of UCSD and Monash. Also to Yoke-Sum Wong and Craig Campbell for inviting me to participate in the "Ex-situ" event at UT Austin, involving a Texas road trip that propelled the book in new directions.

Stretches of time at Dorland Mountain Arts Colony—a magical place presided over by magic makers Janice Cipriani-Willis and Robert Willis—enabled me to make progress with the writing. I was able to finish a good draft of the book in another magical place, Marfa, Texas, thanks to a writing fellowship from the Lannan Foundation.

Lauren Berlant, Saidiya Hartmann, Erica Rand, and Katie Stewart invited *Diary of a Detour* to be part of their series, "Writing Matters!," for Duke University Press. I am honored to be the first book in their series and look forward to more in this terrific initiative. Ken Wissoker has been welcoming, and I am grateful to the entire crew at Duke for making this a pleasurable process.

A version of "Touched by a Whale" was first published in *Feelings of Structure: Explorations in Affect*, edited by Karen Engle and Yoke-Sum Wong (Montreal: McGill-Queen's University Press, 2018), 99–105. "Companion Pieces Written through a Drift" (written with Kathleen Stewart) was first published in *Sensitive Objects: Affects and Material Culture*, edited by Jonas Frykman and Maja Povrzanović (Lund: Nordic Academic Press, 2016), 257–72, and draws on the Texas stories in *Diary*. A version of "Chicken Feet" was published as "Becoming Chicken," in *Vlak: Contemporary Poetics and the Arts* (2015), 532–33.

Chickens Saved My Life

1

Chickens changed my life. Saved my life. Though it is also true to say that as we ride the stormy waves of birth, old age, sickness, and death, many things, people, and events change what we call *life*. A life is merely a conglomeration, a concatenation of effects and affects, often unpredictable, though even when predicted, things seldom turn out as expected.

And it was not by chickens alone that I have been saved. But among all the therapies—chemo, meditation, acupuncture, Feldenkrais, naturopathic treatments, exercise—chickens, four glorious chicklets-becoming-hens, have changed things most dramatically. Holly, Lula Mae, Sabrina, and Funny Face flap, flutter, and jump onto anything that might resemble a perch, including human shoulders and heads. They frequently land together on one side of their feeder and tip it over. They also landed like a miracle, about six weeks ago, on me, and tipped the balance from death to life.

I have an incurable cancer, a form of leukemia called CLL (chronic lymphocytic leukemia), so like everyone else I am going to die but probably not tomorrow. Still, life was becoming rather hard to live. Now, after spending the summer in chemo-and-chicken therapy, I have been given a reprieve. I have been wanting chickens for years, and for years have been putting it off, there were always other things to do, work to get done, fetish desires to satisfy. CLL is one of the slow cancers. For some people it does not progress beyond what used to be called the indolent stage, for others it can race along alarmingly fast for a slow cancer. My symptoms just got gradually worse, though I wanted to defer treatment for as long as possible since once you start treatment you also start damaging your body's ability to fight back.

As my oncologist, Dr. K, says, there are no such things as side effects. All drugs have a range of effects, some good, some not so good (and sometimes the connection between good and not so good is knotted, complicated, measurable only over time). So when he said, I think it's time to start treatment and I saw the summer disappearing into an infusion center, the absolute ghastliness of my condition (so far no treatments have lengthened life for CLL patients) took hold, gloom defeated a habitual Pollyanna-ish reflex. And then, in the midst of gloom, my thoughts turned to chickens. Chickens turned into obsession.

Soon I could think of nothing but breeds of chickens and what color eggs they lay and coops and ventilation and chicken manure and compost and predators and fencing and automatic watering and mites and fleas and worms and herbal remedies, and the chirruping noise that chicks make. I dreamed of collecting fresh eggs from free-ranging chickens fed on weeds and greens and fruit from the garden. I could smell the omelets made from these eggs, buttery and sizzling, sprinkled with herbs. I could also smell the chicken shit and rapturously and endlessly imagined the compost we would have, how contentedly my garden would grow. J, my partner, embraced the idea even more wholeheartedly than I, encouraging a flagrant defiance of budget in order to get the project happening. I spent endless hours on the internet, ordering books from the library, reading back copies of *Backyard Poultry*, visiting friends and perfect strangers with hens in their yard. Planning in minute and exacting detail. My treatment lasted three months, and some of that time was spent backbreakingly (not me) and obsessively (me) assembling *el palacio de las princesas*, so named by my friend Isabel. And then the ordering. And then the arrival one morning, through the mail, of a cardboard box containing four day-old chicks. Through all this demented focusing on chickens I had been feeling not too bad, forgetting the "C" word. And now my forgetfulness morphed into full-blown happiness. We started laughing. The tiny chicks are fluffy and adorable but also absurd in their pomposity. As the chicks grow their absurdity expands, keeping us laughing, tickling a severely compromised immune system, kicking it into gear.

Two weeks ago I saw Dr. K, and he told me what I already knew, could feel, that so far the results are good. This isn't the end of the story; there will be more tests and more treatment sooner or later. But for the moment I'm feeling better than in years and it feels extraordinary, though I guess it's actually normality that I'm feeling.

This book was sprung into being by the chickens, and it will follow, through many detours, the ways that a vague idea becomes focused as a consuming passion. It's also about other things: just as a life can be changed by a chromosome going awry, so it can be transformed by a chicken, or a book that one is reading, or a feral plant that takes root in your garden and slowly grows into an intriguing presence, altering the culture of the garden and making you see and feel differently.

The Time It Takes
(By Way of an Introduction)

2

If I write in order to fend off the feelings of isolation and uncertainty that chronic illness can foster, I write for other reasons too, some merely neurotic, some to do with the pleasure afforded by any addiction, and for some reasons (though *reason* seems far too grand a concept) to do with a sense that putting into words this thing called illness produces a materiality, albeit chimeric and diaphanous, something that can spark recognition, something that can be passed from hand to hand, blown through the air or kicked from one place to another.

Diaries are generally chronological, moving forward in a relatively straight line. This one deviates from the straight and narrow, and is not really a diary, more like a series of meditations, stories, excursions, escapes, tirades, and pirouettes. Nevertheless, it shares some features with the genre of the diary. It began as a blog, written sporadically to inform friends of how treatment was going, asking for a ride to the hospital or setting up a rota for meals. Gradually, as my health improved, some of these entries began to take shape as small essays, or ruminations, they became detached from the blog and morphed into a book. This involved a shifting of the "I," a transition from very personalized and banal reportage to the emergence on stage of a more dramatized, a more fictional "I."

While *Detour* does not, then, follow the path of a disease, step by step, nevertheless a bit of a chronology might be useful, a map, a background against which to read the excursions and meddling with time. I was diagnosed with CLL in 2008. A new primary care physician, MM, asked me about fatigue. Yes, I said, but there are probably reasons for that. Work. Let's do some blood tests, she said. In fact she knew, as she later told me, what to expect because, when she became my doctor she looked over my record and saw that since 2004 my white blood count had been high. This was before you could see your test results online and you (or I) took the doctor's word that everything was fine. I saw a hematologist who referred me to Dr. K, a leading researcher in CLL and very fortunately for me located at the university where I worked in San Diego. Three years later I began my first chemotherapy, a combination of high-dose prednisone, a steroid that slows or stops the immune system processes that trigger inflammation, and Rituximab (both taken as infusions). Rituximab is not actually a chemotherapy, it is an immunotherapy, but generally the treatments are referred to here, and more generally (at the hospital, for instance, by the insurance companies), as chemo. Two years after that, in 2013, I had my second treatment (as part of a trial)—a combination of Rituximab (taken as an infusion) and Revlimid (taken orally, as a pill). Revlimid, an immunomodulatory agent, was seen as a twofer: it was hoped that, in addition to acting on the CLL, it would also promote immunity. There was no expectation that any of these treatments would produce a cure. There was hope, though, that they might provide temporary relief from the symptoms and partial remission.

This book begins with the first treatment in 2011, since at that point something other than medicine entered significantly into the treatment. Call it chickens, or call it obsession, or call it a detouring away from the medicalization of cancer, a deflection from immersion in the idea of illness. The book takes off, however, two years later with my second chemo treatment in 2013. It ends in 2018, ten years after diagnosis (and after fourteen years of living chronically with CLL).

In this account it is illness that determines the march of time, but the chronology is not entirely indicative of the way the book unfolds. People often speak of a cancer journey or, more specifically and in my case, of the CLL journey. Although I recognize that analogy, I bridle against the habit illness has of commandeering attention, and even while this book aims to put into words the experiential dimension of CLL, that very project entails a shadow boxing with the phantoms of illness, a deploying of tricks to nudge the self-importance of cancer, now and then, into the background. There are other backgrounds that sometimes leap forward into sharp relief and speak to obsessives of various stripes—gardeners, for instance, food aficionados, fermentation freaks, travelers and fellow travelers, cat lovers, bookworms, straying Buddhists, and pedantic amateur scientists. Not that it is always a matter of trickery. Once you start writing, the writing escapes your grasp; like an octopus it slithers out of its cage and spreads tentacles in diverse and unexpected directions.

If there is a tension that animates the book, between time as a chronology, where events are narrated sequentially, and time as a time-out, where sensations and feelings expand the experience of the moment, the minute, the hour, there is also a tension between language that evokes and lives in details of the everyday and the language of science. These different registers can be read as speaking to one another, as a blurring of the categories of science and affect or emotion. Or the pieces that privilege one mode or the other can be read entirely separately (though they do have a habit of interrupting each other), you can jump around, skip chunks, circle back.

One way I found of fighting off the imperiousness of the malady was paradoxically to enter further into the lairs of medicine, to try to develop at least a rudimentary grasp of the science of CLL or, more generally, of cancer. Science is mysterious to me, slippery and evasive. So grappling with this, putting it into words, was an invigorating challenge, and needless to say, in the process, I felt that the knowledge I was acquiring was giving me a modicum of decision-making power, power over my future, and a way of communicating with others in the same boat. Is that feeling real or illusory? This is one of the questions threaded in a ghostly form through *Diary of a Detour*. The more I delved into the scientific, the more I found that awe was being ruffled by skepticism. The skepticism is not ranged against science as such, but against the way science can be used and against the extreme medicalization of cancer in our culture. By *medicalization* I mean the impulse to describe its causes, origins, trajectories, and treatments in primarily medical terms. What other language might there be? What ways of evoking the feelings and sensations that one might experience; what ways might there be to think about cancer not in terms of a war waged by the wonders of medicine against a foreign invader, but as something that arises in the body and is a part of life? How to shift or at least shake up the idea of living with a chronic illness, to think about living itself as a chronic condition, not a fortress armed against death?

In a fanciful rather than scientific gesture Plato defined the human being as "a biped without feathers." It tickled my fancy, this aphoristic description of the human being. There are occasions when I experience myself becoming chicken, and there are times when a chicken takes it into their head to become human. This makes for stories. But it also provokes me to think about the process of domestication and how this relates to boundaries, parameters, borders. I was born and grew up in Zimbabwe (though then it was Rhodesia) and lived for many years in Australia. I now live in the U.S. city of San Diego, a city on the border with Mexico, where I also spend time. This peripatetic life has nurtured both a yen for travel and a meditating on borders. Where does one country end and another begin, what is it that makes a difference between a well body and a sick one, how do you distinguish between species that interact and depend on one another in intricate and complex ways, how do the dead speak to the living? During domestication humans change animals and plants through artificial selection, but the process of domestication also changes us, genetically and socially. In some ways my dance with CLL is akin to this reciprocal process of domestication. It begins in wildness and evolves into an attempt to tame and contain the dragon. In some ways the attempt works, in other ways, not. The CLL also tames or shapes me, alerts me to new modes of inquiry. Similarly, I make use of chickens, but as is often the case they turn out to make use of me, to shape the writing and thinking in ways I did not anticipate or envisage.

Being a chronic condition, CLL doesn't go away, but there are quasi remissions when you can up sticks and fly away to new adventures. The book itself can take wing, and on occasion it flies away from San Diego to places far and near. But then there are missteps, the symptoms creep back, gradually the fatigue begins to permeate your every moment, you succumb to infections, some virulent, you dodge death threats, and you realize there's no getting off the bus. On the other hand, here I am, after fourteen years, still going. In the meantime various friends or people who have inspired me on the CLL trip and side trips have died—some suddenly and without warning. The first to go was my friend Miriam, who died after I was diagnosed but a few months before my first treatment began. I wrote a small piece when she died, and I include it in the book, even though it falls outside the time frame, because I learned from her, and from writing about and to her, not exactly how to face death but how to live, how to get on with life. The book is punctuated by addresses to or about friends or people, dead and alive, who have at some stage mattered to me or who shared the journey or parts of it. If there are hungry ghosts haunting this book there are also spirits who inspire. There is no ravine separating the dead and the living, health and illness, animals and humans, chickens and microbes. And so dead ones and animals and plants animate this writing as much as humans and those alive.

The sequence is ruffled because it is not in fact a sequence; or, as one might say, it is not, in the end, the illness that determines the trajectory. Correspondingly, the map encompasses more than lines. The squiggles, veers from the straight and narrow, ideas that grow in the writing and career into obsessional cannonballs— all these excursions embody the energetic impulse of the detour. In the end, and from the beginning, it is the detour rather than the journey that embodies and mobilizes the way time is experienced in this book. Hence: Diary of a Detour.

Secret

3

It is 1958. She is eight years old, bored, waiting in the car on a hot day. They have come into town from the farm, she waits while her mother nips in to see her grandmother in her office. She says she will only be a moment. The moment grows longer and longer, boredom expands like oil in a hot pan, it spreads, the car is cloaked in oily viscosity. She suspects that behind closed doors her mother and grandmother are arguing. She does not know what it is that they argue about, but she does know her mother will return flushed and irritable, frayed, untouchable. Unspeakable to.

Then there is a tap at the window. She has been warned never to wind down the window and talk to strangers, but this woman is not exactly a stranger, she and her husband have a farm in the same part of the country as her family. She is pretty and has two young children. The girl has never seen her like this: distraught, her hair in disarray, cheeks streaked, eyes reddened and mascara smudged. "Where is your mother?" Her voice is jagged; the question, an appeal. "I have to run; everyone is waiting, but tell your mother something for me. Tell her . . . tell her I've got cancer. Do you understand?" She says this—do you understand—in a tone of acerbic despair, as though she knows no one will ever understand, least of all this child. And yet it is important that she understand, she is the one chosen to be the bearer of knowledge, the one charged with a secret. "Don't tell anyone else, just your mother; this is a secret, but you must tell your mother. Only your mother."

The woman leaves, the car turns cold and clammy. Eventually her mother returns, flushed and irritable. "Don't talk to me," she says. The girl rehearses how to say it, she does not know what it is, this thing called *cancer* that the woman has. Where did she get it? Did she buy it, or was it given to her, where does she have it, in her purse, in a safe with her jewels, tucked into her bra with a spare five-pound note for emergencies? But she senses that to say the word entails repercussions. She knows the news she has to impart is lethal. Eventually she whispers to her mother, so as not to crack the brittleness of the air. "I have a secret to tell you," she whispers. "Not now," the mother snaps. Head on the steering wheel, hands in her hair, pulling. Then, more gently, though still exasperated by the demands of the child, "Later, tell me later."

But later never comes. She tries but cannot find the moment, the right moment when she can say the word, pass on the secret. The word becomes cheeselike, heavy and sweaty in her pocket, it grows moldy, accruing guilt. The secret stays with her.

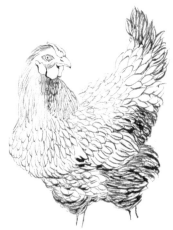

A Possum Fate (Averted)   4

I am woken by a screeching and flapping, the air vibrating, dinosaurs returned to the earth.

Finishing round one of the seven-month regime. I have been taking a daily dose of Revlimid for three weeks (the regime is three weeks on, one week off, during which there are Rituximab infusions). Apart from fatigue, sometimes overwhelming, other things have been manageable, including a rash that came and went. But then last weekend it turned into serious torment. The hospital team determined it was a reaction to either the Revlimid or one of the drugs given to fight the effects of the Revlimid (probably the latter). Since I'd stopped the Revlimid the other drugs were discontinued, but the torment continued. Drinking ginger tea was a comfort, but not a cure. The only thing that gave some relief is a narcotic. This is fine at night, not too good when you have to work. Monday I worked till mid-afternoon, came home, took the drowsy pill, conked out. Surfaced just before Judit, bearing chicken soup, came to fetch me for our Feldenkrais class. The class was, as always, succor for body and soul. I lay on the floor, moved minutely, and every so often dozed off. An hour later at home, heating up the chicken soup, I hear an almighty kerfuffling in the yard, much screeching and flapping, the air vibrating, dinosaurs returned to the earth.

Two of the live chickens (as opposed to the chicken in the soup) were careening around the yard. I grabbed a flashlight and broomstick and staggered out. The door to their run was wide open, and so were all the doors to their little house. One of us had forgotten to lock them in for the night. There in their house taking up most of the floor was a possum, an unusually pretty possum, tan and grey. And just above the possum was Sabrina on her perch, shivering and shaking, silenced. With the aid of a broomstick I edged the possum out. He slipped down the ramp to the ground, gliding with greater elegance than the hens ever do; they slither and hop and stomp down the ramp to freedom every morning. I had to chase the possum into the vegetable garden away from the other two chickens and away from Sabrina, who was now performing in the yard like a yoyo emitting strangled clucks. Then I sat on the ground and lowered my weapons and listened to my own heart emitting strangled clucks. Chickens can't see in the dark, which means it is sometimes very easy to pick them up and sometimes impossible if they are in panic. Holly and Sabrina stopped running, and I cooed to them, making the chicken lullaby sounds they know from nighttime, when we do the final lock and check. Holly is the sook, and so she was, I think, calmed by being picked up and cuddled and stroked and returned to her house. Sabrina next, no problem. Funny Face next. Then Lula Mae, the little wild one who disdains human contact, did not wish to be touched or returned. Every time I approached, crouched and cooing, she would be propelled from her own crouching position into a feathered ball of fury, flying through the air away from the chicken run. Half an hour of cooing, begging, reprimanding, and cursing ensued, half an hour of stalking and stumbling. Adrenalin had expelled all narcotic effects, and the drama suppressed the itching. Eventually I held Lula Mae in my two hands, feathered lightning condensed into a solid little body. Finally they were all back home, all doors sealed, a possum fate averted.

At last I got to eat my chicken soup.

The next day off we go, J and I, to the hospital for the first infusion of Rituximab. I have had this drug before, about eighteen months ago, and tolerated it fairly well. Today it goes slowly but uneventfully. Five hours or so after I arrive, the little packet on the IV stand is nearly empty. Then I start shivering. The PAS (physician assistants) are there straightaway, and lots of nurses and what they call "the kit." Don't worry they say, you've got the chills, it's a common reaction, we are going to give you a drug and then you might sweat and it'll be OK. In a flash something shifts, blackness encroaching, panic, as though there were a possum in the room. I remember saying, I feel really bad. "What sort of bad?" someone asks. But I just feel the tar pits opening up and the possum lurking and can't speak. The next thing I remember is the doctor shouting at me, "Open your eyes! Open your eyes! Look at me!" and all I want to do is sink back into oblivion. Then time seemed to go very slowly, and after a while they said, "You can close your eyes now and relax." When I asked what happened they said, "You gave us a fright, you just lost consciousness, and then you stopped breathing."

So for the next infusion, two days later, they fiddled with the cocktail, added some stuff (steroids), changed the secondaries (the drugs that guard against the side effects). I was really scared this time, like I have never been before. I think that J was even more scared. He said it was really terrifying when I lost consciousness and stopped breathing and the room was suddenly full of doctors, technicians, and machines. It was much more terrifying for him than for me—I didn't know what was happening and couldn't see anything. I am glad he was there.

It went very slowly but without drama. And same yesterday. Yesterday was Sunday, nice and quiet in the infusion center. They had to change me from Saturday to make sure there was an oncologist on duty. My nurse said, "Glad to meet you, you are the Blue Code Lady." Blue code, she tells me, is when a patient stops breathing.

The itching has stopped. I continue the infusions tomorrow. And then restart the Revlimid. We hope the rash and itching will not start up again. If it does it means it's the Revlimid and treatment will have to stop. If it doesn't it means the "side effect" is caused by the anti-side-effect drug. I hope it's not the Revlimid. Despite the horror of all these chemicals and the dubious ways they change your body and the fact that this drug is in the experimental stage for CLL, I remember what it was like to have more than a year of partial remission, to feel normal, to wake each morning with energy. And I want to be there again.

Events Unfold in the Snow

5

(*for Miriam*)

Events unfold in the snow. The bare black winter trees echo the straight edges of the frame, it is a perfect composition in black and white, artistically monochromatic. This prologue is intriguing (we recognize the actor Javier Bardem, but there are no other narrative orientations), and for a few moments, though intrigued, I also feel prickled by the rather precious aestheticism of the setup, the painterliness. A young man, younger than Bardem, walks in out of the blue and into the snow just as Jane Greer walked in out of the sunlight in *Out of the Past*. Who is he? And why are they meeting, here, in a cold and lonely place? There are no smiles, no greetings, no signs of familiarity. Is he a ghost, an assassin, a drug dealer, Alain Delon returned to exact revenge? There is a sliver of icy menace in the scene, a dead owl lying in the snow. The stranger warns Bardem that he should not wear a pony tail because he looks like a fox and will frighten the owls. Ah yes, says Bardem, I heard that story. A glimmer, memories stirring. And then the young man tells Bardem that he can make the sound of the wind. And he does, it is a magical moment as his face changes shape and sounds issue forth, and there is a cut to the snowy expansive space and the sound of the wind whistling through the landscape, through the permeable contours of the film screen, whistling and whirring through the film theater, into our bodies, waking us up. And then he imitates the sound of water, the gurgling gushing whooshing and sucking. Bardem asks him if he can do both sounds together. He can. And when he does, Bardem smiles. The smile cracks open his long granite face and simultaneously sunders the austere aesthetic verticality of the scene—the bare black columnar trees, the standing figures of the two men. The gravitas of his demeanor crumbles into rivulets of pleasure. And we laugh too, involuntarily, as though we have been tickled. We laugh with him, but we laugh too, I think, not simply out of recognition or iden-tification, but because the cinematic technology enervates our senses. The sound is at once human and inhuman, natural and unnatural, and mediated, produced through cinematic technology. We in the audience smile or laugh because we *see* and *sense* the act of making noise.

The smile, like the snow drifting very gently, eddying in small twirls, intro-duces movement, energetic sensation, into this aesthetic scene. It also initiates a discursive dramatization of cinema aesthetics which unfolds throughout this film. This film, *Biutiful*, in which there are very few laughs.

A few weeks before she died Miriam and I walked in the snow near where she lived in Chicago. She walked this route almost every day of her life in Chicago, through the Japanese garden, around the small lake, usually with her husband Michael. It was routine, and yet every time it was new, every time she discovered new things to delight in, new sensuous pleasures. That day was no exception. It was exhilarating and fun, and we laughed at new leaves improbably emerging on dead twigs, the young men improvising a skating rink on the lake, the sound and touch of the softly drifting snow. We argued about the names of the wild flowers that grow in this urban space. And we talked of what would happen to her ashes, and what we would cook for dinner (anticipating a tussle over the exact timing of the beans—*about* three minutes, or, two minutes and forty-five seconds *exactly*), and of the book Miriam had finished, and how her ideas had changed over the years; how, in her close and long and attentively detailed attention to the three old blokes (my term, not hers of course)—Adorno, Kracauer, and Benjamin—her un-derstanding of aesthetics had mutated. Of course, what she has done in this book and in her other work is theorize for us new understandings of cinema aesthetics in a changing and globalized media landscape.

Just before coming to Chicago I had been in a Shambhala workshop in which we had been exploring the icon of the snow lion: on the banner a blue figure—a rather curious rendition of a lion, an Asiatic lion I guess, a lion with a snub nose—against a white background. Suddenly I understood: Miriam embodied this idea, as we walked in the snow—the combination of discipline and joy. And I under-stood her fanaticism or practices that I had often taken to be fanatic: her routines (yoga, diet, a programmed time to take a nap, massage, acupuncture, walking in the fresh air), her insistence, even when ill and feeling lousy and running a tem-perature, on sticking to routine. I understood then how that routine enabled joy and an opening into the world.

It was not a soothing experience to sit through this film, so soon after Miriam's death, this film in which a man dies slowly and painfully of cancer. And that's not all. The film heaps on misery and misfortune in piles, one shovelful after another, in your face. The melodrama is rather extreme. But the sensory excitation of that early snow scene seizes you by the skin and the nails, and reverberates through the film, as various threads unravel, spin out, weave together. Threads that are narrative but also (and not always coincidentally) more like the laughter and the wind and the water: sensations of movement, images that move through you, through the film and that gather like snow, forming new knowledges, ways of knowing.

Biutiful takes place in Barcelona, though not the Barcelona of *Vicky Cristina Barcelona*. It is a contemporary European city. Which is to say: a city no longer clearly defined by Europeanness, but one crossed, often contentiously and violently, by various vectors of migration. In this city Uxbal (Bardem) is a middleman. Living a marginal existence himself, he collects and distributes money, moving between various groups of illegal workers and their bosses and the forces of law and order. But as becomes the role of middleman he is also a mediator. While dodging between the police and the sweatshop owners and the illegal Chinese and African workers, he is a medium, a spirit medium. He can communicate with the dead and is able to ease the passage of a dead child who does not want to leave. Facing his own ghosts, though, turns out to be a bit more difficult.

Facing imminent death himself Uxbal also faces other deaths, or should we say that other deaths, spectral lives, rise up and insinuate themselves into his consciousness and the somatic consciousness of the film? The young man in the snow, it turns out, is the father he never knew who fled to Mexico from the Franco forces before Uxbal was born. In Mexico, where he died, the body was embalmed and then sent back across the sea, back to Spain. In his coffin, moving over the ocean, he hears the sound of the wind and the water. And now, many years later, Uxbal is being offered money for the *nicho*, the space the body occupies. The coffin is opened up so that the body of the father can be cremated. It is a shocking, almost-horror-movie moment in which recognition and misrecognition collide. The body has been uncannily preserved, but when Uxbal puts out a finger to touch the flesh it gives way. I think of Bill telling me how unnerving it was at the funeral to sit so close to the coffin and to (inescapably, involuntarily) think of Miriam's body in there. I think of friends who sat here in San Diego with Arsenio, who died a week before Miriam, the friends who took turns to sit for three days and nights by his body, helping to ease his passage to elsewhere, to reconcile their own feelings of confusion and loss. I hear Ariana in the theater next to me let out an exclamation. Later she tells me that this is the cemetery in which her mother is buried.

The uncanny exchange between body and phantom, flesh and memory, image and flesh. This I think is what haunts us, causes that hollow pain in the solar plexus, the imagining of a body so vividly alive and now not alive. It is as though, like Uxbal, you reach out to touch, but instead of encountering solidity things crumble.

Spain and Mexico. *Biutiful* recasts the old romantic story of the new world and the old. Just as it stirs the pot of hysteria that is materializing all over Europe (and the U.S.) about immigration, it returns to us as a material reminder (a body of proof) of Spain's own migrations and appropriations and enforced exiles and simultaneously complicates the story of a one-way street. Exile, invasion, inversion, appropriation, exploitation, compromise, refuge—all these vectors, and others, mark the globalized urbanity of the twenty-first century.

Uxbal's father emigrates to Mexico and returns as a corpse to Spain. A different Barcelona from the city he left. Miriam's ashes will return to Prague, a different Prague from that which her parents knew.

There is a devastating scene toward the end of the movie in which the bodies of a dozen or so Chinese workers are washed up by the sea, splayed out on a Barcelona beach. They are stone cold dead, all sounds of moving wind and water wrung out of their corpses. They have been dumped into the ocean in order to erase their presence and the crime. They were illegal immigrants employed in a basement sweatshop who die because of inadequate ventilation. Uxbal himself is implicated: in an act of concerned generosity he had provided the space heaters (during a freezing winter) that cause the suffocation. They have no legal status or presence in Barcelona, no families to mourn, it is easy to dump them like trash.

But they return. And Uxbal is wracked by remorse and grief, not only for the political enormity of the crime (and his implication in it, which becomes more contorted as the plot unravels; it is not easy to escape the tangled web of corruption) but also because of a personal relation. Lily, who had babysat his children, is among the dead, washed up on the shore still clutching her young child.

They do not laugh and gurgle and splutter and whistle, but their sounds of silence infiltrate the film. The corruption that sustains illegal immigration is made material in the sound of Uxbal's sobbing. Drowning out my own sobbing, and muffling that of the man behind me in the theater, and others all around.

As I watched this film Miriam was with me, I felt her presence and thought about what I learned from her, the kind of conversations we shared, all the feelings of love and friendship and separation. This is not a bad function for films to perform. But more than this it was Miriam's interest in film aesthetics that spoke to me through the film.

In the film Uxbal's father returns—as a man younger then Uxbal himself—not merely to haunt him, but also to lighten his life. Of course what Uxbal remembers is not a memory, but an imagining. And perhaps it is always this way, the dead haunt and persecute us but also ease the pain we survivors endure in that they lend us their whistling, and their words, out of which we weave new sensations. Part of me feels a terrible loss that I can never again call Miriam up and talk to her—about *Biutiful* for instance. Miriam had the capacity to listen and to read very closely and the tenacity and loyalty to keep conversations alive and lively. And so I will continue to talk to her, to imagine what she might say and to think through with her a whole range of intellectual problems but also shared pleasures of a quotidian kind: swimming, walking, eating, gossiping while driving, choosing colors, picking beans.

Siegfried Kracauer once said that "in a photograph a person's history is buried as if under a layer of snow"; in contrast, films "have an affinity, evidently denied to photography, for the continuum of life or the 'flow of life.'" Snow itself, however, is a very cinematic type of a thing, deployed both for its heaviness—to bury—and its lightness—to flutter; its propensity both to preserve and to instantiate movement, to manifest as a rippling of the air, the passing of time, the dissipation of matter. I think of Walter Benjamin and his collection of snow globes. I think of him dying, stateless, after having lived in exile for seven years in the border town of Portbou, about eighty miles north of Barcelona. I remember Miriam—who has done so much to preserve the spirit of Benjamin and to animate his work in a changing media landscape. I remember her that day we walked and talked in the snow. I wish I could encapsulate that memory in a snow globe, shake it up at will, use it as an antidote to grief. But somehow Miriam won't stay put, in one place, predictably globalized. She has more to say. Her voice, like the sounding of wind and water in *Biutiful*, continues to whistle and whirr through the permeable contours of the snow globe, infiltrating our somatic consciousness, waking us up.

Chicken Feet

Chicken feet. Becoming chicken feet. My hands: scaly, reptilian, taloned. The rash and pustules are drying out and sloughing off, flakes of brittle skin. There is a compulsion to pick and peel, this skin that is me, uncannily so—half dead and half alive. This body—alien, prehistoric. Palms upturned, my hands do not resemble hands. What I see are chicken feet like those bought from Curtis at the Hillcrest Sunday farmers' market, a bonus thrown in with the chicken, along with a few heads and giblets, to add to J's chicken stock.

I imagine how the cats, Elvis and Roxy, felt the first time they encountered the chickens. When we opened the door of their run so that they could range the yard, they stuck together and stayed close to home, moving in a mass, a singular feathery body, delicately pecking at this and that, determining what was tasty, where the bugs were. As the days passed, they grew bolder. Then they saw the cats. Curiosity killed the cat they say, but this time the curiosity was in the chickens. Intrigued by these new creatures they charged—en masse, all four of them—thundering down the yard, wings flapping, huge scaly taloned feet. Dinosaurs in flight. Imagine those talons ripping into flesh.

Layer after layer—though not smoothly, it's not as though there is a layer, as in a ream of paper, where you can shuffle and each piece of paper settles back into its own layer; no it's more like when, in the Los Laureles Canyon in Tijuana, mud—after a churning storm—dries and cracks and flakes when you walk on it, disintegrating. Nothing underneath, no topsoil. Let's stick with the saying anyway—layer after layer my skin peels away. What will be left? My hands will disappear into nothingness. I will be handless. And what will all the peeling away of the body reveal: a complex psyche? Not bloody likely. More likely just a skeletal claw, something resembling a chicken's foot. But without all the gristle and gelatinous support that makes for such delicious chicken soup.

Why Chickens, or Homage to Gloria

7

I remained loyal, as a man would to a bride whom his family received with open ridicule. Now it is my turn to wear the smile, as I listen to the enthusiastic cackling of urbanites, who have suddenly taken up the hen socially and who fill the air with the newfound ecstasy and knowledge and the relative charms of the New Hampshire Red and the Laced Wyandotte. You would think, from their nervous cries of wonder and praise, that the hen was hatched yesterday in the suburbs of New York, instead of in the remote past in the jungles of India.
—E. B. WHITE

Chickens are certainly in the air right now; you can hear them everywhere ruffling their feathers, chirruping and emitting alarmed raucous clucks as they lay their eggs; you can hear them in urban areas as well as farms throughout the country; you can hear and see them in the news, on websites, on Facebook. Forging communities, shaping identities, making people feel good about themselves, validating their farm-to-table authenticity. I like to think I am not merely part of a trend, party to a prevailing home-steady ethos. But such individuating is not new, or rather, the popularity of chickens—and along with it the desire to participate in the party but also simultaneously to set oneself apart as superior in terms of credentials, chicken acquaintance, and history—has happened before in this country.

E. B. White has a marvelous essay, "The Hen (An Appreciation)." I knew of him as the author of *Charlotte's Web* and the husband of Katharine White, a garden writer whom I revere, but I didn't know that, as well as being a quintessential New Yorker (and indeed an essayist at the *New Yorker* for many years), he was also a farmer and a chicken devotee. In this essay, written in 1944, he writes that the chicken has not always been in favor among city-bred people, but "Right now the hen is in favor. The war has deified her and she is the darling of the home front, feted at conference tables, praised in every smoking car, her girlish ways and curious habits the topic of many an excited husbandryman to whom yesterday she was a stranger without honor or allure."

When showing off the chickens, I am often compelled to insinuate into the conversation my long history with chickens, to make it clear that I am not merely a fly-by-night, an arriviste, a devotee of every passing fad. I hear my backyard tour segueing into braggadocio, but even as I hear myself I can't stop the train that's started relentlessly chugging along, assuring my captive audience of my superior credentials. The truth, however, is that although I have been around chickens, off and on, all my life and have indeed nurtured a great fondness for the chicken as a creature and for fresh eggs as one of the great benefits of being a human being (or a raccoon or a snake), I have never before been so involved, engaged, consumed in the project of chickening. Mostly this has been a matter of timing. I had been wanting and hoping for chickens ever since living in San Diego and having more yard space. I arrived here after ten years of living in Bondi Beach, Sydney, surely the most desirable place in the world to live. But there I lived in a small rented apartment, no chicken or garden space. Here, I traded the beach for a garden.

Then I got ill. Or, rather, was diagnosed with CLL that slowly progressed and so began the years of declining energy and fluctuating symptoms. It was when things got a bit worse and I faced the second chemo treatment that I turned to chickens. And at the same time, or perhaps it wasn't coincidental, backyard chickens were coming into vogue. There I was slap bang in the middle of the zeitgeist.

One day I found myself musing upon the two banana trees, gorgeous trees that endowed the garden with tropical opulence and proffered leaves for wrapping tamales and fish. One yielded small red bananas, the other, tasty yellow bananas. Theoretically yielded. In fact we had had very few crops. One day, fixing a tear in the automatic drip system, I sat back on my haunches and gazed upon the banana trees. "You guys take up a lot of space," I said, sadly. And water. And suddenly, like a bolt from the blue, an image appeared to me: a chicken house planted where the banana trees now grew. Curtains for the banana trees. Slowly, over the next months, a chicken plan began evolving. Steve Ilott bought me a subscription to *Backyard Poultry*. The CLL was worsening, and Dr. K had me lined up to start a treatment. Dispirited and drained of energy, I found it hard to summon enthusiasm for research and writing, after teaching. But chickens were a different matter. Somehow the mere mention, a passing thought, of chickens sharpened my mind, focused attention, sent me on a mission to find out *everything*. I was able to focus on the chicken project with obsessive acuity. Bit by bit, week by week, Peggy and

I hacked back the banana trees; J carted the foliage away, uprooted the plants. I paced out the available area and began looking at designs for chicken coops: planning, scheming, imagining a new world.

There is evidence. Small square photos taken by my father with his brownie camera, shots of me as a little girl, among the chickens, gazing at them in wonder and delight. They lived in small A-frame lightweight houses, which were moved around, and during the day they ranged freely. *Free range* was a word that frolicked in the air, danced, a minuet partnered with words like *Rhode Island Reds*. I so clearly recall the adult conversations, the tossing back and forth of possible breeds. Rhode Island Reds were particularly alluring because of their supposed island provenance, the exoticism of islands to a child living in a landlocked country. In the photo, however, the birds are white, not red. These must have been the early experiments. Later there were hundreds of chickens, housed in small pens, each with a small run for ranging. They were situated near the mulberry trees, huge old trees copiously bearing fruit that we would pluck and eat, our bare feet turning purply red as we tramped over the fallen squishy fruit.

It would be nearly twenty years before I would live with chickens again. In Australia, a friend, Doris, whom I had known in Glasgow when I was a graduate student, and I bought a small run-down farm near the town of Toora in South Gippsland, a couple of hours from Melbourne. Rolling hills, a few miles from the ocean and a few miles to a mountain where ancient rain forests grew. It had been a rich dairy farming area, but with the monopolization of the dairy industry small farmers were being squeezed out and weekenders were buying up. There was a small shed behind the house, which sported an old sign, tinny and faded but still legible: TOORA HOLIDAY FLATS. With the help of others, particularly Helen Casey and "the boys" across the road (the farm we bought had been a larger property divided in two, and two local brothers bought the other half) who taught us how, we built a fence around the outhouse, which we smartened up, installed perches, repainted the sign, and planted kiwi fruit and passion fruit vines.

Then the big day came. We went with one of "the boys," our lovely neighbor Peter Danuser, to fetch the dozen white leghorn pullets ordered from a chicken farm in Yarram. Back at Toora, Peter and I clipped one wing on each bird before releasing them from the cage into the run.

Helen was very fond of the chickens. There is an old photo of her proudly holding a chicken as though it were a large but living fish she'd landed. Instead of a man with a fish or a boy with a car: a girl with a chicken. In a comment on my blog, that she titled "Homage to Gloria," Helen recently wrote, "For the curious, the chickens of Toora were all named Gloria as their talents were worthy of a Patti Smith title."

For Charlie Aarons it was different. She had a phobia about birds. She was staying that weekend and came with us to Yarram. Although she was brave, I imagine how she must have felt that time she came with us to buy the chickens. I cannot worm my way into her skin and feel what she feels when in the presence of chickens, yet I have a vague inkling since I too have a phobia. Recently she wrote to me, posting on the blog: "Collecting eggs from a chicken coop is still a serious challenge for me let alone the idea of actually picking up a chook!"

Although it's hard for me to grasp, I do know that you don't have to have a phobia exactly to not be enamored of chickens. And childhood intimacy with the birds does not necessarily guarantee lifetime devotion. I have two friends, Steve Fagin and Allen Shelton, who were sent to collect eggs as kids and found it a terrifying and repulsive experience. Allen, nevertheless, always asks about the chickens, and Steve is my main supplier of chicken stories from all over the internet. He takes delight in the more macabre and bizarre inflections of chicken faddishness. Such as: *Backyard chickens dumped at shelters when hipsters can't cope*, critics say and *ChickensinSweaters* on Etsy. Looking back through the emails I see my response: "Thank you Steve. I would sooner eat my chickens than dress them in such unstylish gear. Get a dog if you want to dress." Always laconic and sardonic, he concluded the exchange: "Glad to hear you ascribe to 'higher values.'"

In Perth I bought a house that came with chickens. Perhaps that is why I bought that house, or maybe it was also the swimming pool. The pool only brought trouble, but the chickens were a joy, especially Miss Fluff, a Chinese bantam with fluffy legs. They used to escape periodically through a hole in the fence to my neighbor's yard, that of Susan Melrose, who was also a colleague. So when I left, the chickens just moved over permanently to live with her.

As a girl I coped once, or rather did not cope exactly, by constructing a project, an obsession, to counteract the humiliations and debilitations endured in the biology classroom. On that occasion it was because of a phobia, and salvation came through poisonous plants. On this occasion it is because of chickens and cancer. Although that girl abandoned science, she learned—through studying poisonous plants—that the category of *poisonous* is relational. Poisonous to whom? When and where is the poison active? And she learned a little bit about botany, about plants in the wild and those that have been domesticated. And in time she would become a fanatical gardener so that when she was diagnosed with leukemia she had a garden to be obsessive about, a garden where she could welcome chickens and build them a *palacio de las princesas*.

Boomerang

8

Why did the Australian go berserk?
Because he got a new boomerang and then he tried to get rid of the old one.

Yesterday—an infusion day—Akos gave me a ride to the hospital. He was euphoric, having just sent off his book manuscript. But, he said, his relief was shadowed by a joke. Akos is married to Judit Herskó, whose father was János Herskó, a Hungarian film director who would often enter his own films to tell a joke. He might for instance materialize on a trolley and, for no very good reason, would tell this boomerang joke. I guess it was at the height of boomerang jokes. I vaguely remember them circulating when I was a kid, round about the time of hula hoops.

Every writer knows this: the sense that your book is never really finished, it will keep coming back, there will be more revisions, and more and more. And now that all the versions are electronic, the old versions, full of typos and one or two crucial mistakes, threaten to reappear in the proofs. It's only when you get the published book—that solid thing—in your hands that it feels finished. Maybe. But of course all that is changing. That solid thing, the book, is disappearing, words materialize and evaporate as you write, as you read. This is not to say that nanopublishing and the drive toward the short bite rather than the long book guarantee the sense of an ending. No, instead there is something far more precarious: ephemeral finality, ghosted by a labyrinthine digital archive. Words are like money. They melt into air and reappear in new configurations.

Akos's book is about plastic money, a history of the credit card in postcommunist countries. Some of these credit cards, linked to the state rather than to banks, are used much more habitually and extensively than in the U.S., for instance. Money in the form of bank notes and coins and written checks scarcely exists. Credit cards have become a form of ID, they store information, can be used to receive, electronically, all sorts of things, like your pension payments. And even as I write, credit cards themselves are disappearing: into cell phones, into thumbprints, into eye scans. Not only in the postcommunist world. You know that dubious item you bought (no didn't even buy, just perused in a browsing sortie late one night)? Well it will reappear for everyone to see on some social networking site as something you "like." Even worse, that aberrant impulse will return to plague you in the form of endless haranguing from cheesy underwear companies. You might forget, but the marketing machine will not. Your secret is never safe with Victoria.

The boomerang joke can manifest in many guises. You could give it a Žižekian spin, which might go something like this. The Australian wants to get away from Australia and start afresh. So he goes to California, say, and sets up an alternative market where he sells tea tree oil and water-wise Australian native plants and a unique new service, surfing therapy (therapy while you surf). . . . No problem with the Californian surfing dudes—they take to therapy like ducks to vodka. But then comes a guy who looks and talks like Bryan Brown. Laconic, gruff, handsome in a chiseled, hard-knocks kind of way. Turns out he himself is a surfing analyst, and the question he asks, which sends the whole new age entrepreneurial enterprise for a loop, is this: "Why did the Australian go berserk?"

For me, in the Moores Cancer Infusion Center later in the day, it bounced back in the spectral form of CLL. In the past week I've been feeling considerably regenerated, exhilarated, hopeful again. The lab results confirmed that the feeling isn't merely illusory, so Dr. C thinks we can now double the oral dose and reduce the infusion to once a month. He warns that things will probably get worse again, before and if they get better. He says they do not know whether the increased dose correlates with increased effectivity (this is a trial; it's one of the things they are trying to determine); it does seem to be the case, but it might be that because patients are improved before the dose is increased their systems are in a better position to deal with the ravages of the drug. In the infusion center, while keeping up a façade of cheerfulness, I experienced again the cul-de-sac sensation. The futility of it all. Although there may be periods of respite, CLL itself will always bounce back. Once it starts progressing, it will move in a relentlessly linear fashion, gathering momentum, working toward a conclusion. But against this teleological drive, as a person who "has" CLL, you (and this applies also, I imagine, to those who have other kinds of chronically incurable diseases) experience periods of optimism, euphoria even. Just when you have forgotten about CLL, are getting on with life in an enjoyable day-to-day fashion, it whizzes through the air and hits you on the back of the head, sending you catapulting back into the ER, back on to antibiotics, back into a funk. The malevolence of repetition.

There is an extraordinary air of cheeriness in the infusion center. At its worst you might think of it as something akin to battery chicken farming. When you close your eyes and try to sleep the noise keeps you awake, the noise of beeping machines, televisions, people talking on cell phones, nurses reading out orders— all these noises merge together and sound like the strangled clucks of a thousand tormented chickens. All of us chickens chained by tubes that run between machines, that run from little packets of clear liquid hanging from hooks, into a multitudinous network of veins, ready and waiting for chemo plumping. But at its best everyone is cheerful in the infusion center, polite even, even as the day wears on. There is much joshing and spinning out of repartee, bits and pieces of verbal exchange are tossed hither and thither, everyone enters into the fiction that this is just an ordinary day, a day like any other. And of course for the nurses and staff it is, which makes it all the more extraordinary that under duress and repetition they are so alert and behave with such good-natured equanimity, remembering names, histories, stories. And through this enactment of an illusion everyone rises to the occasion, enters into the spirit of the performative event, into this compact of civility.

I do appreciate the considerable theatrical skills, as well as the hospital experience, that it takes to generate and sustain a mood. Still, sometimes you want something to puncture the air of equanimity, something that hits the nail on the head, you want a joke that is grim, black, irreverent. The boomerang, as used by Australian Aborigines, was and is a tool and a hunting weapon, some are designed to return (in their flight frightening birds, say), but mostly they are intended to hit and bring down a prey, a moving target. Curiously, when it comes to jokes (and illness), hitting your prey can simultaneously be a way of releasing all those lurgy birds lurking in the wetlands.

A Way of Making Another Egg

9

A chicken is just an egg's way of making another egg.

—SAMUEL BUTLER

We experimented at the weekend with a new way of cooking eggs. It goes by the name of Arzak eggs, and I found out about it reading *Lucky Peach*, a new quarterly magazine edited by David Chang, of Momofuku fame, and Peter Meehan, with whom he wrote the Momofuku cookbook. It is a really fun way of conjuring a roundish poached egg, a sphere swaddled in soft white gauze, a teasing hint of yellow within. Once it's cooked you can slide the slippery ball into a noodle soup or over a puree of some sort (imagine an emerald green pea puree over black rice), gently puncture the roundness with a fork, and watch as the creamy golden yolk oozes into the world.

The Arzak eggs are the final touch, the pièce de résistance, the magical surprise. But it's a long haul to get there. First you have to prepare a bed for the eggs. (Some people might consider this the main dish and the eggs as an accoutrement. Not I, nor Señor Arzak.) Long slow preparation, and then when it comes to it, split-second timing and perfect coordination. Turn it into a ritual, take all day. I invite my friend Steve Ilott, who has been so complicit in the chicken project, to share the play, the sense of craziness, and so we can wander around the garden in between phases of cooking—deadheading flowers, contemplating failures, imagining new plantings, and talking to the chickens.

I went with *Lucky Peach*'s suggestion of serving the Arzak eggs over ramen and a ragu spiced up with a Jamaican mix. The recipe is in the same magazine and comes from Mario Carbone, who serves it in his restaurant P.S.46. To save time I could have prepared the onions—a huge pile of thickly julienned onions cooked down into a sweet, soft, brown-gold mush—the day before, and I could have ground the spices ahead of time, but there wasn't any time in the days before, nor in the days to come. Sunday is the only day we have this kind of time. It was a long, slow, dreamy day of futzing around in the kitchen, wafting through a range of smells, tasting and anticipating. We began at the farmers' markets: from Sage Mountain Farm at Hillcrest we got chuck beef, making sure it was laced with enough fat to flavor the dish, all of the tomatoes came from the garden (the last of the summer crop off the vine and some from the freezer where they were thrown in whole), the spices were ground and roasted, filling the house with delectable smells. The large jalapeño from the garden made for a much more picante dish than anticipated, so we didn't add the chile sauce the recipe suggested (though I did add some crumbled dried anchovies). After hours and hours the ragu was ready.

To make Arzak eggs you first break the eggs, one at a time, into a small bowl lined with plastic wrap that has been sprayed with oil. Steve gathers the wrap and twists it around the runny egg while I tie it with string and hang it off something that serves as a beam to be suspended over a pot of water—a chopstick if the pot is small; we used the handle of a large wooden spoon. Juggling act ensues as we try to keep the wooden spoon steady and attach four swinging egg packages. Then, together—without tangling the string or our ten fingers into a knot—we have to find a way to suspend the balloon shapes into a pot of gently simmering water, making sure that none touch the bottom. Cook gently at the same temperature for four minutes and twenty seconds. Then quickly and deftly (ideally deftly . . .) you remove the balloon, cut it open, and let the round egg roll onto its luscious and delectable edible bed. Our bed was composed of spicy ragu ladled over hot noodles. The egg was nestled in, some finely sliced scallions and dried sardines sprinkled over the surface. J joined us, we broke the eggs with chopsticks, gobbled, slurped, spluttered, then paused, looked at one another and sighed, grinned together and finished our bowls more slowly, slaveringly. What a way to eat an egg.

OK, so talking of therapy, specifically of nutrition, what, you might ask, is someone with cancer doing eating meat laced with fat that melts into and permeates every oozing fiber of the entire dish? And what about the eggs? Moreover, the combination of eggs and red meat? And, perhaps the most edgy question: what about eating eggs cooked in plastic submerged in hot simmering water? So here's the thing. The thing about cancer, or actually about any disturbance of health: you have to play pleasure against wisdom (or if you're a Freudian, maybe you say the death drive). Although diet may not—or at least not alone—cure you of cancer, it will certainly make it much easier for your body to fight and protect against toxins.

Nutrition is therapy. Avoiding pesticides, the residues of antibiotics in produce, the poisons in packaging and preservatives and processing; and, on the positive side, eating foodstuffs that promote energy, all this is foundational. But pleasure, relaxation, bliss, good company, enjoying cooking and eating food—these states are also therapeutic. Stress builds toxins in us humans as well as in the chickens and other animals subjected to ghastly living and dying conditions.

So, because I'm fortunate to have a reasonably large (though never of course large enough) backyard, I grow, and buy where I can and when I can afford it, organic vegetables and meats, try to minimize eating processed and canned foods and sugar and saturated fats. Though there's quite a bit of stumbling and tripping along the path of good intentions. I don't eat much red meat, but wow is it sometimes fantastic. Phil and Juany Noble who own Sage Mountain Farm graze their cattle entirely on grass and also feed them all the surplus pumpkins and other vegetables from the market stands. Eggs, if they are fresh and organic, are good for you, the cholesterol beneficent.

Cooking eggs in plastic wrap though, that is kind of crazy. The combination of heat and plastic is horrible. You wouldn't want to do it every day, probably you wouldn't want to do it more than very occasionally, if ever. And you can surely arrive at a similar kind of poached egg a number of different ways. At all costs, however, you always want to avoid the kind of ineptly poached egg that haunts me still, the rubbery look and the sulphuric smell, from boarding school days, so vividly evoked by Kate Atkinson as "a sickly jellyfish deposited on toast to die." But the Arzak way is experimental, fun, and in the end beautiful and texturally divine. The original handwritten and drawn recipe in Spanish (where the eggs are part of a larger concoction involving chorizo and bacon) is from Juan Mari Arzak and is reproduced in the magazine.

I have to admit my feelings about the magazine are mixed. The insistently bad-boy braggadocio of Chang, Bourdain, and cronies gets a bit tiring. Beneath the exultant enthusiasm you can hear a muffled whining refrain: kill the mother! kill the mother! Alice Waters and Judy Rodgers run for cover. Nevertheless, there is a welcome verve to the Lucky Peach project, a combination of irreverence and inventiveness, terrific graphics, and a refreshing refusal to divide the world of food into haute and fast.

When all is said and done, the thing about eggs is their versatility, the remarkably different ways they can taste, how they are incorporated, deployed, displayed in different cultural cuisines. The humble hen, call her Holly, Lula Mae, Sabrina, or Funny Face, embodies all this potential.

Shivers and Shakes   10

Cold. One moment everything is normal and then—fast and without warning—an iciness zips into the world. I ask Amie if she's cold, she says no and brings me another blanket and calls Brenda, the nurse. The danger signals dart through me, and just at that moment the shivering starts. Terror, somatic memories, sensations repeated. Anticipating that perception of blackness, of slipping away, out of this life.

A month ago she had a code blue episode during an infusion of Rituxin, where she stopped breathing. It began with shivers.

Now, she is again in the infusion center, though at a different hospital and for a different reason. She is having an ivIg, an intravenous infusion of immunoglobulin: white blood plasma which will top up her depleted supplies and strengthen her compromised immune system.

The nurses, Marcie and Brenda, are there with a stopwatch, timing the shivers that shake her body as though someone, some creature, has reached up out of the black lagoon, has her in a steel grip, and is shaking. She tries breathing very slowly to see if she can stop it, perhaps it is just a hysterical reaction. But the hiccoughs are demonic, involuntary. Brenda stops the infusion. The shivers get worse, not better. She pages Dr. K, and then Dr. C. Brenda was there during the code blue episode and senses her terror, is calm and comforting. The kit is here she says, we can give you Demerol. But Demerol might have been the problem last time, she says, it might have lowered my blood pressure too much. Dr. C responds to the page in a minute. He says no Demerol. Benadryl and some steroids. 25 mm Benadryl is shot into her veins, through the port, and almost immediately she starts feeling woozy and the shivers and shakes feel as though they are happening to someone else, to a facsimile of her, a paper doll. Then gradually everything subsides, her body floats. She falls asleep.

I wake fuzzily to J arriving. He has brought me a sandwich for lunch and is greeted by the news of another adverse reaction. I can vaguely hear Brenda and him talking, isolated words—chills . . . Choi . . . cheese . . . cheery. Cheery that the creature from the black lagoon has lessened its grip and let me float to the surface, float on air. No thanks I say, not now, and drift back into sleep. Am vaguely aware of the world since Amie is taking my vitals it seems like constantly. Someone has switched on the TV, the word *bombs* echoes through the room, wending in and out of my brain. And *wounded* and *hundreds*, as the world woozes back. The Boston Marathon. A world of images, and terror, a world mediated by television.

In here: cocooned and safe. Out there: chaos and terror. Safe in my blankets, J there at the bottom of the bed, quiet on his iPad, the murmur of familiar faces and voices. Images and sounds sidle in and out of consciousness: bodies bleeding, bodies running, explosions, death. Words torn loose from sentences, limbs torn loose from bodies, images—fragmented and bleeding—struggle to surface.

One aspect of CLL, as it progresses, marches, or ambles along, is that your immune system is weakened. This can become serious if and when your body's capacity to produce antibodies (to fight infections) stops or severely slows down. IVIg is given as a plasma replacement therapy to boost and maintain adequate antibody levels, conferring what is called a passive immunity. Immunoglobulin is an antibody, a protein, used by the immune system to identify and neutralize foreign objects, such as bacteria and viruses (the infusion is very specific, however; it does not fully protect peripheral tissues, such as the eyes, lungs, gut, and urinary tract). I have an infusion once a month, and it generally takes three to four hours. But it takes much longer to get all the stuff into the two little bottles that are hung upside down and delivered in a carefully measured way into my veins. "All the stuff" is immunoglobulin extracted from over one thousand blood donors, tested, and then preserved in detergent.

A few days after this adverse reaction I'm back home chatting away with my neighbor, the doctor, chatting away about this and that, and I happen to tell her what happened. She says that IVIg varies from batch to batch (produced by different companies) and that people who have had adverse reactions are usually OK after changing to another product. I do some research, which corroborates Barbara's advice. I call Sheila and ask her to ask the doctor to change the brand. This is done, and the next time I hold my breath for almost the whole of the three hours, but everything is fine. The month after that I'm relaxed, and we are two-thirds of the way through the infusion; I'm telling Lisa C, who is sitting with me, about the allergic reaction. Risa, my nurse, suddenly looks pale and starts checking something on her computer. She disappears but returns quickly. I am so so sorry, Lesley, she says. We are giving you the old brand. I just filled the order from the doctor, but I should have checked more closely, I know about your adverse reaction. She says, we can stop right now. Or if you want to risk it (reaction would more than likely have happened much earlier) we can keep going; we'll monitor you very closely, and we'll catch any suspicious changes. I decide to keep going, but it's a bit nerve wracking. We get to the last drop, however, without any incidents.

It is extremely expensive, at this time about seventy-five dollars per gram, which puts the cost of those two little bottles at about seven thousand dollars a pop. And that's just the drug; the price escalates when you add in the needles, ancillary drugs, hospital expenses, etc. CLL is on the list of approved conditions to receive this treatment, though for the insurance company you have to have proof of almost dying (which I have after several very serious infections landing me in hospital). CLL is not the only illness that results in immunoglobulin deficiency, and certainly not everyone who needs it gets it. I am extremely lucky to have good insurance, a tenacious medical team who fight for coverage and probably, as a research hospital, have more experience and leverage than some doctors. But I do wonder how many people are dying because they do not have access. And I wonder why it is so expensive. I can see that it is time-consuming and labor-intensive. But seven thousand dollars. Really? Yes, really. In large part I imagine because of (not very regulated) competition between the different private companies who produce the different brands.

Between warm and cold, dead and alive, betwixt the pen and the page: a series of chance happenings. It wasn't Risa's fault, she was following the orders on the chart, but I appreciate her concern and honesty. It is rare in the medical realm that anyone says sorry since it immediately lays them open to litigation. The nurses and aides in this unit are simply marvelous, and as I write this, after about four years of monthly visits, I feel affection for them all and look forward to seeing them, exchanging chitchat and banter. It is a small unit, and their predominant mode is drollery. They treat everyone with the same courteous, reassuring attention, but there are challenges, not always visible to us. Bill tells me, with a wry expression and dry tone, A patient said to me, why do you nurses hate us so? And I replied, Oh no does it show?

The doctor, also, was just doing what he was asked to do—he changed the order (the brand), but he did it for one treatment, not permanently. So easy for this to happen. In a hurry, on the way to an emergency, thinking about those research results, you put in the order and it's done. And just chance chatting with a neighbor, who happens to be a doctor, alerts me to the brand issue (the offensive brand—probably also varying batch by batch so a bit of a lottery as to its immediate effects—was soon discontinued by the pharmacy after several incidents like mine). Because of specialization, different doctors and specialists don't know what's going on with patients in the other areas and don't or can't keep track. The system of modern Western medicine is not conducive to integration. As is so often said it's almost a truism: you gotta be your own advocate.

Just chance that those runners and spectators at the Boston Marathon were in the line of fire. Back home after the adverse reaction, in the garden, images of limbs torn loose and the sound of screaming are imprinted on the lettuces and herbs. I'm craving greenery, freshness. I've survived. This adverse reaction was not as severe as the code blue episode, I was really in little danger, the nurses are trained for these emergencies. But it felt frightening. How to make sense of terror, my survival, weighed against the Boston body count? There is no sense. I think about how to weigh the isolation and safety of U.S. citizens against the aggressive wars that have been waged in the name of U.S. democracy. All I know is I am lucky. This, this garden, is a way back into the world. Picking stuff in the garden and making a salad. The smell of a lemon, just plucked, when you cut and squeeze it, the sense of weight and heft when you pull beets from the earth, the cradling in your hand of a perfect blue egg from Lula Mae.

The Chicken or the Egg 11

It's time to get up, it's time, it's time, it's time to get up. But you cannot move, inertia spreads through your veins, leaks into the air, blankets the room. Your body is a loaf of unleavened bread, heavy, sinking.

She knows that if her limbs were liftable, if she could only summon enough spirit to rise up out of the morass, to become a person moving out into the world, she knows that then she would be OK. She imagines the early morning just as light starts filtering through the darkness. The world then, for a short time, is new and unknowable. Roxy streaks through the dark—a pale furry flash. Elvis scruffles along, dragging his useless back leg, wheezing. Then there is a noise on the roof, and there he is. He saunters along the roof top, a silhouette. A mighty hunter, he pauses and surveys the view below—not just our yard, but the whole of North Park, he sees the ocean to the west and Mexico to the southeast, and he grows large and filled with pride and contentment. He lifts his nose into the air and sniffs, testing, taking the pulse of his kingdom.

The white flowers of the potato creeper on the chicken run. The chickens cooing, hungry not just for their food, but for light. The more light, the longer the days, the more eggs.

She conjures these sensations into being, imagines herself there in the backyard in her dressing gown and slippers as light infiltrates, as the world takes shape, as shapes become things. No good. She cannot counter the blackness, can't get out of bed. What she wants is to disappear into the blackness, for this residual sensation of despair to disappear her.

Kirsten Dunst as Justine in *Melancholia*, weighted down by her intolerably heavy wedding dress, a beautiful encumbrance sinking her into the ground, trailing behind her, pulling her back and down, gathering twigs and branches and the world's debris. The dress embodies the dominant affective modality of the film: depression. The planet Melancholia in Von Trier's film echoes Julia Kristeva's *Black Sun*. In her book, a meditation on depression, Kristeva poses the "thing" as always "something" massive, ineffable and unspoken. Justine often experiences her own body as unbearably heavy, herself as imprisoned corpse-like in a crypt, and the great achievement of the film is to convey this affective sensation as a state—of being between dead and alive—rather than a character trait. Justine and her body: an alien interaction. Her body, like the wedding dress, is attached by a malevolent magnetic force to the dark center of existence.

She talks with S, who has come through a harsh cancer treatment and now is clear. S tells her that she has only just realized that the sense of paralysis currently afflicting her is depression. Why, she asks, now when I'm free? She knows, however, that it is related to the cancer experience. The sensation that invades her is the same but different as that which often gripped her when she was undergoing chemo treatment. The same but different. Then it would begin as a tangible sense of dread, it would start as a heavy painful sensation in her stomach. Then there was a tumor, then there was a thing, and the thing radiated pain and fear. Now there is no thing, the fear is attenuated, melancholia of a sort.

A chicken-and-egg question. Which comes first: psyche or soma? Depression, which induces a physical sensation of sickness, an inability to move? Or bodily illness, which induces deep incapacitating misery?

Eventually she knows she will somehow just do it: get up, get dressed, go to work. And when she's talking and doing, her body somehow generates enough adrenalin to perform like a normal being. But there will be moments in between when the terrible weight of exhaustion seems unbearable and there is only a slow silent weeping, a seeping out of spirit.

Strawberry / Fetish

Last night was a party to celebrate Milane, who died four nights ago. She loved a good story, a wicked joke, a gathering of friends. And so we gathered, a small party hosted by Nina MacConnel and Tom Chino. All of us shell-shocked, seized in passing moments by grimness, but mostly there was conviviality and the sharing of food and drink, particularly gin and tonics, Milane's favorite.

There was a gift for each of us. Before she died Milane sorted through her photos, and there was a little bundle for each of us with our name on it. Moments forgotten: memories returned. There I was in a celebrating group at a Christmas party at The Book Works, the bookshop Milane once owned, there in the Getty Villa garden, a trip made when the renovated villa opened. At book signings. When we left the party that night Tom and Nina gave each of us a large white paper Japanese lantern to take home and light for Milane.

. . .

In our garden, hung on the fence where apples are espaliered, close to the chicken run, the lantern has refused to stay put. It dances wildly, a white ghost cavorting in the dark swell of the night.

. . .

Milane had a gift for gift giving and an eye for things. She took great pleasure in choosing just the right thing. Around my garden there are various Milane manifestations, but the one I love the most is a cement dove, a garden ornament migrated from another era, cast aside, I imagine, at some swap meet where her anachronistic beauty caught Milane's eye. I love to hold the dove, her solidity fits perfectly into the shape of a hand, her lines are simple, her proportions just right.

I knew Milane was dying when she gave me a clay icon of Ganesha that she had brought many years ago from India. She told me that his dharma is to place and remove obstacles and also that he is honored at the beginning of rituals and ceremonies and invoked as the patron of letters during writing sessions. As part elephant, he likes to eat flowers, fresh ones every day, she told me. At first, and for a while after Milane died, I did make an offering every day of fresh flowers, but the punctiliousness of the habit has waned, the offerings sporadic and whimsical. Like my efforts at writing, at meditation.

The dove sat for several years on a rock in the white garden (so grandly named, more for aspiration than actuality, all kinds of colors creep in, some muted, others garish like the scarlet and orange nasturtiums). Then came the chickens. In their frenzied searching for bugs, in their rampaging destruction, they knocked the dove to the ground, and she broke in two. Distraught, I was ready to send the chickens to the pot. But Milane cocked an eyebrow and laughed. We jammed the two pieces together and wedged her high up in a corner of the bower where the grapes and wisteria grow. In summer you cannot see her, but in winter when the foliage dies back, when the garden mutates, you can see her there, up high, looking down at the chickens.

. . .

Nina's chickens were asleep that night, the night of the party. I imagined them dreaming of Milane, carousing together in their sleep, a communal feathery dreaming. I hold Nina responsible in part for the coming of chickens to Herman Avenue. Steve, sensing a whiff of chicken desire in the air, had been waging a gentle campaign that began by the mysterious monthly appearance in my letter box of *Backyard Poultry*. Gorgeous full-page spreads of birds: the Silver Spangled Hamburg, white feathers adorned by black crescent and V-shaped spangles; the Bearded Buff Laced Polish, creamy white and golden buff laced together, sporting an extravagant feathery top knot; the Mottled Houdan Bantam—lustrous greenish-black feathers, with one of every two or three tipped in white. My dreams were infiltrated by Porcelain Bearded d'Uccle Bantam cockerels from Belgium, Black Breasted Red Aseels from India, and Old English Creles. And then, almost every time I saw him, Steve would suggest that I visit Nina and take a look at her chickens. So eventually I succumbed, and Nina invited us to lunch. Us was me and Helen Barnes, or Helen B as she is sometimes referred to, as two Australian friends called Helen weave their way through this book (the other is Helen Casey, or Helen C). She and J were continent swapping: while J was visiting Australia she had traveled from Melbourne to keep me company in San Diego. I had a bone marrow biopsy scheduled for that morning and had forgotten what an ordeal it can be (forgetting is part of the game, selective memory a survival device). It took a long time, and then there were all sorts of bureaucratic hospital diversions and waiting and waiting and waiting. So by the time we got to Nina's—stopping by the farm to see Tom and gather some vegetables from the farm stand—it was long past the lunch hour. But the sight of the chickens was restorative, to see them roaming, pecking, zigzagging around, following one trail only to be distracted, tempted by a posse of insects over there, a potential worm in the woodwork over here. To examine their coop, how the perches were composed and food distributed, how their shelter was organized—all of this was inspiring.

And then there were the eggs. The eggs did it. Helen and I watched spellbound as Nina conjured from the eggs an omelet, so effortlessly, breaking the eggs with one hand, flicking a wrist and twirling a fork and then on our plates: yellowness, the taste of yellow in our mouths.

. . .

The transmutation of matter. How an egg becomes something else. You look at an egg; there it sits on the kitchen counter, self-contained, perfect in its ovality. Perhaps it is a deep speckled brown, maybe pale blue or green. When you crack the shell, break the oval perfection, you release into the world a magical potential.

. . .

At the party on the 24th of April I could not eat much. Nausea was settling in. Stomach cramps. I could not resist Nina's couscous and Tom's vegetables, the mellow spices that tickled the tongue but did not obscure the taste of Chino carrots and peas and fava beans. But when it came to the dessert I could not manage a single spoonful. I was sitting next to John Alexander, who was entertaining our end of the table with hilarious stories of gardening mishaps. At one point he looked quizzically at me and said, "What about strawberries? How do you like them?" Oh I like them, I said. "How about I bring you a plate just of strawberries, no cake or cream?" It almost broke my heart to say no. It wasn't that I didn't want those strawberries that come from the garden of the gods. It wasn't even that I couldn't imagine the taste. It wasn't that they made me feel sick. It's just that there was a nausea right through me, not just in the stomach. John's hilarious stories had made me forget for a while, or, rather, the storytelling and ripples of laughter had absorbed the yucky sensation.

I do not think I would have felt this way if they were other sorts of strawberries. But Tom's strawberries are something else. For several years the graduate seminar I taught on gardens and public space, a peripatetic seminar, would visit Chino's farm, and Tom would fire up the tractor, load everyone on the trailer, and off we would go into the fields. But before that we would sit at the trestle table where the workers have their lunch and discuss the reading, and someone would present a paper. And Tom would send out two large bowls heaped with strawberries. Sounds of ecstasy, inappropriate sounds of swooning. I thought then that you would have to be on your deathbed to ever refuse a Chino strawberry. In the field Tom would stop occasionally and encourage people to pick from the plants in the field, strawberries, for instance. And he would talk about the culture of strawberries, the particularities of the plant, selection for this region, how they grow, how they need to be nurtured. I have pages and pages of notes from Tom's field discourses. He talks too about water, where it comes from, the price of water in San Diego, this virtually desert region, how he uses expensive domestic water on the strawberries because the municipal farm water contains too many salts. You might think of this as coddling, but Tom, I imagine, thinks of it as farming.

Farming is work, practical, you get up each day at 4 AM, and by the end of the day you have to balance the books. You have to weigh up what comes in against what goes out and figure out how to make a living. The process is practical yes, but there is something mysterious, alchemical about the way in which water—clear liquid that flows, that has no color—is transformed into scarlet heart-shaped succulence. Water, labor, knowledge, money: the condensation of a process into a succulent jewel.

. . .

Clear liquid that looks like water drips into my veins during infusions, and some kind of transmutation happens, equally mysterious to me. Even when you check the science it doesn't all add up. Even the oncologists say, we don't really know exactly how it works. Drip by drip by slow drip it disappears into my body. A week later my lab results change; many of the danger flags disappear.

. . .

Saying no to those strawberries last night at Milane's party felt to me for a moment like the approach of death. I wanted to howl for Milane. I thought to myself: she would never have refused a strawberry. Her ALS, once diagnosed, progressed fast, but she continued to party with friends, a few at a time. Not long before she died, when speaking was difficult, she wrote on her writing app a version of an old W. C. Fields saying, "Who put tonic in my gin and tonic?"

. . .

A few weeks later. I am beginning to emerge from that nauseous miasma, a shout at the back gate, and there is Alex Kershaw, a graduate student from Australia.

A little sheepish looking, the way Australians sometimes are when performing an act of generosity. A self-deprecating shrug that says, Oh it was just something that fell off the back of a truck. He is bearing a cardboard box, in which gleam vegetable gems: round yellow and green striped squash, candy red radishes, and strawberries, deep scarlet strawberries. Around the vegetables he has tucked a Humboldt Fog cheese, a slab of dark spicy chocolate, a pack of organic Yerba mate.

Immediately I picked out a strawberry and bit into it. As that strawberry dissolved in my mouth, the juice dribbling down my chin, I knew it was a Chino strawberry.

The chickens, too, love strawberries. Though *love* is too tender a word to describe what happens when a chicken encounters a strawberry. They are not particular, any strawberries from anywhere will send them over the moon, it's the color red that attracts. Never go near them in open-toed sandals if your toe nails are painted crimson, or they will dive-bomb, pecking mercilessly. They play dirty football with spoiled cherry tomatoes or mushy squished strawberries. We always keep the hulls for them, they go berserk when tossed the green bits with juicy red entrails slurping out.

. . .

Today, I will feed Ganesha some flowers. My daily ritual is to rise early, feed the cats, let the chickens out of their house as the sky lightens. They hear me approaching and set up a mighty hullabaloo, hurling themselves against the door and scratching at the wire window. As I open the door they come flying down from their roosts and cavort down the ramp, fluffing and huffing and preening. Then I make a pot of tea and bring it back to bed, set it over the tea candle warmer, and sip as I write on my magical writing machine, the Mac Air. This is a ritual. It sets me in motion for the day. Later I will meditate. Really I should start the day by meditating, but I'm greedy for writing opportunities, for using that early morning energy before it dissipates. As I describe this early morning ritual it takes on a life, seems orderly and calm. But the truth is there are many mornings when I can't rouse myself, when the chickens remain in prison, many mornings when I can't get writing, read a detective novel instead, or feel sorry for myself, or find distractions like email or the newspaper, which reveals all sorts of hyperlinks, passages into other worlds. And then of course there are too many other things to do, and so meditation slips away. I'll do it tomorrow. . . .

. . .

Between habit and ritual a thin line: between therapeutic and spiritual practices, between the gracious and orderly lighting of candles and the compulsive repetition of obsessive desire, between routine and observance. Many ritualistic practices—from the quotidian and idiosyncratic to those more formally prescribed—serve to preserve the way things are, to protect us against change, transformation, difference, grief. And yet, and yet . . . there is always the possibility of something mysterious happening. Rituals might be ways of channeling and bolstering obsessive impulses, but also they are often mechanisms for structuring pathways and passages, for enabling transformation. Lighting lanterns to guide the dead in their journey, to ease the transition from one state to another, not merely for those who are passed but for those of us who remain. Making a pot of tea in order to write. Sometimes though the pot of tea is not enough. And so today I will feed Ganesha some flowers.

. . .

Gifts circulate, chemo too. And in the circulation: transformation. Of course gifts seldom come without ramification, this we know. If I offer flowers to Ganesha it is in the hope that he will, in eating them, keep Milane alive even though she is no longer here. The flowers are at once food and fetish and gift, not unlike the strawberry. Superstition, ritual, faith. In offering Ganesha flowers, day after day (punctuated by desultory periods of neglect), I believe that the gods in general will be appeased. Of course I also hope that Ganesha in particular will preside over a writing session and kick my ass into gear.

Life after Life

13

Life after Life is Kate Atkinson's new novel—it's long and gratifying. I have read a lot during the past three weeks, mostly though not exclusively novels, the reading matter overseen and sat upon by Elvis. Reading is one of the things you can do while keeping your head very still so the world doesn't spin, and if it's engrossing you can be transported. You might think that the "second" life in the title is a replacement of the word and concept of *death*. Not really. On the most simple level the novel plays with the idea of the novel. The novel as a progression of seemingly inevitable events, of teleology, of the crocheting of character and description into the momentum of plot. But life too, as we live it day by day, entails plotting, dramatization, and anticipation. Atkinson asks, "what if?" What if, for instance, the baby had lived instead of dying? What if—that old chestnut—Hitler had been assassinated? What if the dog had a different name? What if the girl had kicked back? A writer can mess with events, and this is what she does, giving us multiple versions or possibilities or, more accurately, unfoldings. But philosophically, she also spins a meditation—upon the eternal return. The idea that what exists after life is not death but more life or, more prosaically, we could say people go on living and the dead reemerge in various incarnations according to different beliefs and modes of representation and through the intricacies of memory. As always she is preoccupied with the concepts of *déjà vu* and *amor fati*, of history and the future, of memory and delusion. A minor but key character whose presence is woven through the book is a Buddhistic (come Nietzschean) psychoanalyst. In one of her incarnations, as a ten-year-old girl, Ursula is sent to see him.

> He had trained in Vienna ("where else?") but trod, he said, his own path.
> He was no one's disciple, he said, although he had studied "at the feet of all

the teachers. One must nose forward," he said. "Nudge one's way through the chaos of our thoughts. Unite the divided self." Ursula had no idea what he was talking about.

Atkinson also plays with the idea of the novel as a bourgeois form. *Life after Life* begins with a long idyllic evocation of upper-middle-class English life. She has said it was Forster always at her back, but to me the angel at her back is Virginia Woolf, particularly *Mrs. Dalloway*. As the story begins again and again on that snowy night in 1910, so the Merchant and Ivory scenario disintegrates and nostalgia is untethered, teased out, floats like seaweed in a bloody sea. Not just the Virginia Woolf of the novels, but also the essayist and the woman who kept a diary full of quotidian details. While it is undoubtedly false to pose quotidian detail against the sweep of history, the trick is surely to understand and craft scale, through writing to mobilize that precarious, never stable, relation between scale and perspective. What the most intriguing novels and biographies do is illuminate not just details within the large sweep of history, but the sweep of history in the details. The new biography of Marx by Jonathan Sperber does this. I dipped in and out of it while out of it. J read it voraciously from cover to cover (when it could be pried away from Elvis) and would relay the revelations, day by day, in between making endless supplies of chicken soup, a ministering Scheherazade.

I always find myself (again, time after time, life after life) a better Buddhist when things are going well. *Better* of course is the wrong word, no, I mean more inclined to be philosophically calm and accepting of fate, unperturbed by death. The past few days, before this awful smothering black blanket of nausea lifted, I felt very despairing, as though I would never get better, even for a while. A "this is it!" kind of feeling. There is a simple line in *Life after Life*: "How sorry she felt for herself, as if she were someone else." Somehow, as almost everyone must know, illness induces this as you see time falling through all the cracks in your life, never to be retrieved. Today, though, I feel grandiosely like a besieged city that has been liberated. I woke up this morning feeling transformed, the nausea almost gone, euphoric. I hadn't quite finished the Kate Atkinson and so got up, fed the cats (without experiencing that usual vomit-inducing odor as the tin of grain-free chicken-and-herring delight is prized open), let the chickens out in the dawn light, made a pot of tea, and went back to bed and finished the novel—it felt so luxurious, reading not to allay sickness, but for pure pleasure. And of course I should know from the novel that after a besieged city is liberated (London and Berlin during the Second World War bombing) there isn't immediate relief, what follows may be starvation, suicide, old age, mundanity. And yet . . . and yet I loved the novel, it filled me with a peculiar happiness like Mrs. Dalloway with her flowers. Atkinson has said you cannot write about happiness, that's not what life is. It's true the novel is not about finding happiness, I wept in parts and had to gloss over others that were too grim, and yet happiness is no less complex an emotion than, say, despair or misery, it's just as implicated in the devious trajectories of desire. I'm glad I finished the novel on a high so I don't always have it snuggled into bed, in a semi-illicit association with sickness.

Today I feel quite different, not sorry for myself at all, actually rather overwhelmed by the wonderful world I awoke into but more convinced than ever that the self, though experienced materially, bodily, is a fiction.

And what is it that constitutes feeling OK? Being drug-free is undoubtedly a big part of it. It surely must have been the combination of antibiotics with the Revlimid that made for such awfulness. Because of the initial searing gut pain and fever I diagnosed myself with a flare-up of diverticulitis, and my primary care doctor agreed, insisted on the antibiotics, and since the fever and pain were subsiding, succumbed to my resistance to yet another CAT scan with contrast (time after time, too much radiation). I thought the antibiotics were working, but not really, the pain came and went. And the worst thing was the unrelenting nausea, dizziness, sensation of fainting even when lying still in bed. Dr. K is inclined to think that this could have been because of the piling up of chemicals ("we don't know how the body will protest") but also that the pain was not in fact provoked by an infection (hence no need for antibiotics) but caused by tumor lysis. This refers to metabolic complications that can occur during cancer treatment, particularly in leukemia and lymphoma. Although the treatment is meant to reduce, say, the size and number of lymph nodes, in fact it can do the opposite for a while. The lymph nodes in my gut area are increased, and he guesses that this has put pressure on the colon. This makes sense, but nevertheless I have a gut feeling (so apt a truism) that the chemicals are also ravaging my gut and so am drinking aloe vera juice an hour before eating and also taking L-glutamin powder, both of which restore the mucous membrane of the colon stripped away by antibiotics, as we know, but also by the other drugs. Acupuncture provided miraculous relief, but only for a short time (though it was amazing to see how color returned to my face during those sessions). However, my skin is so thin now. Thicker emotionally perhaps, but in the end there is just that thin penumbra between you and the world.

Now I'm into the fourth round. Dr. K decided not to up the dose because of the complications, though he is reluctant, feeling that it is only with an increased dose that some of the symptoms will abate and improvement register (white and red blood counts are miraculously in the normal zone, but others are wonky). Still, it is underway, and I am feeling almost fine. Phew! With trepidation I have another immunoglobulin infusion this week, since an adverse reaction during the last one. . . .

. . .

There are other things besides acupuncture that provided relief and forgetfulness. I thought I could drive myself to acupuncture one time, but when I got out of bed realized that this wasn't going to work. I called Tershia, and she came and fetched me in her 1969 Porsche. It was originally sand colored, but Tershia turned it antique apple green. Just looking at it is a joy. It registers beauty—in its design, but also in that color, that delicious green that seems otherwise to have disappeared from the world, a green of mahjong pieces, of bathroom tiles and my grandmother's kitchen. Nothing grandmotherly about that ride to the acupuncturist, however. Tershia drives her ancient racing car as though it were a racing car. You might think that this would exacerbate nausea, but it was rather like entering into a dream. I loved being inside that greenness, whizzing through the city.

And then there was the poppy. Steve Ilott gave me, months ago, some white poppies he had started. We planted them out and waited and waited as they grew in a spindly fashion. Then one day as I lay languishing, feeling sorry for myself, Peggy—who was working in the garden, fighting the weeds which have gone berserk since people on the street started planting "low-maintenance native" grasses—took a picture of the blooming poppy on her phone and sent it to me in the house. It was a totally unexpected apparition: a glorious white pom-pom. I had been assuming that an old-fashioned and elegant poppy would eventually bloom. Instead: the sheer exuberance and excess of that Swansdown startled me into delight. On the morning when I awoke feeling OK, I opened the front door in the early morning, and there were four white pom-poms, gleaming among the irises and salvia, roses and fennel, brash colors muted momentarily in the dawn, ceding glory to Swansdown.

In the infusion center at Hillcrest Nurse Marcie entertains us with stories about her weekend in LA and the meals she had. She went to the restaurant Animal and ate a pig's ear.

Time passes.

Then, maybe twenty minutes later, a voice from one of the other infusion chairs speaks:

not everywhere
can you eat
a pig's ear.

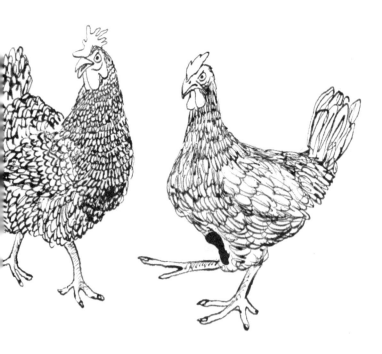

Some Musings on Metaphor

Looking at my lab results on the computer each week is like watching a soccer ball, soaring in slow motion, peaking and then descending. You hold your breath: where will it land, inside or outside the line? Before I started treatment red flags plastered the screen. Now there are few, many items that were flagged too high or too low have settled into the normal category. June has been a good month, I am feeling considerably better, with miles more energy.

My white blood cell count fell into the normal range fairly soon after starting treatment. But actually there are many kinds of white blood cells, and at least two kinds are crucial indicators for CLL, or since each case is idiosyncratic, let's say for me at the moment. My neutrophils are slightly low—most likely induced by the Revlimid. If they go much lower it means likely neutropenia (when you are dangerously at risk of infection, when you have to eat only cooked vegetables and fruit, wear a mask, etc. . . . everyone probably knows someone who has had cancer and endured a period of neutropenia, induced by the chemo), but so far it's very borderline. Then there are lymphocytes. In the past month the absolute lympho-cyte count has normalized.

MM, my primary care physician, said no wonder you are feeling better, when your lymphocyte count is up it's like you have a constant virus you are fighting day in and day out. My first reaction was, Whoa, how would you know what it *feels* like? Stick to science, Doctor; don't presume to tell me how it *feels*. A flashback to hot flashes and the gynecologist (young, compassionate, efficient, female) who said, Just think of it as a normal part of life; everyone gets hot, I get hot some-times, and I just take a deep breath and drink some water and it passes. Well bully for you, lady, may you wake one day in your best silk blouse suddenly sweating swinishly as you address a room full of bright-eyed and bushy-tailed gynecology students. A moment ago they were hanging on your every word, now their eyes are fixed on the sweaty, stained blouse clinging to your breasts. But MM is not that gynecologist. She is tough and vigilant and frank. She is also a go-between, mediating between the various specialists I encounter, ping-ponging from one to another. She was the one who really kicked me into treatment the first time. "You have put it off for long enough, and now you are saying, Well I think I'll wait a while. You really need to start treatment *now*." She must be about half my age, but she calls me "sweetie." "Well done, sweetie," she will say when she thinks I have conquered the denial impulse and recognized some danger signal and given her a call. I find it very endearing to be called sweetie. Bittersweet like the Jane Campion movie.

. . .

Friends are curious and always asking: What is it like? Much of the time we look quite normal, when you go to the CLL support group you might think you were in a room of perfectly healthy people, the swollen lymph nodes and spleens are not visible, nor the haywire white blood cells, cavorting platelets, nor the havoc being played in bone marrow. Nor the sense of utter exhaustion and fluishness. People often say to me, "How are you? You look great!" On bad days this can be irritating because typically they ask a question and answer it themselves, pronouncing you well and fine. This was a refrain after my dance with death just before our Boxing Day party, though on this occasion not in the least irritating. Boxing Day is the day after Christmas, and this past year it was also the day after I came out of hospital. The cause was an infection that went haywire overnight, landing me in the ER. Four nights in hospital, and then I was fine, immensely relieved, and we went ahead with our Boxing Day tamale party. Teddy Cruz brings the most delicious Guatemalan tamales. They are wrapped in banana leaves and steamed. Unwrapping is at once a delaying mechanism, a stringing out of anticipation, and a process of revelation. As you unwrap the smells start swirling, not just one smell but many. The masa (or corn dough) inside the banana leaf wrapping is in turn wrapped around the filling—pork or chicken or vegetarian—and a sauce that is beginning to ooze out so you have to lick your fingers to get a taste of what is to come. You pause, fingers in your mouth, imagining. And then you break into the tamale. Inside there is pork and a piece of fruit, an olive perhaps, and even though there is a melting moment flavors are distinct—sharp, sweet, meaty. You scoop a bite of tamale into your mouth and enter heaven.

I have never met this woman who works in her kitchen at home and conjures these magical tamales into being. Teddy is the go-between. But I do know something about her. A week before Christmas her husband, who had been living and working in San Diego for years, was walking along the street not far from our house when a Homeland Security van pulled up and stopped him, requesting his papers. He had none. He was pulled into the van and deported from the country.

Although I sometimes find the "you look great" refrain irritating, receiving it as vacuous routine politeness, actually I know that when people say this they are more often than not performing an act of sympathetic magic: they are wishing that all is well, they want you to be well, they want to believe that everything is fine. And you participate in the performance. You are relieved to be alive and want to look as normal as possible. On Boxing Day I was particularly glad to be alive and celebrating. But the scary thing is the knowledge that it could be something like this that will take me out. Many CLL deaths (because CLL is a disease of the immune system) are from simple infections that flare up quickly and can't be controlled. This is what MM has always been trying to impress upon me: be alert to the signals, act immediately, don't be so cavalier. She was pregnant and on leave when this happened, but when she came back she said, "Well done, sweetie, you got yourself to ER in time."

. . .

MM offered the metaphor of living with a virus. There is an aptness to it, it's graspable, something one can offer to others. Dr. K offered another. After my first treatment I said to him, It's like a miracle. I had no idea how awful I had been feeling. For years. This is the real normal, and it's a great sensation! Dr. K said, Many patients say exactly the same thing. And he offered a metaphor: It's like hiking up a hill with a backpack on your back. You start with a few pebbles in your pack, and after a while you add a few more, and then after another few miles the gremlin at your back tosses in just one more stone, but this one is a little larger, heavier. And so it goes, and as you climb you accommodate to the weight and the difficulty, and you come to imagine this as normal.

Rather than being affronted by Dr. K's simile, or his presumption in describing my sensations, I experienced a surprising sense of gratitude. His image was not exactly intricate or poetic, and certainly was far from scientific. Perhaps though this is precisely the key to understanding how it works. How a simple metaphor describing an illness can spark delight. Why? I wonder. Clearly, on one level it's because of recognition. It offers a mirror image, a confirmation of identity. Thus, it might be argued, it doesn't do much to shift anything, it simply confirms the way things are, the way you *feel*. And though I abhor the kind of feel-good triumphalism that validates *every* feeling as evidence of self-worth, nevertheless I think there is something crucial that happens when the language of medicine or science is blurred by the poetic impulse of metaphor. Many illnesses, particularly chronic ones, as well as many psychological states, are isolating, for the patient it's hard to situate what they *feel* as anything other than ultra-personal. There are times when you think maybe it's all in my head, or maybe I am inducing this illness because of the way I feel. So to have an image flashed up, from elsewhere, from someone else, that is evocative and feels accurate, this is gratifying. You want to shout out, Yes! That's it! Something surges through your system, is energizing, and it isn't a drug. This kind of metaphor differs from the destructive metaphors that Susan Sontag so brilliantly described in *Illness as Metaphor*.

Metaphor literally means a bridge between two things, two words, two images. The more unlikely the linkage the more powerful the metaphor, and the more it can be spun out the greater its capacity to inspire intrigue and wonder. But in addition to confirming the way you feel, metaphor has the potential to perform an intricate dance of difference. There is always that space of difference, of something incommensurate that stretches between the two unlikely images. A patient *is* and *is not* a hiker. In that tension, in the surprise, in the fact that the image flashes up from elsewhere—it is in this process that metaphor has the capacity to open your eyes, to introduce not just sameness and recognition, but newness. The drugs serve to lighten the load, but words too.

. . .

Newness and surprise are great medicines.

. . .

Much of the time I swim through Dr. K's language, feeling an idiot because I haven't done my homework and there is still so much I do not understand, and sometimes despair that I ever will. And there's not much time. And how will I ever make the right decisions about which therapy if I'm so clueless? He has a lot of patients to see on this one day of the week when he isn't doing research or flying around the world talking about CLL. Often I call up Sheila Hoff, our CLL research nurse and case manager, and she patiently spends hours going over it all, translating, helping with decisions by giving examples, and always she says, Think about what kind of a person you are, how you want to live your life, which treatment will suit you best. Or I turn to a patient advocate site on the internet, like that of Chaya Venkat. Sadly she has announced this week that she is retiring. Her husband died of CLL. Though not a medical doctor, she is a science writer and started the site to link her husband's journey with that of others, to mediate between the scientific community (and scientific language) and patients. For twelve years (eight while her husband was alive, four after, by herself) she has done a quite amazing job as a patient advocate and as a magician of words. Understanding the language, yes, but something more. Finding the words. Saying the words. Her retirement blog is very poignant.

. . .

When I was looking for good crime novels (when not?), the kind you can lose yourself in, Patricia Montoya, my friend and neighbor (who has herself recently been through hell, survived a rough stem cell transplant, now back for the summer in her bittersweet home, Medellin), suggested I read *Tijuana Straits*. It's a surf-noir novel set primarily in the Tijuana River Valley, the area that stretches from Imperial Beach in the northeast corner of the valley and along the U.S. border with Mexico. Twenty minutes from where I live. It begins in the estuary, with the main protagonist, whose charge is protecting certain migratory birds (most notably the western snowy plover and the light-footed clapper rail), discovering in the early morning dawn a woman in distress, who seems to have crossed by an illegal route where the border fence cuts the valley in half. Kem Nunn evokes the area vividly: the crashing surf, the lighthouse in Las Playas on the Mexican side of the fence, Yogurt Canyon, Smuggler's Gulch, the routes through the valley on this side—Monument Road at the edge of Border Field State Park, Hollister Drive, Dairy Mart Road—and the maze of dirt roads and horse trails. I started reading the novel after a particularly hairy infusion and experienced a peculiar delight in recognizing these places, even seeing these names in print, saying them out loud. There is the comfort of familiarity of course, but also there is always a slight, maybe infinitesimal, mismatch between the image offered and your memories. There is a pleasure in puzzling out how the images cohere, form a landscape, in imagining even when you can't be there. Nunn wrote this novel shortly before Homeland Security hacked into the landscape in 2003 so brutally, demolishing a mesa, filling in a canyon, and building a new, second wall flanked by a perfectly asphalted wide road, a road where no one drives except the occasional border patrol vehicle. So sometimes he describes a landscape I hardly knew, and I try to conjure it, ripping out the new steel fence, and the asphalt road, and restoring the canyon in my mind.

. . .

You picture and imagine a landscape, a configuration of space shadowed always by various histories, some quite personal, others social, unfolding, oblivious to your personal existence. It is like this too with simple metaphors, thrown up in the haze of misrecognition, when you do not know how to make sense of this place where you find yourself.

. . .

For me the Boxing Day party was a celebration of being alive, of having escaped again, of friendship. The house was packed, the air was festive, people drifted in and out of the garden, unlikely people became entranced by the chickens and entered into chicken conversations. The tamales, however, as well as being delicious were a reminder that cancer is a card you can carry, it's like having papers, if you are lucky enough to have medical care people are basically on your side, want everything to be fine, want you to be well. Of course you live with the fear of sudden, or slow, death. But as people who have cancer and Buddhists and even total strangers with whom you strike up a conversation in the long line at the pharmacy remark: We are all going to die, death is a part of life, and, anyway, who knows? You might walk under a bus tomorrow. True no doubt. But it is also the case that many people in this country live without any papers at all, let alone a cancer card, and they live in real and daily fear of a chasm opening up when and if the Homeland Security van pulls up one day as they stroll to work, to the shop, to the neighborhood park.

Tricking the Body

16

There are all kinds of ways of tricking the body. Working is one way, if you can find ways to make working work. These long cancers (any cancer of course) have psychic effects too, and after my body encountered crisis at Christmas, and then the prospect of this long treatment, a black hole opened up. Having a commitment to carry out all the duties I'd signed up for at work has been a way of dodging not just the hole, but all the puddles of gloom. One foot in front of the other, and every time you have to be at a meeting or in a classroom and are called upon to perform somehow the energy arises. In particular, teaching has been energizing. Even though at the end of the day you feel drained, during the day you're buzzing.

But in two weeks' time I will stop working. *Work* work, that is. Not just a pause for medical leave; no, I've made a radical, anxiety-fraught decision—to retire. On the one hand, this is an acknowledgment that time is running out, on the other hand, it's a hedging of bets: that this way you can stretch time, make more of it, more time of your own choosing, less time whittled away in academic responsibilities and more time spent on a different kind of work—writing. Gardening too, and cooking, and being with friends. It is with mixed feelings that I tie or sever the knot. MM is relieved, she thinks I should have done this long ago, but it is hard to break with habits of a lifetime, with an identity and way of being in the world. I will surely miss teaching, and many friends, and the possibility that university life—at its best—offers: the possibility of encountering strange ideas and compelling arguments and idiosyncratic characters. But the bottom line, the murky truth, is that I'm afraid I will miss the structure and the institutional status that makes you visible in the world. I do not fancy describing myself as retired, but Sylvia, the indomitable, pulls the rug from under my mousiness; she writes from Australia saying, "You are not retiring! Writers never retire!"

With a group of graduate students I've been working on a small project constructing viable miniature mobile gardens with a community living in a canyon in Tijuana, where the combination of polluted soil, water scarcity, and poverty has made it impossible to grow nutritious vegetables. It's a modest experiment, in collaboration as much as anything, in entering into a learning process with the community. It is the students, though, who are undertaking the liaison and the traveling and the hard work, as the area is too toxic for me to venture into right now. Of course it is doubly toxic for the people who live there, and they have no escape; it is their home. For many who are squatting, it is a transitory home, but many others have established ingenious dwellings on the precarious slopes. I hope the project will continue and that I will be able to return to the canyon, but perhaps it will take different forms than expected. In the meantime I continue to meet for long sessions with the group at my house, where we are reading, writing, planning, budgeting, arguing over ethics and pragmatics. They are motivated, brave, and inspiring. It feels as though both Los Laureles and CLL will be lengthy projects, but each meeting with the students offers a moment of drama, of performance, a gathering of forces, a distillation of knowledge and desire. An infusion of resilience.

While it is true to say that work is a way of tricking the body, it is also true that I would not have managed to keep on working without supportive colleagues; the rides and gourmet meals delivered to the door by friends; the messages, tapes, books, and Buddha machines that came from far afield. I could not have kept working without J looking after me, and me looking after the chickens and Elvis and Roxy. Collaborations take many forms.

Chicken Joke

17

A man believes he is a grain of seed. He is taken to a mental institution, where the doctors do their best finally to convince him that he is not a grain, but a man. No sooner has he left the hospital than he comes back, very scared, claiming that there is a chicken outside the door, and he is afraid that it will eat him. "Dear fellow," says his doctor, "you know very well that you are not a grain of seed, but a man." "Of course I know that," replies the patient, "but does the chicken?"

This joke is told by Alenka Zupančič in *The Odd One In: On Comedy*. She says that what is at stake here is the post-Enlightenment assertion: I know very well, but nevertheless . . . (I know very well that there is no God, nevertheless I pray that God will save me from this awful situation, pluck me out of this shithole). She traces a thread of connection between Hegel and Lacan, between the phenomenology of spirit and the concept of the Other. Her twisting of the skeins is provocative; she takes a paradox and plays it as though it were a queen of hearts or seven of spades, the paradoxes proliferate, the tricks are blindingly spectacular. Is it sleight of hand or logic refined to the nth degree?

Yet there is something left over for me, something that she doesn't directly address, though perhaps it lurks and swims around in the lower depths of the joke. What is left over is fear, a kind of fear embedded in category confusion and realized most obviously in phobias but also in simple fears like the fear of dying. It's not just me and the chicken, me and the other, but there is a third term: this thing, this grain of seed, or let's call it a corn kernel. *Self* and *Other*, these terms are mobilized in a circuit of exchange involving Other Things, and at some stage this circuit involves (or threatens) consumption and disappearance or annihilation.

. . .

I came to chickens and to Buddhism at roughly the same time. Not entirely true, I grew up with chickens and as an adult have had chickens in my life whenever possible, so in part I was enacting a repetition of the familiar (rather than the sense of discovery implied in the notion of *coming to*). But my relation to chickens has been very different this time. Buddhism was not familiar. After coming to political consciousness as a teenager I settled into a habitual semiconscious cynicism about religion, or let's just say faith or spirit with either a small or large *S*. But in Shambhala I have found myself sometimes in a not-unfamiliar place. Not the place of religion, but of therapy, specifically psychotherapy. Another form of repetition, therefore.

Chickens became an obsession when I was pretty unwell and heading into my first treatment. Obsession, I'm convinced, is potentially curative. It is a form of denial certainly, a delusional projection, an enactment of repetition in the face of death. But it works. Sometimes it works. It takes your mind off things, prevents you from succumbing to another competing repetition, to the mantra of despair or, worse, of resignation.

If we want to use the language of psychoanalysis we might say that chickens are the way the subject's unconscious (and her relation to herself) are externalized.

Cancer brought me to meditation. I signed up to Shambhala (a version of Buddhism) in order to learn some techniques for meditation. There is no doubt that meditation is a way of calming the body, reducing stress, promoting the antitoxins, giving energy. Science tells us this, though anyone who has meditated can tell you the same thing. But when I started going to Shambhala I found that the *techniques* of meditation were not so separable from the *ethos* of this version of Buddhism. One way of looking at this is to say that you bring into meditation a whole lot of baggage, and meditation itself shakes loose the careful packing (or repression), interferes with habitual patterns, throws into the unconscious—in slow motion—a Molotov cocktail. *Baggage* has become a remarkably familiar term in everyday parlance, it's the kind of language that makes me squeamish. And indeed there are aspects of the Shambhala training that have induced squeamishness (many new age therapeutic models, such as mindfulness training, draw on and are heavily influenced by varieties of Buddhism, and then in turn varieties of Buddhism have adapted to a Western environment and borrow familiar new age language). Sometimes I have yearned for a more severe practice, for what I imagine the spartanness of Zen to be. But then I remind myself that after all I am not Tibetan, like others in the room I am a predictable Westerner looking to Buddhism to change something. So I tell myself this: Suck it up, darling.

I came to meditation hoping to find a way of being more at peace in the world (and therefore healthier, better able to fight the cancer). Of course, once you start shaking that can of hope, all the worms come squirming out. And you find that you are faced with the phantoms of repetition. And you would like to change, quite simply (and even though it makes me squirm to say it), you would like to be a better person. Being more at peace might also have payoffs—for those around you, those who suffer the importunate blasts of bad temper, inveterate quibbling, acerbic barbs exploded randomly, not to mention hardly muted envy.

Squirm and quease. Buddhism has in common with psychotherapy a serious engagement with the unconscious (even though the word *unconscious* may not occur). Often the distinction is made between acknowledgment (just letting it come to the surface, letting it be) and analysis (analyzing dreams, jokes, stories, memories, and so on). This distinction is hard to maintain, but let us put the difficulty on hold for the moment. Some of the Shambhala trainings are built on a dyadic structure. In a workshop you are given a question, or situation, and then the group divides into pairs. The first person has five minutes to speak (or not). The other person listens, they are not to respond in any way, they should not smile or offer encouragement, express agreement or approval or disagreement. And then you swap positions. And then there is five minutes for dialogue. The hard thing, the really hard thing, is not speaking, but listening in such a way as to resist solicitation.

Over and over again we repeat the same moves. We enter analysis (let's say analysis, but perhaps we enter into other therapeutic spaces too—the sangha, the garden, the yoga studio, the church). You do this because you want to change, you want to break old habits, alter the way you relate to others or to the Other. Or you want to face life (and death) more fearlessly. Or both these things. You are prone to believing that when the therapy or retreat is over you will reemerge into the world and be liberated, *cured*, able to act differently. But actually, as we are repeatedly warned, nothing will change until you fully recognize the Other as something *other* than a projection of self. And this has to take place in the world.

In short, it is not simply that in analysis the subject has to shift her position (or even adapt herself); the major part of the analytic work consists precisely in shifting the external practices, in moving all those "chickens" in which the subject's unconscious (and her relation to herself) are externalized.

I wonder sometimes if I am not becoming chicken, clucking and cooing and chirruping, grubbing around in the hedgerows looking for worms. Flapping around like Charlie Chaplin in *The Gold Rush*. Holly, Lula Mae, Sabrina, and Funny Face have coaxed from me a much more intimate relationship than I have ever before experienced with chickens. Is this identification? Have I wormed my way successfully into the being of the chicken? Or perhaps more profoundly found a way of acknowledging the otherness of chicken-being, realizing how the chicken thinks and feels, out there in the world, independent of my consciousness. Often, as I sit in the garden at the end of the day and the chickens pick and peck and scratch, I feel remarkably contented, at one with the world, grateful to have passed through the repetitive obsessive phase. And then Sabrina will suddenly extend her neck, cock her head, and stare. Eyes glinting blackly she will dive at my leg and peck. It hurts. She thinks I am a corn kernel.

I know very well of course that I am not a kernel of corn. Nevertheless . . .

Nice Paint Job

18

At a farewell party Matt Savitsky gave back to me as a gift a story I once told him, a story about writing. It was when you were living, he said, on the Lower East Side of Manhattan, late eighties I think. You used to walk past this wall which was always covered with graffiti. One day you were ambling along and came to the wall and it had been painted white. A great expanse of whiteness. And across the wall someone had painted, in black paint: NICE PAINT JOB.

. . .

I'm into the fifth round (the fifth month) of the chemo. The dose has been upped again. And it's going OK so far. Seem to have a handle on managing the GI issues. There has been low-grade neutropenia (common with chemo, it makes you very vulnerable to bacterial infection), but it could be much worse. And tomorrow I have another immunoglobulin infusion that will strengthen the immune system and should counter the neutropenia somewhat. As I finish up at work, time and space seem to be opening up—for writing, more gardening, more time to do the healthy things like juicing and walking and meditation and bread baking.

The stupid thing is that I twisted my ankle pretty badly. Picking peaches, looking at the peaches instead of the step, thinking about peaches rather than where to put my foot. Have resisted X-rays because of all the radiation. This is the thing once you start going down the cancer road: Each therapeutic mechanism or drug carries its own dangers, very often dangers that expose you to other cancers. Anyway, now it's over a week and they are concerned about the swelling and bruising that persists and want an X-ray to see if there are fractures and an ultrasound to see if there are blood clots. This is the vicious circle: Revlimid can cause blood clots, so I take a baby aspirin every day. This thins the blood, makes the internal bleeding from the ankle twist worse, potentially exacerbating clots.

On the bright side: visitors. Eileen Myles came to visit from New York, a great sparkle in the sky. Adriene Jenik also came through town and paused for a long reverie, and Leslie Dick visited for a day, and we talked nonstop for eight hours, and instead of feeling drained I felt charged by light. A lovely encomium from dear Norman Bryson at a faculty send-off. A tiny part of me has always felt ever-so-slightly frightened of Norman, as though I could never measure up to his intellectual standards. So I was very touched. Trying to accept praise graciously I told myself: Grow up already! Yet, even as I uttered the reprimand it seemed time to acknowledge that perhaps it will never happen, never be reached, that mythical state of being grown up.

Frenzied Calm   19

The obsession grows slowly, building in momentum. In the beginning it tickles, a feather playing whimsically over the surface of your skin, a pleasurable sensation. Delicately a world opens up, a world of the imagination, a "what if" universe.

It begins as a stray thought, a meandering fantasy. You are into your sixth month of chemo treatment, have decided to throw in the sponge at work, and are contemplating time stretching out like a desert before you. Fueled by a fantasy of slow time and slow food you nevertheless imagine rapidity: What if you had a stove that heats up more quickly, that cooks more speedily, that responds to your touch the way his car anticipates James Bond's every tactile desire? What if there were gas burners that could alternate between flames shooting into the sky and the merest whisper of heat? Imagine not having to get down on your knees to use the broiler. Imagine having all four rings that work, tossing that pair of pliers you use in place of a missing knob.

And then you think, well why not? Why not give myself a retirement present? An idle thought.

You start dreaming, in a desultory way, about kitchen ranges. Just occasionally, while waiting for the clothes to dry, the water to boil, the chickens to lay an egg. The thought starts idling, seldom switches off, purrs away this side of consciousness. You encounter some beautiful ranges online. Italian. Far too expensive. Gorgeous primary colors and great design—chunky yet streamlined. Suddenly kitchen ranges seem to pop up in conversation everywhere. Everyone has an opinion. Even people you'd always imagined as rat runners, always eating out, grabbing fast food with the works, and eating on the run, they too have range stories. Every house you visit lures you into the kitchen, every kitchen range you encounter elicits a story, a saga of mishaps, opinionated suggestions, alarming anecdotes. In

Nasser's kitchen you come face-to-face with the desired Italian range, magnetic, gleaming redly. You feel that this undoubtedly is it, the decision is made. Then you open the oven and it's the size of a shoebox. So that puts a kibosh on that, and the search is on. You start visiting showrooms, department stores, specialty appliance shops, talking to the sales people and experts, reading reviews and users' comments on cooking sites. And all the information you receive is totally contradictory. Nevertheless there is some pleasure in the exercise. It takes up time, time that could be devoted to other things. It takes up space in your head and on your desk where bits of paper are strewn, scraps on which are scrawled notes about ranges, scraps mixed up with insurance elective forms, with thick booklets on how to fill out retirement forms, and receipts for drugs that have to be checked against the FAS list, and lists of foods that are poisonous to chickens. You chuck that list, the chickens eat everything. You start a folder called "ranges."

It seems you might have to stretch the budget a bit to get the kind of range you want.

The horizon of desire expands. Eating your breakfast you imagine your beautiful new stove, you imagine it orange. You look at the timber floor, scratched, worn down to paper thinness. You look at the dingy walls. You look at the grungy grayish cabinets, painted an eon ago. You look at the bulky energy-guzzling lights. They look back at you.

So you start researching sustainable flooring. Seized by nostalgia you are seduced into the world of linoleum, bewitched by the range of colors and patterns, Play-Doh colors, gorgeously marbled, slightly unreal. You order samples and they come in great big boxes and take up lots of space. You start cruising around paint shops picking up swatches, speculating, merely speculating, what color walls, you wonder, would set off a Pop Rocket floor. Idly. Just for fun.

And so it begins. You rename your ranges file: "kitchen." The idling revs up. You imagine a creamy color for the walls, not quite white, off-white perhaps, though your purchase on color is clearly precarious. The descriptive confusion, however, is just beginning, you are about to enter a forest, a delirious entanglement of names and colors that seemingly bear no relation to one another and yet are always presented categorically in columns and rows, or in families, as though they accord to genre specificity, to taxonomic logic: puppy paws, French manicure, cappuccino froth, papaya, frappe, squish-squash, little angel, pineapple fizz, Havana cream. The difference between moonlight and morning sunshine is infinitesimal, if it exists at all. You wake in the gloom of indeterminacy, gathering strength to face the forms, the endless insurance forms in which you have to find exactly the right words to describe your disability, make elections, decide once and for all how much income you'll get each month versus payouts to your partner when you die. The more you get now, the less he gets when you pop off. You put the forms away, unfilled-in. Nevertheless you feel pleased with yourself, your capacity to make at least a few decisions, today you will narrow the range of possible kitchen paint colors. You cruise around the city collecting paint samples. You get home and try them out and they all look different in situ, all wrong. Start again. Like a lepidopterist organizing their butterfly collection, you are completely immersed in the project, captivated by detail, utterly content.

Details, ah yes, the myriad swarming details, such as knobs for the cabinets. On the industrial edges of the city you find Knob Heaven and float amid the offerings, a Holly Golightly buoyed by treasure in this Tiffanys of Hardware. eBay opens up even further opportunities and choices. You spend hours and hours there, discover a glass color called Coke bottle green, aka depression green. It is warm ice: clear, pale, translucent. You purchase samples to compare, one or two here another few there, you will send them back if they aren't right. Now the house is full of boxes of knobs. Most aren't right. It seems translucent green is a difficult color to render, and not all depression green glass is created equal.

And another detail—those bulky dim energy-guzzling lights, they have to go, cannot survive in your new streamlined gourmet paradise. LED ceiling lights, this you can get a handle on, but under-the-cabinet lights, this is mysterious. What is the difference between strips, tapes, and diffusers? You find an environmental lighting place and a charming engineer who is happy to explain it all to a dumbass Martha Stewart wannabe.

Could it be that the knobs are a way of screwing down anxiety? It's true that the more you screw the more a calm seeps into the kitchen, but it is a calm infiltrated by willowy strands of frenzy.

This frenzied calm is not unfamiliar. It comes with fixation, especially a new one, a new one displacing or not inconceivably augmenting old obsessions. It brings pleasure: You wallow luxuriously in endless rolling waves of choice.

. . .

Painters come, inspect, frown, and then smile and say: This is easy, will take no time. They estimate a week, ten days at the most. We choose a guy called Jack, he's worked with a lot of old houses, he flatters our small Californian bungalow, he says that when he's finished it will look like an original craftsman. He is reassuring. He tells us he teams with an electrician, a whiz at working with old houses, at figuring things out. He's Jack too. The painter says, "I'm Little Jack, he's Big Jack." Big Jack, when he comes on board, tells me that he taught Little Jack everything he knows.

To compensate for the mid-high-end range it will be a modest remodel—no tearing down of walls or installing new cabinets. You will keep the deep green Formica counter and the old wooden cabinets even though the Jacks have called them "carcasses." Just a simple paint job, new flooring, new stove. Oh and what about the rusty chugging fridge? You narrow your choices, make decisions about things, use this opportunity to expunge the clutter. There is a long list of things, big things like a commercial stove (heavy but petite, adapted to a small domestic space), a new bisque fridge, a shiny hood, and small things like hooks and knobs and icy glass splash-back tiles. All these things will make your kitchen cleaner, sleeker, more streamlined, easier to work in.

. . .

Speaking of things, this is a period of transition. As a retiring Buddhist, or a Buddhist retiring, I am in the process of letting go, infinitesimally, of material things. This relinquishing isn't like renouncing pleasurable things for Lent. It isn't really about things as things, it's more about a state of mind. It's OK to love plants and cultivate them but not to lust after the cerise blossoms of the peach called Red Baron. It's OK to raise chickens in your backyard but not to love them immoderately. It's a question of proportion. This I know.

I think of this kitchen adventure as a last fling with things, a slow waltz with the sensuous cushioning of daily life.

I had no idea how slow that slow waltz would be.

. . .

It begins with a rearrangement of the whole house. Everything has to be taken out of the kitchen. It's a small kitchen. Not much stuff, you'd think. Yet box after box after box fills up. We start by labeling scrupulously, in the end the garlic press and paintings and the iron and cans of cat food are flung into the same box. At two o'clock in the morning we run out of boxes, so stuff is just carried through to the spare room, where the bed is upended to make space. Cookbooks are all over the living room. You have to step over large containers of vinegar, toilet rolls, cans of tuna.

The house has to be entirely rearranged. The entry to the attic is through my minuscule closet overcrowded with clothes, with fantasies of a more fashionable life than I get to lead in my mundane chicken-bound existence. The Jacks have to enter the attic in order to ascertain where the beams are in the kitchen, to construct a duct from the newly installed hood out through the ceiling. They return through the attic and into the bedroom in clouds of spurious gray matter. So I have to drag all my clothes out. It begins systematically, but in the end, or very soon, I start throwing things randomly into black plastic trash bags. For the next six weeks I will wear the same three articles of clothing again and again, day in, day out.

We are all discombobulated but the cats most of all. Elvis and Roxy are freaked and suspicious. Nothing is in its right place. They cannot enter the house through their normal way—a cat door that leads from the back garden into the kitchen. We have to rig up a ramp to the back bedroom and leave the window wide open. The chickens take this as an open invitation: *Mi casa es tu casa.* Chickens and cats pick their way over a forest floor of things—boxes of kitchen items and bags of clothes, a blender, toaster, food processor, quesadilla maker, cake tins, wooden spoons, my mother's fish knives: the detritus of human hubris. Elvis, who has ignored J for twelve years, turns his back on me each night and curls up in the crook of J's leg. He holds me responsible. He is right, and my heart is crumbling.

As work begins on the kitchen clouds of dust, shards of dried (old and toxic) paint, globules of grouting, slivers of rotten wood fly into the air and spread through the open doors and windows into the rest of the house. You fight your way through a fog of filth, space travelers entering an alien planet. Big Jack and Little Jack, and J too, are all indifferent to what I consider filth. And all three are indifferent to the difference between open and closed doors. You cough and splutter and seethe and go around closing doors and windows. Two minutes later they are open again. You close them. You watch the dust settle daily over the few bowls and plates that have been secreted in the living room for eating off laps, over clothes, CDs, plants, the cats' food, tea towels, books, bread. My skin is scaly. Irritation and stress fester and bubble. I cannot comprehend this indifference to filth. The three men no doubt consider me fanatical, and as Buddhists and painters and electricians and husbands know, fanaticism is pointless. What does it matter? Well, to me, matter out of place is dirt. The more displaced the more alarming. I imagine the filth as endemic, the project of cleanliness never-ending. I have become a suburban Woman of the Dunes, endlessly removing sand that seeps back through the cracks, rising up, engulfing the universe.

· · ·

If only I were a chicken. The greatest joy for a chicken is to take a dust bath, to hunker down into the earth under the pepper tree, to scrabble and scratch and hurl the body around and fluff the feathers and make sure grit infiltrates every feathery layer, and then to shake and shimmy and fill the air with clouds of dust.

· · ·

For meals we have to perch on the edge of chairs clutching our plastic bowls of cereal, or hard-boiled eggs, or sandwiches bought down the road. At lunch we turn on the TV and we are in a courtroom drama. Today, June 10, 2013, the trial of George Zimmerman begins. Trayvon Martin was shot and killed by George Zimmerman on February 26, 2012, in Sanford, Florida, while visiting his father in a gated community in which Zimmerman was a neighborhood watch volunteer. Trayvon Martin was carrying Skittles and a can of iced tea. He was not carrying a gun.

We aren't the only people in this country, and in the world, to be drawn to the TV today, to cell phones, to laptops, to radios. This trial has been much anticipated, preceded by protest and by media debate about racial profiling, vigilantism, and, given the proliferation of guns in this country, laws governing the use of deadly force. The protests were prompted by the failure of the Sanford police to arrest Zimmerman. Before a special prosecutor assigned to the case ordered Zimmerman's arrest, thousands of protesters gathered in Sanford, Miami, New York, and elsewhere, many wearing hoodies like the one Martin had on the night he died. President Barack Obama said that if he had a son, "he'd look like Trayvon."

Forty-four days passed before Zimmerman was arrested and charged with second-degree murder, to which he is pleading not guilty. In order to secure a conviction, prosecutors must show that Zimmerman acted with ill will, hatred, spite, or evil intent.

. . .

One day follows another, dates crop up and fall into line, stories follow a sequence, history is narrated. Sometimes, however, the flow of time is barbed. Time spins furiously in slow motion, in Spartacus time spinning wheels are intercepted by spurs, spokes, foreign bodies. Collisions occur: Time is derailed.

. . .

Perhaps I have grown more particular, sensitive to dirt, to alien microscopic creatures, since having CLL. With a damaged immune system you get to be more cautious. Neurotic even. You imagine things: You imagine the state of Jack's lungs and skin as he scorns to wear a mask, you ask yourself, What if those lurgies glom onto my wonky immune system? What if Elvis's asthma is exacerbated and he has a fit and dies? The line between pathology and realism is fragile. One thing leads to another. What if the colors are all wrong and Big Jack and Little Jack become fixtures in the kitchen, here to stay forever, forever never-ending, never-completing. The what-if universe in which you wallowed, purring, fed by and feeding a luxuriously obsessive fantasy, has changed its contours and tones. What-if is now a perpetual unrelenting anticipation of disaster.

Conceivably, it has nothing to do with CLL, is simply a matter of categorical dissonance. Mary Douglas speaks to me in magisterial tones: Categories, she says, are in and of themselves spurious. There is no absolute distinction between clean and dirty, no invincible boundary, what is dirty in certain societies or circumstances may be clean in another. The point is not any absolute difference but, rather, the processes and attempts and elaborate rituals erected to instantiate those distinctions, to make sense of the world, to ensure order. Mary Douglas speaks to me and I listen, and it makes no difference. Or put it this way: The fault line between filth and cleanliness, purity and danger, opens an invincible crack of opportunity for that night stalker: obsession.

. . .

Again, we find ourselves in front of the television. Every lunch time we turn our backs on the chaos in our house and enter the public courtroom. The trial begins with jury selection, a process that, as it turns out, will take nine days. Prosecutors and defense lawyers cannot overtly use race as a reason to challenge a juror. But jury selection is a space where the insularity and focused particularity of the court is haunted by ghosts and demons that infest the larger location and culture. Animated, those ghosts invade the courtroom: invisible, but not nameless. Emmett Till, the Scottsboro Boys, Martin Lee Anderson . . . Remember Rodney King—an African American man brutally beaten by white cops in Los Angeles in 1991, an incident vividly captured on videotape. Nevertheless, a jury without black representation (after the venue was moved from Los Angeles to the virtually all-white Simi Valley) acquitted the officers of state criminal charges.

On day five of jury selection a middle-aged black man who works in a school describes his family and friends' reaction to Martin's death as "typical," given a history of violence against African American men in the U.S.

Day nine. A six-woman jury is selected, five are white, and the other is of mixed black and Hispanic ancestry.

At the end of the day we turn to the news and analysis and interviews. It is becoming a habit, a fixation, an obsession.

. . .

Every so often, randomly it seems, Word announces that it's in incompatibility mode. What, I wonder, is incompatibility mode? Computer dumb, relationship savvy (or battle scarred), I can say with some confidence what incompatibility mode is in a relationship. It occurs in the kitchen. J and I, after some years of frustration in a shared kitchen, worked out a modus operandi or compatibility mode. The key is not-sharing. He is easygoing, unmindful, nonjudgmental, a great cook, full of invention and surprise. I'm the sort who cleans up as they go and can't help offering generous dollops of free advice—albeit well considered, based on many years of perfecting a range of kitchen techniques, of doing things just so, this way precisely, and no other. He's the sort of person who produces utter chaos in the kitchen, using every available pan and pot and utensil, several different kinds of oil and flour and sugar, much of which lands up on the floor along with vegetable peelings and a few fugitive oily anchovies. All squished and trodden underfoot. Out of all this apparent chaos and disorder J invariably produces a marvelous meal, a wondrous alchemical concoction. But then, afterward, replete and sated, I would be left to face the chaos and would have to spend many hours washing, cleaning, sorting. There would be moaning, whinging, recriminations. For him, after my turn at cooking, cleanup would be a breeze. Moaning, whinging, and recriminations would follow—from me. The solution we found was to reconfigure the division of labor: whoever cooks, cleans—the kitchen is theirs for the night. Peace ensued.

. . .

"Fucking punks. These assholes always get away." Prosecutor John Guy quotes Zimmerman from a tape of a call he made to a nonemergency police number after he spotted Martin walking around the gated community where he lived. We are riveted to the television for the first day of testimony. The opposing attorneys set the scene today. "We think that this is a simple case," says Benjamin Crump, the Martin family's solicitor, outside court. "There are two important facts in this case. Number one, George Zimmerman was a grown man with a gun, and number two, Trayvon Martin was a minor who had no blood on his hands. Literally he had no blood on his hands." Defense attorney West: "George Zimmerman is not guilty of murder. He shot Trayvon Martin in self-defense after being viciously attacked." The claim is that, after the two got into a scuffle Martin was slamming Zimmerman's head into the concrete pavement when he fired his semi-automatic pistol and shot him in the chest.

"Stand your ground" is not mentioned today—and indeed the 2005 law will not be mentioned or actively invoked in court during the entire trial. But it is this law that provides the scaffolding, that makes it easy to plead self-defense in a killing in Florida, and it is what will put the onus of proof in this case on the prosecution. The state will have to prove beyond a reasonable doubt that Zimmerman did not act in self-defense. Zimmerman's team will merely have to argue that Zimmerman felt threatened.

Prior to 2005 most states required you to retreat from a confrontation unless you were inside your own home. But in 2005 Florida, urged on by the extremely powerful gun lobby headed by the National Rifle Association, became the first state to pass a "stand your ground" law. Now twenty-five states have these "shoot first" laws.

Imagine Jack arrives at my house one day while I am in the garden planting bulbs, dibber tucked into one side of my belt, handgun on the other side. I refuse him entry, say I've had enough, cannot bear this home invasion a moment longer. He becomes abusive, starts cursing, and lunges at me. I feel threatened and so, in self-defense, pull my gun and shoot. He falls to the ground, dead. Painter dead as a dodo. Under protection of "shoot first" laws I am authorized to use deadly force even if the person who makes me feel threatened, let's call him Jack, is—like Martin—unarmed. An upright and righteous citizen-sheriff I am safe from prosecution.

The fact that Jack is white might make it less automatic; it would be easier I imagine if the hoody that Jack habitually wears were pulled low over a black face. My sense of threat would be more believable to a jury. Or then again, maybe not. What if gender enters into the picture? Remember the Florida case of Marissa Alexander, who last year cited the "stand your ground" law to justify firing what she said was a warning shot to protect herself from her abusive husband. No one was killed or injured. But that defense was rejected, and she was convicted by the same state attorney's office prosecuting the killing of Trayvon Martin. She is currently serving a twenty-year sentence.

No doubt there are many legal complications, loopholes, and explanations to be taken into account (mandatory-minimum sentencing not the least of it in this case). Nevertheless, U.S. Rep. Corrine Brown, of Jacksonville, an advocate for Alexander, seemed to have touched a nerve when she said at the time of sentencing, "The Florida criminal justice system has sent two clear messages today. One is that if women who are victims of domestic violence try to protect themselves, the 'Stand Your Ground Law' will not apply to them. . . . The second message is that if you are black, the system will treat you differently."

Brown is a woman not afraid to exercise rhetorical flair and not afraid to say the "R" word. During the Haiti crisis in 2004 she referred to the Bush administration policies on Haiti as "racist" and called his representatives a "bunch of white men." When Assistant Secretary of State Roger Noriega said that, as a Mexican American, he deeply resented "being called a racist and branded a white man," Brown lobbed back: "You all look alike to me."

. . .

Peace ensued. But now, in the domain of the kitchen, our orbits collide, a ferocious incompatibility reigns.

Exchanges might go something like this:

"These light switches looked elegantly off-white, in their packaging in Home Depot," I say to J, "but up on the wall, here in the kitchen, they look gray and murky. We'll have to go back and change them."

"Oh, they aren't so bad. I can live with them."

"Live with them! For the rest of your life you can get up every day and face this ugliness and live with it?"

Or like this:

"Do you have any receipts?"

"Receipts for what?"

"Well, for instance, the wax furniture paste we had to buy to fix the scratches on the countertop the painters made? Or the extra primer, or the screws for the knobs, or the drill we had to buy to cut the glass tiles . . ."

"Hmmm. I wonder where they are. Don't worry, they are somewhere, they'll turn up."

Or

"Everything went well today, it's looking great!" Thus J entices you into the kitchen. You look, nothing seems to have changed. You look closely, peering into every corner, into the back of every cupboard. Aha! There's only one coat of paint on this shelf. "Oh, I didn't notice. Do you think it matters? When there are things on the shelf no one will notice." No one? Who is this phantom "no one"? This No One reconciled to half-assed mediocrity.

. . .

"Through time, in this country, what I like to call bleeding-heart criminal coddlers want you to give a criminal an even break, so that when you're attacked, you're supposed to turn around and run, rather than standing your ground and protecting yourself and your family and your property." These are the words of former NRA president and long-time Florida gun lobbyist Marion Hammer, championing the "stand your ground" law.

. . .

You feel you are losing your kitchen and it may never come back to you. I don't want to leave the house because there's always something left undone, overlooked, incomplete, botched. But I have to leave the house, have to keep returning to the paint shop because we can cut costs this way. Big Jack and Little Jack get paid by the hour and run by the seat of their pants, fixated on the job, unmindful of how the future unfurls. We are always running out of primer, out of this, out of that: rollers, paint trays, rolls of plastic, sandpaper, buckets, primer, more primer, just another quart of trim. You also have to keep returning to the environmental lights shop to consult and get advice. Big Jack, who is also Old Jack, knows nothing—it turns out—about LEDs. When I try tentatively to explain the difference in voltage he looks at me contemptuously and says, "I've been installing lights for sixty years." He proceeds to fuck up grandly. So over the weekend we call in another electrician, a green guy J knows through yoga circles, who unearths the problem, fixes it, and charges a lot. You are nervous about raising this with Big Jack, so you raise it with Little Jack, who says he'll sort it. And then he adds, "Big Jack's not as young as he once was. But he taught me everything I know."

. . .

Day seven. Detective Chris Serino takes the stand, and audio and video recordings of police interviews with Zimmerman in the days following the shooting (made public during the discovery phase of the case) were replayed in court today. In these interviews Serino appears skeptical and pushes Zimmerman, suggests that he was running after Martin before the confrontation, suggests that he shouldn't have followed Martin after a police operator had told him he did not need to, asks Zimmerman if it hadn't occurred to him to ask Martin what he was doing there. Racial profiling aside, the cops seem not entirely happy with these law enforcement mavericks who take it upon themselves to do a job the police can do quite well themselves. Yet today, very calm and considered in the box, Serino explains that the questioning was tactical, a "challenge interview" where detectives try to break someone's story to make sure they're telling the truth. He was persuaded that Zimmerman was indeed telling the truth. "In this particular case, he could have been considered a victim, also," he concluded.

There is, however, one interesting moment in the interviews that contests the (not without foundation) stereotype of the profiling proclivities of the Florida police.

SERINO: What is that you're whispering? Fucking what?
ZIMMERMAN: Punks.
SERINO: Fucking punks. He wasn't a fucking punk. [*clears throat*]

Serino had initially recommended a charge of manslaughter, which most legal experts agree would have had a much greater chance of conviction than second-degree murder. Why did he change his mind? What pressures and negotiations and deals occurred? This we might never know, but for sure we can assume that the judiciary and the police and the neighborhood watches and various political pressures intermesh in complex and contorted ways.

. . .

How electricity is generated and how it moves in circuits from the sun and through a dwelling is hard to imagine but not as complicated as circuits of indebtedness, circuits of giving and receiving, owing and repaying, commissioning and paying by the hour for services received, for immediate labor embodied in skills accumulated over years of experience. Priming—this is tough and meticulous work, tedious and slow. You are appreciative of the Jacks' attentiveness to this part of the process, you bear witness to the pain in a sprained wrist, the back that's a bit crooked, the legs that buckle occasionally. You know that even though Little Jack in a moment of exasperation told you your cabinets were a piece of crap and should be trashed this hasn't prevented his patient persistence, pride in a job well done, in cabinets that begin to gleam as the final coats of filtered sunlight slither on. You forget sometimes to ask them what they think, to show appreciation, you don't want to behave like a madam, but you want the guys to know that you know what you want. Yet the more the job progresses and drags on the less you feel you know what you want, and the more perfection bays at your heels, aggravating everyone's anxiety.

. . .

Day fifteen. It has felt as though this trial will never end. Day after day we pull the plastic shroud off the television, dust cloths off the sofa, prepare our feast of hard-boiled eggs and switch on the cable news. Now, after almost three weeks of testimony, after the interrogation of fifty-eight witnesses, it is over. July 13. Zimmerman is declared NOT GUILTY. Race has hardly been mentioned in court.

The processes and attempts and elaborate rituals erected to instantiate and often to blur boundaries, to make sense of the world, to ensure order. Clean and dirty, black and white, a threatening act and an act of self-defense. Lines of continuity, jagged lines of differentiation. Consider the line of continuity between the old lawless South and the South today, where racial violence might enjoy legal sanction. Boundaries. Categories. Where are the fault lines?

There has been one witness who's rocked the boat, who's raised the issue of race. Rachel Jeantel—spiky and insolent, contemptuous of protocol, uneasy in court, ungroomed for public appearance—was Trayvon Martin's friend. He called her just before he died. Over nearly two days, days three and four, Jeantel's testimony was broadcast live, nonstop, on cable news. It was riveting, not just because of revelations and certainly not because of her persuasive powers, but because of the dissonance she introduced into the proceedings, her disturbance of the tacit agreement to not discuss race or gun laws. In her reluctant laconic sullenness she danced into the court, out through the television set, into the world and into my dusty house like a skirmishing corkscrew. Jeantel said she overheard Martin demand, "What are you following me for?" and then yell, "Get off! Get off!" before his cellphone went dead. She testified that he described being followed by a "creepy-ass cracker" as he walked through the neighborhood.

"Do people that you live around and with call white people 'creepy-ass crackers'?" the defense asked.

"Not creepy. But cracker, yeah," Jeantel said.

"You're saying that in the culture that you live in, in your community, people there call white people crackers?"

"Yes, sir," she said.

When the defense suggested that Martin attacked Zimmerman she blurted out, "That's retarded, sir." It was the conjunction of these two words—"sir" and "retarded"—that sparked a macabre levity, for the first time in weeks J and I roared with laughter. It was as though the unconscious of half the U.S. erupted for a moment, shattering the precarious compact of civility, exposing how frenzied is the calm.

. . .

You imagine a deep dark hole in this country into which all the puddles, all the rivers of heartache and injustice perpetrated by the judicial system trickle and disappear. They don't always mesh: justice and the efficiency of the system.

. . .

The chickens are neglected. They are fed and watered, let out in the morning, and locked up at night. There is no time that isn't kitchen time, or Trayvon time, no time to pick up Holly and stroke her neck, watch her eyelids flutter and close as she sinks into sleep.

So when Katie and Susan visit they pick up the chickens and murmur sweet nothings. I am thrilled that they are here, not only because they are who they are but, also, because it gives me license to shut the door on the kitchen for three days, walk away from it, not think about it. But Katie and Susan discern a cranky demeanor and try shucking, teasing, easing out the oysterish story. To deflect their attention from my fixations I tell them a story about my maternal grandmother who lived in the inner suburbs of Salisbury in colonial Rhodesia. Every night she drank a lot of whisky. But her drinking was not random. It was ordered, repetitive, and ritualized. She would never touch a drop during the day, would only begin at six o'clock in the evening, just as the television news came on, though the news was preceded by preparations, undertaken by the cook but overseen by her: ensuring that the soda siphon was full, the tray laid with her special glass, a tumbler of ice, and a decanter of whisky. Two minutes before six she would rush from the veranda into the living room, settle into her armchair, switch the TV on, and as the news began, take her first sip of whisky and soda. After the news she would continue sipping, dreamily edging into blotto land. I remember how she would regularly complain to my father about the weekend shebeens held by all the servants who lived in the neighborhood, they would produce stills of illegal *skokiaan* during the week and have loud parties on Saturday night. "You simply can't imagine, Jack," she would say, "how strong *skokiaan* is, how it induces violence, it shouldn't be allowed." And he would roll his eyes, and say, "And what about whisky?"

Katie and Susan look at me, incredulous, and they say, in unison: "Jack? Your father's name was Jack?"

. . .

You imagine a small but deep and dark hole opening up in the middle of the kitchen, a deep dark hole which sucks, dollar by dollar, all your retirement savings.

. . .

The obsession grows slowly. At first a feather stroking your skin, teasing. Then you start making decisions, a mix of torture and delight. Then the renovations begin, and the obsession takes a turn. For the worse. No longer in control of a fantasy world, the world starts intruding, making demands, taking up time, insisting. The feather insidiously sprouts razor teeth, becomes a baby shark nibbling, nosing you into a corner, drawing blood.

Tokhm-e Morgh

Eggs: a bowl of hand-painted, intricately designed and colored eggs at Brian and Parastou's wedding. They are part of the Sofreh Aghd, a special cloth on which are placed a number of symbolic objects, facing east, where the sun rises. Here the wedding is outdoors, behind is the ocean. The Sofreh Aghd includes as well as the decorated eggs (Tokhm-e Morgh), a basket of walnuts, almonds, and hazelnuts, a mirror, two candelabras, flatbread, and a tray of multicolored herbs and spices.

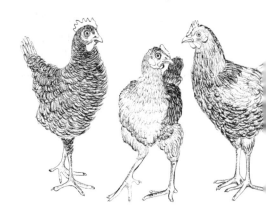

Disability

Negotiating the rapids and snarls of disability retirement these days I often find myself adrift.

Isn't it enough just to have to cope with cancer, not to mention the insurance? As you enter the cancer world there are so many alien words, concepts, drugs, treatments, diagnoses, choices, and decisions to be made. You stagger through mostly in the dark. When and if you are up to it, you do research, go to lectures, interrogate your doctors; if you are a control freak you try to understand everything, and this makes you feel a bit better even though you know this knowledge is illusory and the feeling of knowing even more so, and the decisions you make somewhat arbitrary. Sometimes you just want to get on with other things and do not want all your head space taken up with this new vocabulary.

Then, on top of everything, you are faced with the bureaucracy and paperwork and incomprehensible rules of disability. But compared to others I'm on a gravy train. For most people in this country disability benefits are akin to a slow death sentence. There are only two exits from the disability route for most people—back to a crummy job that probably caused the disability in the first place or, more commonly, death. You get a paltry check in the mail each month but no therapy or remediation or home help or medical assistance or job retraining. On public radio yesterday I heard a number of people on disability benefits interviewed about what would be their ideal job if they were able to go back to work. Most said they would like a job where they would not have to stand. But they were unable to identify any such jobs.

Why Me, Lord?

A leper, on crutches and with only one arm, enters a church. He looks up and asks, "Why me, Lord?" There is no response, and so he shuffles in. One of his legs shrivels up and drops off. "Why me, Lord?" he wails. No answer. He struggles on, down the aisle toward the altar, until his other leg plops off. "Why me, Lord?" he beseeches. Still no response. At last he reaches the altar and as he does so his remaining arm detaches itself from his body. Not much left. "Why me, Lord?" he whines. A big thumb comes out of the air and squashes what remains. "Because you give me the shits," says the Lord.

Anyone who has had a cancer diagnosis (and now that seems to be half the people I know) knows (though what would I know? I haven't a clue really what other people know or how we confuse, each in our own way, knowing and feeling) that moment when the diagnosis is delivered as a moment when the earth opens up and there is nothing there, you are suspended, no solidity, no light. It comes at you, the diagnosis or verdict or pronouncement, straight at YOU. Or ME. *Straight at you* (or me) and no one else.

I once heard Doris Lessing being interviewed on the radio. It was after Zimbabwe gained independence (after a long civil war, at the end of which Rhodesia became Zimbabwe), and she was free to return to the country of her birth, from which she had been banned for many years. Her books had been so profoundly a part of my youth, of coming to political consciousness in Rhodesia. For a generation across the world, mostly though not exclusively women, Lessing was a medium of exchange, common currency, embedded in the milieu. Familiar, and at the same time an exotic inspiration. As a graduate student in Glasgow—cold, depressed, culture-shocked, shakily married—I took to bed with *The Bell Jar, Children of Violence, The Golden Notebook*, Freud, and scotch. Joan Didion once wrote:

"To read a great deal of Doris Lessing over a short time span is to feel that the original hound of heaven has commandeered the attic." Yes. I overdosed. And so for a long time after the Glasgow descent I didn't read much of her, but then, listening to the radio, I experienced a jolt.

Lessing was asked why she had turned to science fiction. There was a long pause. And then she said, "I just got fed up with threshing around in the personal." A lot of murky water under the bridge. A lot of threshing around in the personal went on in those Lessing years, in a time when "the personal is political" motivated so many encounters in groups, so much confession, so many accusations, so many hours of shared soul-searching. Now, it seems to me, there's an awful lot of threshing going on again. The self, the self, is everywhere in social media: self-esteem, self-knowledge, self-help, self-branding, selfies.

When I was diagnosed and went into slow spiraling shock I felt a need to know why. Why me? DDT immediately presented itself as a prime culprit. Growing up on a farm DDT was used all the time for all sorts of purposes. In the fifties, before Rachel Carson published *Silent Spring* (1962), we kids would spray the horses for ticks in our bathing suits, gleefully drenching both the horses and ourselves. Perhaps my memory has wrongfully conflated the hosing down of the horses with the spraying. But anyway there was extensive use of DDT without protection. Many years later I shared a small farm in Victoria, Australia. A neighboring farmer, Brian, grazed his cows on the land, and in exchange he kept the invasive blackberries (brought originally by the British colonists) under control. Immersed in our permaculture gardening we did not pay attention to how he tamed the savage invaders. When I went to Japan I had to share a secret with B and M who were staying at the farm, they were the only ones in the world who knew that I was growing a small crop of marijuana hidden in a large defunct rain tank. Brian certainly didn't know. In Japan I received a sad letter. It seemed that when Brian sprayed the blackberries on top of the hill above the house and vegetable garden, the spray (2,4,5-T, a derivative of DDT) drifted down the hill and all the marijuana plants keeled over, dead as dodos. It is true that they were higher up the hill than the vegetables, but if you can see the spray drifting slowly you might imagine it permeating the fruit and vegetables. We kept eating.

Amid the flashing lights and urban excitement of Shinjuku my brittle heart broke into little pieces: all that care and nurturing and delicious secrecy. But now all I can think about is what kind of cognitive dissonance was operating that somehow separated out organic whole earth surety from all that we should have learned from Rachel Carson. What an idiot. Who else can I blame for getting leukemia?

Or perhaps it was genetic, perhaps it was CLL that killed my mother. This possibility is more painful. I knew she was tired, unusually tired, but did not pay enough attention. And then one night I am woken in Sydney with the news that she is dead. The medical resources in Zimbabwe were stretched and she was never given the attention she needed. To say there were many even worse off is no comfort. How did I not see this coming? Why was I not there with her? I could not face a postmortem, but that was foolish. And from a selfish, albeit more responsible perspective, even if we had found out that she had CLL it wouldn't have stopped me from getting it. I would just have been in shock ten years earlier, ten years more anxiety, a decade longer, waiting for the symptoms to materialize.

The most common answer to the question of why me, lord?, the answer we give ourselves at some stage or another, is this: I brought it on myself, though usually it is voiced as a punitive self-accusatory question rather than a definitive answer. Could I have created hospitable conditions for the cancer to take root: through stress, overwork, ambition, ignorance, repression, bad diet, lack of exercise, corrosive immersion in envy, jealousy, not looking after myself . . . ? You name it, there is a sin lying in wait. When I screw my head back on again I know that even if medicine is aiming to become more predictive, more targeted (largely through the development and utilization of big data), it is unlikely that the occurrence of every cancer can be pinpointed to a single cause. And even if this were the case, cancers are likely to continue mutating, both generically and within individuals. There surely are connections between environment and cancer, the unleashing and leaking of industrial chemicals, especially since the Second World War but in fact throughout history. We can always do something somehow about this. But to start burrowing down the rabbit hole of doubt and self-blame and querulous uncertainty simply consigns one to an exhausting and ultimately futile game of threshing around in the personal. You'll land up losing an arm and a leg and more, like a slow and dumb mosquito you'll land up squashed, squished to a paltry pulp by a gigantic gleeful thumb, by a malicious god finally exasperated beyond whimsy, incited to end the whining chorus of why me's.

. . .

After being diagnosed I was threshing around in search of some sort of therapeutic/psychic support. I couldn't, however, face the specter of more talk schrifts and shrunk at the idea of a support group, a forced encounter with an inevitably grizzly future, with people whose CLL was more advanced than mine, a group where everyone sat around talking about their feelings and symptoms and grizzly experiences. I wanted to escape this me me me feeling.

I wanted, I guess without knowing it consciously, to find a way to connect this profoundly self-centered revelation—you are going to die of cancer (though since it's a chronic form, and the therapies are improving, you might die of something else first)—with some form of engagement beyond the self. Beyond everyday encounters and exchanges. How to get on with the business of living?

Eventually I found my way into the support group organized by Sheila, the research nurse and case manager for Dr. K. This is not a support group in the usual sense: Sheila conceives of it as an educational group, she organizes lectures once a month, by oncologists, researchers, alternative health practitioners. After the talk we have a brief period to exchange notes, about experiences, drugs, mutations. It totally changed my engagement with CLL. It got me interested in science: That obtuse, opaque, previously incomprehensible area of knowledge opened up. New things to learn, a new language, new obsessions . . . Strangely, although the talks are all focused narrowly in the sense that they are about CLL, about "our condition," in fact they serve to situate CLL and its different manifestations within a continuum. A continuum of cancers but also of that between health and illness. There is no ravine separating health and illness, complete bodies from incomplete, the nadir of self-blame from the exaltation of self-esteem. For the flip side of self-blame is self-exaltation. Why I'm special. How I entered the valley of death and came out with self-esteem.

Then one day Ruth suggested that since I was meditating I could visit the Shambhala Center at the end of my street. Entering the meditation space for the first time the colors surprised me. I was entranced by the iconic figures depicted in orange, white, red, and purple: Tiger, Lion, Garuda, Dragon. A poetic space, not a literal space. I was intrigued by slogans framed on the wall, written in beautiful black brush strokes, slogans that invoked the warrior. Some people, I would come to discover, are uneasy with this warrior aspect and say we should be emphasizing peace, but I see it as a dramatic staging of the encounter of the individual and the world and a welcome alternative to an inward dwelling on the personal.

. . .

This staging of an encounter was being played out as the blog that I was writing began to mutate into a book. "My blog" is the exemplary staging ground for this generic journey from persecution to enlightenment, from defeat to victory. Many blogs, like mine, mutate from acutely personalized and self-obsessed banal reportage, for a restricted group of friends, to something more public, to a memoir. The problem, as I see it (or perhaps I should say the challenge of putting into writing, as I experience it), is that the mode of the memoir can operate as a lure, seducing one into conjuring answers to the question, Why me, Lord? If one tries to swim out of the sewer of abjection then the answers tend toward the preposterously perky. And there are other dangers you encounter as you paddle out into the reefy shores of memoir: the aggrandizing of a personal story (subjective trauma, say, cast in the language of universal ethics) or ontological pontification (a story which narrates a grand theory) or quotidian fetishization (all truth is in, and only in, the details).

I ponder these issues, but just as I'm about to sink into that great big fish tank where a superfluity of egos are threshing around in circles, I hear a voice murmuring in the background, my animating spirit if you like. It is that of the great essayist Montaigne, who pondered, so lightly, so slightly, and yet through idiosyncrasy opened a passageway for all future essayists, the question of how to live, and responded—practically and in his writing—by saying, Don't worry about Death. Don't worry about that great big thumb in the sky. Just get on with living.

Five Down, Two to Go 23

I have now started on the sixth cycle (five months down, two to go). The Rituximab infusion went fine on Tuesday. As always it was a long day, Judy fetched me and stayed at the hospital for the first three hours, and then Steve took over, reading while I slept, taking notes when Dr. C came round. I perfectly remember him saying, Not only are you a bit groggy, but there can be amnesia, so it's good Steve is taking notes. He refrained from raising the Revlimid dose, since it could tip things into toxicity. I anticipate a good month ahead with the ankle—broken pruning the peach tree, not feeling the ground beneath my feet—much improved, am starting to walk, get into shape, though putting the brakes on excessive ebullience. There are many things to factor in—lymph nodes are reduced in size but still swollen, spleen seems to have shrunk back, yet even if all the signs are clear the final test will be the bone marrow. But here's something to really be ebullient about: It seems that a trip to Australia in the antipodean summer (during December and January probably) will be fine, even if it's necessary to continue with the Revlimid—We can find ways to accommodate this, Dr. C said.

The Warrior Song of King Gesar 24

The walls are colored: tones of green and burgundy, orange and gold. There is a simple shrine, five candles burning, a densely intricate mandala, photos of two robed men; pale chartreuse blowsy chrysanthemums rather austerely arranged in a composition together with spiky reeds on each side of the shrine; the main room is separated from the entrance by a curtain of white shot silk, which shimmies in the breeze blowing in from the garden. Along one wall large banners hang: a tiger striped in red against a brilliant orange background, a pug-faced lion outlined in blue on a snowy white background, a scarlet Garuda, and a soaring purple dragon.

So many years exercising disdain, crinkling my nose at the slightest whiff of religiosity. And where am I now if not within the belly of the beast, as happy as a pig in shit? It does not seem to me like worship, not in a monotheistic sense. But the question of faith certainly arises. Is it the ritual that appeals, or the routine itself, or on the contrary, the drama of mobilizing a struggle to recognize and break with routine, with habit, with the familiar?

When we were students in Harare I witnessed my friend Molly's bipolar (though then we called it manic depressive) swinging between the Society of Friends and Catholicism, between puritan impulses and grandiose extravagant gestures. I happened at that time to also know someone becoming a priest (I think Franciscan, though perhaps I am wrong about that; my friend Stephen, a Catholic lay preacher here in San Diego, has gently suggested that perhaps my entire memory of this episode is somewhat screwy) and to be invited to his ordination. For someone who had never set foot in a high church of any denomination, it was a revelation, a spectacular staged performance in which the elaborate costume changes were stunning. Peter appeared and walked down the aisle and did various arcane things and then disappeared and then reappeared. Each time he came out in a costume more elaborate than before. He began in ordinary dull simple attire, an approximation I suppose of sackcloth, and eventually emerged in splendor, in rich gleaming silks, in purple, white, and gold. Or was it the other way around? Maybe my memory betrays me yet again and in fact he landed up in sackcloth.

This ostentatiously orchestrated scenario bore little obvious relation to the Peter I knew. It seemed, also, an incongruous display in a country where priests like Peter were politically engaged and often served in very poor rural communities. In the cathedral in Harare I was awestruck (even in the moment of skepticism), yet now I discern a logical chain of substitutions, a link between elaborate ritual and the quotidian. The ordination, it seems to me now, was a highly charged ritual of abstraction, a process of stripping away the self, individual identity, and simultaneously a celebration, through analogy and metaphor, of instantiation.

. . .

I love the banners, and colors, and stories of warriors like Gesu and am grateful to Jeff Glatstein for so gently, sardonically, and persistently encouraging me to read *The Warrior Song of King Gesar*. I love it when Ryoko sings at festivities, Ryoko who brings together Basho and Bach, who improvises songs for the occasion— somewhere between Kabuki and cabaret. I love the way that she dresses up, like my friend Page, she treats every day as an occasion for splendor, both have an eye for high design and also a love of thrift shops. Page gave me for my last birthday a brilliant orange shawl. It is immense, you can wrap yourself in it and disappear, luxuriating in the feel of raw silk. It is the color of the tiger. I drape it over my shoulders at sitting practice, the color seems to detach itself from its material ground, vibrates, the air is charged, the room becomes a jungle. The tiger is here, sinewy, gliding, moving among us.

. . .

One day, serendipitously not long after I had read *The Warrior Song of King Gesar*, I drove to Los Angeles and met Leslie Dick in Long Beach, where we ate at a Greek restaurant and then went, as the sun set, to see a performance by the Long Beach Opera Company of Peter Lieberson's *King Gesar*. This opera company, scaled down in elaborate pomposity and scaled up in ambitious experimentation, has so often saved me from the doldrums. A pleasure often shared with both Eileen Myles and J. Once the three of us went to Long Beach for a weekend to see a shortened version of Wagner's *Ring Cycle*, dubbed *The Ringlet*, and stayed in the Holiday Inn near the freeway, the one I always eyed, loving the circular design. I'm glad we did (though it's better to look at than to sleep with, as might be said of many buildings and men) because those Holiday Inns are all disappearing from the world or being turned into expensive boutique hotels.

This production of *The Warrior Song* was staged on a grassy knoll by the water, with a submarine and the *Queen Mary* in the background, and with the sounds of a police helicopter circling overhead and a lobster festival drifting over the water, through the air, and into the operatic refrains.

It gave me particular pleasure to visit Long Beach again with Leslie, for when I first visited Los Angeles thirty-odd years earlier she and Peter Wollen had taken me on a speedy tour, whizzing all over the city, visiting sites popular and obscure. What I remember most about Long Beach and San Pedro was the shock of the industrial seascape, the docks, the sense of Los Angeles as a port city, a major hub of international capital. Allan Sekula has vividly, through many photographic works and writing, conveyed and analyzed this but most wonderfully to my mind in the film he made with Noël Burch, *The Forgotten Space*.

I was curious about how Andreas Mitisek would stage this great epic, filled with fantastical appearances and disappearances, changing identities, alchemical wonder and dirty tricks, battles and magical steeds racing across the sky, deserts and mountains. Peter Lieberson scored the epic as a chamber opera for a narrator and small instrumental ensemble, based on the poetry of Douglas Penick's text. Mitisek simplified even further. He divided the narration between two singers (ranging from shamanistic declamation to rhythmic patter to song) and the action between two dancers. The stage was a small, two-tiered platform with the dancers atop—their job was to convey a sense of ritual or, behind a sheet, provide a shadow play for a battle scene.

It was a little hokey. And at moments transcendental.

Not a transcendence of daily life but a part of it, in it. A tension between, on the one hand, the ceremonial aspects, the formalized and ritualistic; and, on the other hand, the concrete, the ordinary, the sound of the police helicopters, the smell of lobsters, the discomfort of sitting on hard bleachers. For me this is what Shambhala itself offers. On the one hand there is formality, abstraction, ceremony, the emphasis on decorum, eating well, dressing with respect, orderly progression through the stages of warriorship. But on the other hand, it also encourages and provides the tools for cultivating careful attention to details, to being in the body, to being in the moment and in the world. Between here and there, between the world and this thing called me.

How surprising that I have come to like the formality. This tension between stricture, straightness, formality, and something that escapes, can't be precisely reproduced. Even though it might feel that authentic self-expression only arises spontaneously out of unconstrained gut feelings, actually passion, intensity, wisdom even are often generated out of a structure where there are constraints. Think of Robert Bresson, think of Chantal Akerman, Maya Deren, Samuel Beckett, Johann Sebastian Bach, Laurie Anderson.

I once found Ikebana distasteful, rigid, the antinomy of natural flower arranging. But during walking meditation in the sangha the colors would call out: the red, for instance, of a lily or gerbera (we used to call them Barberton daisies; my aunt Irene cried when, learning to ride a bicycle, I careened into her bed of Barbertons). That red would lasso the gaze and slither into the red of the cushions, sashay into the splotchy redness of the T-shirt worn by Ken walking in front of me, and bloom in the dragon. The moment would yield a quality of redness, detached from individual things, but then too the redness would encourage an attention to detail and particularity. And so, after a while, I became one of the flower arrangers taking my turn every month or so, and together with others in the sangha I've taken classes with Sensei Donna. Doing the flowers is a special form of meditation.

Judy Glattstein's flowers imbued the room with peace and perkiness. A fuchsia-colored arrangement, and on the Saturday of the Memorial Day weekend in each vase a wispy greenish gray stalk or two with a prick of blue at the wavery end. Sunday the blue became bulbous, and on Monday there were blue cornflowers.

Talking of blue, after spending some time here I will discover that the purple dragon should be blue. Something went wrong somewhere, either the person sewing the banners got confused, or the intense blue faded to a sort-of-purple, or the sangha was shortchanged. Anyway, it doesn't seem to worry anyone inordinately, we refer to the blue of the dragon and imagine that our purple is blue.

Where did they come from these creatures, these icons, these colors? Where does the story of Gesu come from? They come, I believe, from the shamanistic element of Shambhala.

I did not go in search of a spiritual path. The only belief that I hewed to was the belief that I did not have a religious bone in my body. Nevertheless, I was less inclined to disdain Buddhism than other spiritual domains because of some hazy idea that it did not involve worshipping a god and also valued as fundamental the connection between all sentient beings.

And so it came about that after much muddling, scuffling around in the thickets of mindfulness training, I found myself at Shambhala. Or rather, this is where I fetched up. It is where I still today, so many years after Peter's ordination, continue to bob around between skepticism and awe. Yet it isn't accidental of course (even though most of the time it feels rather like happenchance) that I've stayed. What is surprising to me is the fact that what really attracted me was the sensory richness in the shrine room, the inkling of ritual and formality that I sensed, as well as the peacefulness afforded by meditating in that space with others.

Euphoria   25

You wake up feeling normal, and the feeling lasts and the evening comes and you still seem, amazingly, to be functioning fairly brightly. Today, August 20, 2013, is the final, jubilant, day of the seven-month trial. There have been ups and downs in the past month. The feeling of euphoria, though, is so overwhelming you tend not to care.

There have been ups and downs, close monitoring because of borderline toxicity, an infection, antibiotics inducing their own brand of awfulness. Lab results are good, not perfect (the CLL still lurks), but it's rather amazing to open up my chart online and see so few red danger flags. Dr. K says I've tolerated a reasonably high dose, better than many in the trial, and hopefully this indicates that the CLL can be kept at bay for a while, perhaps by continuing the Revlimid at a much lower dose. He did report on a trial in Europe which was stopped (like the trial I'm in, combining Retuximab and Revlimid) because a few people died. He doesn't know the details yet but suspects they might have started everyone on the same high dose rather than starting low and slowly increasing for individuals if and only if there's a tolerance. This news was rather sobering. But hardly a revelation, all these drugs are dicey, you play the game of dicing with death and gamble that the treatment will do more good than damage. You know that Revlimid isn't as damaging to every cell in your body as traditional chemo. You cross fingers that the other, so far unknown, effects won't be too destructive.

. . .

But now I am feeling great, energized, revving up for a new world out there.

. . .

I told Dr. K I've started a new book (during the last partial remission, which lasted a year, I wrote a short book). He was enthusiastic, said, "If you write this book it will be a testament to the efficacy of the treatment, as valid as any scientific data." Looking back I wonder if he really said this or if it was a projection by me, a wish fulfilment: that writing itself could cure cancer.

. . .

I thank the goddess of mercy (Anne Freadman posted on my blog a photo of her from the Kenchō-ji Temple) for friendship: Katie Stewart, with her daughter Ariana, and Susan Harding bringing a typhoon of energy. Helen Barnes is here now, from Melbourne, while J is in Australia. She has cleared the vegetable garden of all the jungly mess that happened while I couldn't garden, and this has made time for me to write. Helen dug up dahlia tubers, given by Steve Ilott, growing near the Italian dandelion, and we planted them in the front garden where they can show off more extravagantly. The passion fruit, given by Brian two years ago as a small spindly plant, an offshoot from his vine, is blooming this year, festooned over the chicken run, promising fruit.

. . .

Travel: vistas are opening up. A short trip to Baja for Elana's birthday. We rented a house on the coast and cooked each night on a barbecue overlooking the ocean. I was cautious this time with a still-fragile system and didn't touch any street food even though it has never made me ill, and there is nothing like those *maravillosos* street tacos in Ensenada. But we had two extraordinarily long slow lunches—at Muelle3 on the wharf in Ensenada next to the Mercado Negro, the fish market, and on the way home at the open air Finca Altozano in the Guadalupe Valley overlooking a vineyard. The drive back: through the valley I love, up into Tecate on the border (a long and insufferable and stupid border wait), and then down through the mountains into San Diego County.

. . .

I've booked a ticket to spend Christmas and New Year's in Australia.

A Fern Romance

26

From up near the Oregon border down to San Francisco, driving and hiking along the coast and through the redwood forests of Northern California. J and I have just returned from this trip, for so long just a dream. Having researched the early save-the-redwoods movement and its murky entanglement with the racist fringe of the eugenics movement (via a particular figure, Charles Goethe, who wrote gardening books as well as anti-immigration tirades), I have been itching to actually walk in these forests. It is a stunning part of the country, of any country—wild erratic coastline, forests that induce a sense of otherworldliness. But of course this sensation is carefully nurtured by the worldliness of the state and national parks. During the trip I became immensely grateful for their intervention, their custodianship, for their maintaining of the trails, for the way they juggle and balance the claims of public access and wilderness preservation, for the incredible knowledge of the park rangers. The highlight was a hike through Fern Canyon in Prairie Creek Redwoods State Park. There are many fern canyons in this part of the world, but this is the most spectacular. You clamber back and forth over the stream, on each side of which rise the canyon walls, fifty- to eighty-feet high, densely carpeted in green ferns and mosses and waterfalls.

I live in an urban area, sprawling across two countries, built on canyons. They are not delectably green, our canyons. No, they are dry, brown for most of the year, and malformed by urban development. Immersed in the moist velvety greenness of Fern Canyon my thoughts turn to the canyon with which I am most familiar, Los Laureles, the endangered dusty toxic canyon that runs from Tijuana, where it is an informal settlement, into the estuary in San Diego. My thoughts and sensations turn to the question of why certain landscapes are deemed worthy of preservation and others not. I am far from yearning for restoration to some hypothetically natural origin, but it had never quite hit me before, the extent to which conservation is shaped by romantic and aesthetic considerations. Of course one knows this intellectually. But hiking through the forests, and through Fern Canyon, feeling blissed out, did provoke me to reflect on my own environment. You can live in San Diego and hardly realize that you are living in and out of canyons.

Now, back home, my resolution (particularly since my immune system makes the return to Los Laureles more and more risky) is to hike each week in a different canyon in San Diego, particularly the lesser known, less spectacular but no doubt fascinating, ones.

Weeding

27

NOVEMBER 2013

The trial is over, and traveling has begun. The trial is over, including the time-to-settle and then a bone marrow biopsy and the barrage of tests. The news is mostly good. The long and the short of it is that I am still feeling great and have what will probably be at least a few months' respite from symptoms and most drugs. Cancer is still in the bone marrow and will seep back into the system. My immunoglobulin reserves are exhausted, and this won't change, but I can luckily have an infusion each month to help the immune system.

The CLL landscape is changing; there are new drugs being approved, so we will reassess which way to go in a few months.

The garden landscape too is changing. The garden, of course, like any garden, is inconstant, mutable, unpredictable. Despite all the planning, the drawing up of diagrams and charts and maps, despite the documentation month by month and year by year.

After Helen left the vegetable garden was bare, ready for planting, inviting. So I resurrected the seeds stored in a small fridge in the garage, ordered new untried seeds, and over a few weeks scoured the nurseries of San Diego to buy the best seedlings. Suddenly our Northern California hiking trip was on the horizon, and so the planting was done in a frenzied manner, for days and days, from sunup to sundown. All that immersion, through the long months of treatment, in deliciously illustrated seed catalogs, all that anticipation of color through the long dark months: now the time had come to plant those promises, to prepare for fall and winter. Small cauliflower seedlings, cheddar orange and Sicilian purple and bright chartreuse; cabbages red and green; purple sprouting broccoli. All kinds of radish and turnip varieties, their seeds so similar, yet each variety evolving so distinctly: daikon from Japan—tiny seeds that will, months later, emerge long and snowy white from the dark soil; from China "red meat" and bright "green lobo" radishes; long black Dutch heirlooms, and round black ones from Spain; from India Pusa Jumini, soft lavender streaked with deep purple. Bull's Blood beets, heirloom rainbow chard, variegated sage, and the climbers: peas and fava beans, reaching for the sky, tossing out delicate shimmering blooms before forming plump pods.

When we return the garden is carpeted in green. Every seed that ever fell there seems to have sprouted, but they are not all vegetables. How could I forget that it isn't only seeds which sprout and plants that grow in the fall, but also weeds? Weeds weeds weeds have colonized every corner of cultivated earth. Frenzied again I spend days weeding out the unwanted, the greedy interlopers, the mimics and impersonators and blatant bullies. But it isn't straightforward. Many of these tiny green, un-spiraling hopefuls have become weeds by default, by going rogue. A few seeds were once sown, a few grew into plants, and the plants produced hundreds of seeds that blew in the wind and landed on the earth, multiplying, becoming a problem. Thus nasturtiums and amaranth and fennel and borage. I leave a few borage and nasturtium plantlets, as they will grow and produce edible flowers—garish orange and yellow in the case of nasturtiums, the borage throwing sprays of small sapphire blue flowers. The amaranth leaves are left for a while to grow between the lettuces and cabbages, they will be pulled soon, when the young leaves, growing on burgundy stalks, are still tender and nutty. Fennel will be left selectively, where there is space, for their wondrous bulbs that grow above ground but also to sprout their yellow umbrils and to provide fodder for the anise swallowtail caterpillars that will gorge themselves and then turn into butterflies. Although fennel plants take up a lot of space above the ground, beneath the ground they grow long taproots that work to cultivate the soil, preparing a propitious bed for future vegetables and flowers. There are a few tenacious savages, like dandelion, that are pulled and fed to rapturous chickens. The chickens also love stinging nettles, but so do we, though mostly it is the color that entrances as the weedy leaves are heated and turn a brilliant emerald green.

Today I gather heaps and heaps of small borage plants. The young leaves taste of spring even though here in California it is fall, they are bright like cucumber but with a lettucey edge. I make some ricotta and then fold into it the lightly mashed leaves with some shallots and thyme. From the Vietnamese store I buy dumpling wrappers that I fill with this mixture, fold the wrapper over diagonally, and there we have a dinner of improvised ravioli. But as I feed weeds to the chickens, I hear their reproachful refrain: "What's the point of us, our eggs, if—given the gift of tender young borage leaves and fresh ricotta—you are not prepared to pay homage by conjuring the queen of ravioli?" And so I make, in my fumbling inexpert way, pasta dough: watching the eggs turn the dough yellow, kneading and rolling, kneading and rolling. And then I invite some friends over for a glass of wine and a single ravioli. Each large round ravioli is filled with the borage and ricotta mixture and an egg yolk. No more than a few minutes in the simmering water and they rise to the surface, are transferred to a plate, dribbled with browned butter and a few shavings of parmigiano, then pierced with a fork so that the yolk spills, gloriously golden, over the blue plate.

The body is not a garden. The CLL landscape is not analogous to the familiar but changing landscape around my house. Yet the garden gives me clues, suggests ways of envisaging the future. Cancer cells are not invasive foreigners (though they often feel like this) but cells of your own body that have gone rogue. When you are young your body feels volatile, permeable, separated from the world by a membrane as thin and pliable as a sheet of fresh pasta draped over a rolling pin and stretched through the air. Older, your body feels more shaped, solid and stolid. But the body too, like the garden, is inconstant, mutable, unpredictable. Where some weeds are tasty, I doubt that cancer cells are delicious; but just as there are ways to deal with weeds that are less toxic, so too the recalcitrance of cancer might provoke more inventive and experimental modes of treatment.

You turn your back on the garden for a moment and the weeds take over. Yet that moment when you are gone, a moment of vacation and adventure, gives you the energy to weed, and replant, and turn the weeds into sustenance for the compost heap or the body.

Next stop: Australia.

Untimely

28

We find her lying on the straw. Ungainly, inert, the shimmer of her black feathers fading, her iridescent greenness smudged. Oh Funny Face, dear Funny Face: What happened? You gave us no clue, you were eating and drinking and scruffling around the yard as usual yesterday. You are too young, too young to die, to leave us.

. . .

We place her in a shoebox in which we have folded up an old but clean kitchen towel so that she may be gently cradled. We take her to the Avian and Exotic Animals Hospital for an autopsy, in case she has anything contagious that might have endangered the other chickens. The vet rings up a few hours later, very excited because he has found indications of a very rare and undiagnosable condition. Over the next three days he keeps calling, brimming over with enthusiasm, full of new theories about what caused Funny Face's demise. Later I realize that he is starved of chicken patients and corpses since most people who live with chickens know that they are prone to drop dead without rhyme or reason.

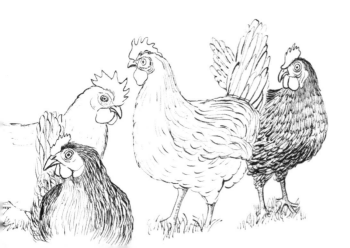

Blue / Shimmer

Blue, Sydney blue, blue sky, blue sea.

Through the glass, a flash of blue. Material calling out to be touched, a frock waiting to be slipped into. Although it is composed of different fabrics, they shimmy together, stretchy T-shirt cotton and scalloped silky edges. Deep indigo, patterned like African prints, and delicate ribbon inserts: a splash of burnt orange and a streak of perfect ultramarine. You could wear it to the beach or to the opera. A Sydney frock, incarnating the blueness of Sydney.

We are in the Queen Victoria Arcade in Sydney, a flaneuring paradise, ornate and elegant. We have moved from yum cha in Chinatown into this late Victorian Romanesque phantasmagoria of delights. I am in search of a shop called Von Troska, which was not there when I went this time to gaze in its window in Oxford Street. The door and windows were closed, the interior empty. Oxford Street: once glitzy and gay and buzzing, old-fashioned greengrocers rubbing shoulders with shiny bars and bookshops and old pubs and chic boutiques and the aroma of coffee. Now Oxford Street is tawdry and sad, I presume because of the gigantic Westfield mall built in Bondi Junction. When I lived in Sydney here is something that often happened: after seeing a movie in the Chauvel cinema located in the old Paddington town hall, or visiting Ruark around the corner, and gossiping and arguing with him, and before hopping on the 380 bus and heading back to Bondi, I would find myself before Von Troska, gazing in the window. Then, skating on air, I would slither in to fondle the fabrics, bury my face in luxurious silky folds, try-on-for-fun dresses designed on the cross, falling in folds, or cut austerely, marveling at how Von Troska conjured unlikely colors and textures into a simple frock or scarf. I have a silver jacket from Von Troska, bought long ago, it shimmers, at once excessive and austere, singular, no adornments or tricky curlicues. Now I find that Von Troska herself died of cancer a few years ago, but her shop continues, relocated to the Victoria Arcade. And there is a sale. So Julie and I peel off from the large Chinatown yum cha gathering and after a stop for Julie to purchase dried pandanus leaves at a Thai market, we enter the fray of hopeful, pugilistic shoppers thronging the streets. It is Boxing Day, and thousands are fighting to get to the sales. In the Victoria Arcade the crowds are slightly subdued, and when we find and enter tiny Von Troska it is like entering a shady luxuriant fern canyon.

I try the frock on, it's perfect. I look in the mirror and see a blue woman who has never known a day's illness in all her long life.

Sydney blue, quintessentially captured in Brett Whiteley's painting *Sydney by Night*, also called *The Balcony 2* (1975). You might say it represents a scene, a sort of seascape, a bay view. But it's blue, the blueness of Sydney, that the painting lets rip. Blueness flies out of the painting into the world. "Windsor and Newton Deep Ultramarine oil colour has an obsessive, ecstasy-like effect upon my nervous system quite unlike any other colour," said Whiteley. And he found a way—through lashing on the paint, in this work over a base layer of black—to effect a transfer, to transfer effect into affect. When I visit the Art Gallery of New South Wales to see another show, with Rosemary, I sneak a peek at *Sydney by Night*, overwhelmed by its hugeness and by the way that, in the flesh, framed, the blue is concentrated and distilled. Wherever I live away from Australia I have a postcard of this painting propped by the computer, but the colors are fading in the San Diego light, and so in the gallery shop I buy a new supply to take home.

Sea and sky—a continuous saturated blueness. A heron zips across the blueness of Whiteley's painting, leaving a trace, a flurry of whiteness. A small wrought iron balcony protrudes into the frame, suggesting a perspective, someone looking out from inside, out at the water, beyond the skyline. No sense of direction. Although, if you know Sydney, if you know that feeling of looking out on the harbor, perhaps you imagine looking southeast.

I replenish too my Margaret Prestons, postcards of her woodcuts "Harbour Foreshore" and "Sydney Heads." Preston made these woodcuts in 1925 after a visit to Japan to learn the craft of wood-block printing. She quotes Hokusai and others in her blue washes, but against the subtlety of the Japanese model her blueness is intense, visceral. "The colours," she said, "should not be put on subtly. It is better to use them in simple crude masses to match the key blocks." Norman Lindsay accused her of "violent crudities of pure colour." Where Whiteley's painting is huge and made for a gallery wall, Preston's woodcuts were small, sold at a price that flat-dwellers could afford. As postcards, the Whiteley and the Prestons are the same size.

I grew particularly fond of Whiteley and sought out more of his oeuvre as I got to know Thirroul, a lovely seaside town on the south coast of New South Wales. Whiteley killed himself here in a seedy motel in 1992. Then Thirroul was just a name to me, but some years later a friend had a shacky cottage on the cliff where I would go to write. And now Sarah and Derek live close by, and so I got to spend a night there in December, to watch a sulphur-crested cockatoo attacking with great vigor the magnificent gymea blooming in their garden, to walk down to the beach past chickens for a swim before breakfast.

I was introduced to Margaret Preston by Meredith Counihan, who took me to see her (her prints and paintings) in the National Gallery of Victoria when I first came to Australia in 1976. This is where I saw my first gymea, Australian rock lilies, wheel flowers, Manly pines, flannel flowers, Banksias, Sturt's Desert peas, waratahs, Australian tea trees, Western Australian gum blossoms, Australian coral flowers, Australian glory flowers, Christmas bells, bottle brush trees, and Angophoras—not in the bush but in the prints and paintings of Margaret Preston. The harbor paintings represent one tendency in Preston's work: a modernist tendency that looked to the city, its industry and views as well as to the domestic realm. But there is another tendency that existed in tension with this, against the internationalist and urban impulse of modernism, a turn toward the nationalist, to Australianness, to an affiliation with the bush, a desire to bring the bush into the apartment. But above all, manifested in an increasing incorporation of what she perceived to be Aboriginal colors and designs. An unusual embracing of indigenous culture this, at that time in white Australia. But not without problems, and over time this impulse for incorporation, viewed as an act of appropriation, has provoked considerable criticism.

"It's like speaking in a French accent without speaking French. The accent is there, the intonation is there, but the meaning is not." This is what Hetti Perkins, the curator of Aboriginal and Torres Strait Islander art at the gallery, says about Preston's borrowing of images. "The narrative [in Preston's work] isn't clear for an indigenous person."

I sneak a peek at the Whiteley but am actually at the gallery to see another show. We walk through the cool and magisterial, even pompous, halls of the gallery and into another, utterly unexpected world, the world of the Yirrkala drawings. Color explodes here, shimmers, in arresting patterns and shapes—blue, brilliant blue, but also red, yellow, green, and black. These drawings were done in 1947 by a group of senior ceremonial leaders and bark painters in Arnhem Land, in collaboration with two anthropologists, Ronald and Catherine Berndt. The anthropologists provided butcher paper and colored wax crayons, and the artists adapted their skill at working with pigments on bark to the process of drawing on paper, to illustrate and elaborate their *wangarr* (dreaming) stories. As a depiction of their country and the details of Yolngu life, the drawings were an extension of songs and oral stories—a material manifestation of Yolngu culture. This, some years before the transfer of traditional skills to working with acrylic paints and the development of dot painting.

To my untrained eye these are mostly abstract drawings, though more like paintings, combining an extraordinarily vivid color palette and stunning design sense. Although there are occasional representational and figurative elements (turtles, fish, water, human forms . . .), my eye is drawn by the sheen of the crayons, by the geometric patterning, by the intricate and varied combination of diamonds, triangles, straight lines and curved, circles, squares, zigzags. But the narrative isn't clear to me, a nonindigenous person. "If you can understand the paintings, you can understand the landscape," says Baluka Maymuru, son of Nän-yin' Maymuru, an artist in the show. But I can't understand the paintings, they are marvelous to me, but they also confront me with what I do not know.

Luckily, however, I don't have to swim around in the abstract quotation of Preston's era. The show has been curated in close collaboration with the Yirrkala community and is attentive, through a range of documentation, to the context and location of the drawings, to the individual artists, to the mapping not just of place, but also and simultaneously of cultural inheritance. This show, occurring in a different century and after Margaret Preston worked, is alert to difference as well as to continuities. The show includes, for instance, a display of contemporary bark paintings, *larrakitj* (hollow logs) by the descendants of the crayon drawers, which throws into relief the fine crosshatching in graphite pencil which some of the Yirrkala artists deploy in their crayon drawings (Narritjin Maymuru, in *Connecting Munyuku and Manggalili Estates*, for instance, uses sharp-pointed lead and color pencils to outline and to produce fine-lined crosshatching).

Rosemary and I leave the gallery. Nothing looks the same as it did before we entered the world of the Yirrkala drawings. We have experienced a flash of light: This we know, though what to make of it we do not know. I return to San Diego and try to write about the show but cannot find the words, the language. The sensations, attenuated ideas, simmer as I pore over the beautiful catalog. Then, five months later, I hear Deborah Bird Rose at a conference speak about "shimmer."

Bir'yun, brilliance or shimmer, is the word used by Yolngu artists to describe an aesthetic effect and to evoke the process and ancestral power summoned in that effect. The process of making a painting (and to some degree of perceiving it) involves an initial elaboration of a base design—underlying patterns and figuration over a single-color wash. At this stage the painting looks dull. Then comes the crosshatched infill, and suddenly the painting shimmers. *Bir'yun* refers to intense sources and refractions of light, the sun's rays, and to light sparkling in bubbling fresh water, as in

gong ngayi waltı bir'yu-bir'yun marritji ray

[its sun scintillate-scintillate go the sun's rays scintillate]

As applied to paintings, *bir'yun* is the flash of light, the sensation of light one gets and carries away in one's mind's eye.

Although much of the explication of the term *shimmer* is used in relation to process and the key component of crosshatching, shimmer can be evoked through many shiny materials and through the intensity of effect that is achieved when various techniques and systems are brought into a relation. The creative transformation of matter that occurs when wax crayons are used clearly generates a sense of brilliance, a sensation of light.

The artists used the potential of the new medium to produce bold geometric patterns, a clarity of form and brilliance of color patterning so that the paintings seem to vibrate, to dance on the surface, to scintillate. But it is not just a matter of technique, and nor do the crayon drawings materialize out of the blue. They continue a tradition in which painting (it could be on bark, on a body, on a coffin lid, or incorporated into performance) is a manifestation of spirit, of ancestral power, of nature, of country. At once a complex incarnation and emanation. As Waka Mununggurr writes in the preface to the catalog, "Our art is not just a bark painting or a crayon drawing—it talks about the relations between land, sea and people. When you look at this art, it is not just a thing of beauty—it discusses the environment and nature, the secret areas for Yolngu."

The complexity, the semiotic richness of these paintings, of the world they incarnate, is fascinating to me but also, and necessarily so, elusive. I mostly don't get the narrative, even when it is explained, but I begin to grasp the play between figuration and abstraction, the sense of a different kind of storytelling that is nonlinear, that interfolds presence, mapping, and a totally different kind of time.

Water and land, images and sensations, linear time and Dreamtime, words and things.

"You can hear their language within our own."

A surprising and intriguing element of the show is the strong presence within the drawings and supporting documentation of Makassan (Macassan) culture, words, things. "You can hear their language within our own," says Laklak Ganambarr, a female descendant of the artist Munggurrawuy Yunupingu. She is referring to the Macassans. The Yolngu people have a long history of trade and intermarriage with the Macassans, people from the land we now call Indonesia. Before European settlement of Australia, from as early as 1640, the seafaring Macassan from southwest Sulawesi established trading contact with indigenous communities in northern Australia, arriving with the monsoon season each December. They constructed outdoor factories to process trepang, a type of sea cucumber (which they took back to Indonesia to trade with the Chinese) but did not establish permanent settlements in Australia. It is estimated that as many as one thousand trepangers arrived each year.

Until 1906, when the South Australian Government, then responsible for the Northern Territory, passed legislation effectively banning Macassan mariners from entering Australian waters by imposing oppressive license fees. But some of the Yolngu men who drew of the Macassan presence are said to have first-hand memories, and some are thought to have made return visits to the Port of Macassar. The schema of the Macassan port and the Macassan exchanges remained alive in memory, through reenactment, through ceremony, and through art. Words from the Makassarese language (related to the Javanese and Indonesian languages) can still be found in Aboriginal language varieties of the north coast. Elements of Macassan culture remain today, including ceremonial flags and dances, stones, coins, pots, swords, songs, steel knives, rupiah (money).

"Their story is still alive today as it was from the old times. . . . You can hear their language within our own, and the Yolngu taught them ours," says Laklak Ganambarr. "We can call up the things that Macassans give us—calico, eyeglasses, hats, machetes—all of the names were incorporated into our language and young people know these as such. The Macassans showed us how to make the canoe." Whereas, "White people came and teach Yolngu people a word called Australia." Macassan culture was incorporated into Aboriginal Dreamtime, the past, affiliated to moieties and clans and given a place in the kinship system. Yolngu art, in various media, materialized the Macassan presence in ceremonial performance as well as everyday life. Yalpi Yunupingu, in an interview, speaks of the way his father (Bununggu Yunupingu, whose *Ceremony with Macassan Influence* is densely imagistic) used crayons to depict spirits with names from both Yolngu and Macassar ancestry: "These beings had the power to travel over deep waters of the ocean."

Most popular histories of Australia represent first contact as an encounter with the whites from the South: Captain Cook and his fleet arriving in tall ships, with weapons, from across immense oceans stretching between incommensurate land masses. The sea: a conduit, providing a way to get from one place to another, rather than being a place, a place continuous with the land. As though Australia only ever existed in the southeast, in this encounter. As though there never were people inhabiting the top end, living by the sea, a sea that linked them with the land and also with another country, at its closest point only a hundred and twenty-five miles away.

blue/shimmer

In a drawing called *Port of Macassar* by Munggurrawuy Yunupingu, there are ships, at once huge and smaller than people. The ships are blue. When I tell Fabian about this he says perhaps this is an example of hypalagia, a rhetorical trope where the quality of one object is transferred to another: the blue of the water to the ships. He sends me lines from Neruda where the poet writes of sadness:

. . . *La noche está estrellada,*
y tiritan, azules, los astros, a lo lejos.

[. . . The night is starry,
and the stars are blue and shiver in the distance.]

The stars are blue. The people are blue too, actually. In various drawings fish and shark and platypus and crocodile are blue, but people too, or rather—figures that are humanlike. Although sometimes, and sometimes in the same drawing, there are also red figures, as in "Canoe travel from a distant island," and black, as in "Influence from a distant island" (both drawings by Bunung Yun). I don't know whether blue is associated with water, or if color is detached from a referent, or has a materiality of its own, though in a different schema. Perhaps the colors serve to differentiate spirits and human beings, Aborigines and Macassans. But then why are animals blue too on occasion? While it is surely a stretch of the imagination to think of these paintings in terms of a Western rhetorical trope, deployed mostly in poetry, nevertheless Fabian's suggestion opens a way to thinking about what happens, what sparks fly, what scintillations occur when colors are indeed detached from customary referents, when ways of seeing the world are reconfigured. When, for instance, patterning (genealogical patterning, say) matters more than classification, as in *Ceremony with Macassan Influence*. Intricate networks, in which freshwater and saltwater interflow and are connected, are interconnected with the land and all creatures (as in the marvelously evocative for me *Larvae of the Rhinoceros beetle at Ngyapinya*, a tracing out of something like the web of life in paler, delicate colors).

Blue/shimmer. Is the sky always blue? Does blueness invariably signify water? I begin very tentatively to discern the presence of water in the drawings (supplemented by videos incorporated within the show), an element integrated into the country. But it is not Sydney Blue. No, it is the blueness of the sea and the sky over the Timor and Arafura seas and the waterways meandering through land.

"We are all connected through the mixing of waters there at the river."

Water water everywhere: dams, water holes, rivers (on occasion green, as in Birrikitji Gumana's *River at Gängan*), fish traps, saltwater country, spring-fed flood plains. Water creatures and things: dugong, fish, trees, lizards, goannas, turtles, possums, sharks, platypuses, Macassan ships (*praus*), canoes, the ancestral whale (who, dying, came in to freshwater and, furious, destroyed a fish trap). Yalpi Yunupingu says, "So, two different styles to our sacred paintings: saltwater and freshwater." Yet these distinctions generate further variations. Water is not just water. And not just blue. In Wonggu Mununggurr's many grid-like paintings of fish traps and floodplains, in particular in *Differing States of Freshwater*, where "differing colors signify the differing states of water: running, still, low, agitated." In Marawili's *Fish Trap at Baraltja* there is "a sense of movement, that has references to the interwoven structure of the dam and the water flowing down stream."

The sea, the sea. The land, the land. The Timor Sea and the Indian Ocean, the Arafura Sea and the Gulf of Carpentaria.

Where does the sea begin? Where does the land end? Who has rights to land, to sea?

In the Yirrkala drawings land and sea are connected in a single cycle of life. The sacred designs in the crayon drawings, integral to Yolngu society and for the first time—through extensive regional negotiation and agreement—brought into the open, represented the clans' rights in land. They were an important stepping stone in the process that eventually resulted in the Yolngu gaining recognition in the rights of land, a precursor to the Yirrkala Church Panels (1963), but also a precursor to the Saltwater Collection of large bark paintings, which were instrumental in the Yolngu gaining recognition in the rights of sea.

The Saltwater Collection consists of eighty bark paintings made by Yolngu artists that share their sacred knowledge of sea country. The catalyst for this collection was an incident in 1996: the illegal intrusion of a barramundi fishing party at Garrangali, sacred home of Bäru, the ancestral crocodile. The fishing party had not obtained permission to go to this special place and had further offended by leaving rubbish lying around. But the thing which upset Yolngu custodians most of all was the discovery of the severed head of a crocodile, left to rot in a hessian bag.

After this desecration of Bäru, Yolngu people began painting a series of barks that demonstrated the rules, philosophies, and stories of their region that related to the coast, rivers, and waters.

A selection of these barks was presented as evidence of Yolngu connections to saltwater country in a 2008 High Court case. The court verdict gave precedence to Indigenous rights and use of the Arnhem Land coastline and coastal waters over commercial interests and fishing.

The Yirrkala drawings and the saltwater barks bridge two very different traditions of law by explaining and sharing ancestral stories with nonindigenous people.

. . .

Here, where I live, the border between the U.S. and Mexico, San Diego and Tijuana, seems solid, but at Playas the border fence simply runs into the ocean, disappears in the water. There used to be a park that spanned each side of the fence at the beach, called Friendship Park. People—often families, separated—could speak through holes in the fence and touch fingers, but when the new fence was built the area between the two fences, the old and the new, formerly Friendship Park, became a no man's land.

. . .

"We are all connected through the mixing of waters." Six centuries of trade and intermarriage spanning sea and land. Boats have come and gone carrying people and goods.

. . .

But even earlier than this, as long as forty or fifty thousand years ago, the first crossings were made from Indonesia to Australia. Imagine an archaic time when the sea represented a barrier, an uncrossable expanse between landmasses. And then something happens unprecedented in the annals of human history. An Afro-Asian group of people from the area of Indonesia develop new technologies and skills for building and navigating seagoing crafts. The people of this first seafaring society become fishermen, and long distance explorers, and traders. These skills enable them to reach and settle Australia, to become the original human inhabitants of the continent.

But now the boats carry items that cannot be traded. Between Indonesia and Australia the sea is highly contested.

The recent history of relations between the two countries has been fraught to say the least. At the end of 2013, just before I arrived in Australia, a scandal rocked the country when Indonesia recalled its ambassador and suspended security cooperation with Australia after revelations by the former CIA analyst Edward Snowden included evidence that the Australian government had been spying on the Indonesian president, Susilo Bambang Yudhoyono. Shock and horror. Of course, but surprise? Governments, even allies, gather intelligence and routinely spy on one another. Such is the nature of spying. In fact the spying imbroglio is symptomatic of a much more festering tension played out on the ocean, and the scandal is less about spying than about Australia's conception of land and sea rights, of human rights, and less obviously but nevertheless implicated, the rights of whales and other creatures that live in the ocean.

Think of all the praus in the Yirrkala drawings, boats that would come regularly from parts of the Indonesia archipelago, to the northern part of Australia. Today boats that arrive from Indonesia are being towed back by Australian naval vessels to the edge of Indonesian waters. Indonesia refuses to accept these boats. These boats—old, leaky, overcrowded, improvised vessels—are dangerous to travel in. They carry people: asylum seekers who are prepared to undertake a dangerous journey in order to escape persecution and unbearable conditions at "home." The asylum seekers come mostly from South Asia, the Middle East, and Africa; they use Indonesia as a transit point to make the dangerous boat voyage to Australia.

The asylum seekers are also called, in Australia, "boat people" and "illegal immigrants."

Where does the sea begin? Where does the land end?

. . .

A maritime boundary exists between Australia and Indonesia, and both countries have been concerned to definitively delimit that boundary. It exists within a larger schema of agreements between the two countries: concerning trade, fishing, aid, defense, security. The term *boat people* entered the Australian lexicon in the 1970s, in the wake of the Vietnam War, when boats carrying refugees from Indochina began arriving in Australia. The asylum seekers who arrived by boat were processed on Australian soil, and many were resettled in Australia (though not welcomed by all—the Darwin branch of the Australian Waterside Workers Federation called for strikes to protest the "preferential treatment of refugees"). There were no substantial changes until Paul Keating's Labour government introduced mandatory detention of noncitizens arriving by boat without a valid visa in 1992.

And then came, in 2001, the dubiously titled Pacific Solution.

In August of that year a red ship appeared on the horizon—a great hulking red presence, there day after day, never getting any closer. This was the Norwegian freighter MV *Tampa* that had on board four hundred and thirty-eight refugees (mostly Afghani) who had been rescued from a stranded twenty-meter Indonesian wooden fishing boat. What ensued is referred to as the Tampa Affair. The Australian government would not allow the media or even the Red Cross on board, and so "the image remained that of a large imposing red hulk, often shimmering in the heat on the horizon." An affective image to be sure, but one that also raises the question of when and how shimmer emerges, how its affective force circulates, how it may be exploited.

The Australian government refused the ship entry to Australian territorial waters. The ship's captain, questioning the legality of the order, refused to comply. The Australian government responded by dispatching Australian troops to board the ship. As the crisis escalated the government enacted the Pacific Solution (and its popularity ratings rose within the Australian electorate).

The "solution" incorporated a number of policies, but the linchpin was the disallowing of asylum seekers to set foot on Australian soil. Instead they were transported, using Australian naval vessels, to detention centers set up on Christmas Island, an Australian territory in the Indian Ocean (2,600 kilometers northwest of Perth, 500 kilometers south of Jakarta, Indonesia), on Manus Island in Papua New Guinea, east of Indonesia and northeast of Australia, and on the island nation of Nauru in the South Pacific. The transporting of asylum seekers to detention centers was enabled, in the first instance, by excising islands around Australia from the migration zone, effectively meaning that any asylum seekers who did not reach the Australian mainland would not be able to apply for refugee status. In the second instance, it was enabled by Operation Relex, which authorized the Australian Defence Force to intercept vessels carrying asylum seekers and turn them back to Indonesia.

The Pacific Solution was largely dismantled with the election of a Labour government under Kevin Rudd in 2008. But four years later there was a changing of the ALP (Australian Labour Party) guard, a coup which installed Julia Gillard as prime minister. The Solution was back. The Gillard Labour government reopened the Nauru detention center and the Manus Island detention center for offshore processing. Then, in 2013, there was another changing of the Labour guard. Kevin Rudd was back as prime minister and this time announced that "asylum seekers who come here by boat without a visa will never be settled in Australia." Asylum seekers arriving by boat to Australia were now to be detained indefinitely.

The other place under Western jurisdiction where this—indefinite detention—happens is Guantanamo Bay.

Rudd's government did not last long. In a national election Labour was defeated and Tony Abbott, leader of the conservative Liberal Party, formed a coalition government in August 2013. This government sees the boats issue as a central matter of Australian sovereignty and national interest. Operation Sovereign Borders was an election policy and a vote winner, and commenced on September 18, 2013. The operation is a military-led attempt to address issues surrounding "people smuggling." The emphasis is on turning back the boats.

As I write this (February 25, 2015) Australia has returned its seventh boatload of asylum seekers to Indonesia since the coalition's policy was enacted.

After three days and nights at sea the boat entered Australian waters and was intercepted by an Australian warship; the twenty-six people aboard were transferred to an orange lifeboat and turned back to the southern coast of Java. Indonesia's foreign minister, Marty Natalegawa, has repeatedly attacked the Abbott government's policy of boat turn-backs, warning the practice would damage relations between the two countries.

"As I write this . . ." I write these words over and over again, and each time the date is different, the present tense belies coherence. "Now" was February, and now "now" is August. Over the course of eight months I search for words, and the grizzly scenario keeps unfolding. It is not as though I am waiting to see what the future brings. But neither can I write definitively in the past tense. Jenny Lloyd writes to me from Sydney a few days ago (August 4): "Asylum seeker policy continues to get worse even as it seems that surely there is no 'worse' to reach. But I seem to have been saying that for a long time. I'm reading a biography of Hannah Arendt and am struck by the repetitions of history in refugee policy."

Maritime law experts have voiced concern about the legality of Operation Sovereign Borders. If Indonesia wanted to, it would be within its rights to take Australia to the International Court of Justice over the matter. Although, as of yet Indonesia has not indicated that they are considering a case. Interestingly, Australia is no stranger to the International Court of Justice in relation to maritime issues; as recently as March 2014, it won a highly publicized case against Japan for whaling offenses (hailed, internationally, as an environmental victory).

I'm all for the whales. But the narrative isn't clear to me. I can't figure out how whales and asylum seekers fit together into a broader canvas, where there are also boats and islands, natives and foreigners, and different kinds of waters, seawater and freshwater.

It is not only maritime law that is at issue. Amnesty International, refugee rights groups, and sections of the public concerned about humanitarian issues have said that Australia is failing to meet its international obligations, both moral and legal, and have questioned whether it is the Australian government that is in fact breaking a number of international laws.

Here the word future is not a word.

These words—"Here the word future is not a word"—are spoken by a refugee on Nauru island. What language is there to describe the inhumane conditions in these offshore processing centers? From the beginning facilities have been appalling, but as time passes overcrowding exacerbates conditions. A law enforcement approach to asylum policy guarantees poor services, including intermittent electricity and freshwater, poor medical facilities, inadequate protection from the heat. The impact of detention on people in these conditions is exacerbated by the sentence of uncertainty, not knowing when and if they will be given a hearing. A friend who works with survivors of torture and trauma writes that even if people were not traumatized when they arrived in boats, they undoubtedly become so after spending time in these detention centers.

Between Australia and Indonesia, over the centuries, boats come and go.

"We may have all come on different ships, but we're in the same boat now." Asylum Seeker Resource Centre. Painted in black handwriting on a wooden board. Posted Tuesday, March 11, 2014.

Under the blue of the painting there is black paint. The grotesque flip side of the Saltwater Collection of Yirrkala Bark Paintings of Sea Country is this conception of a land-sea continuity, one couched in terms of sovereignty and prevention, of legality and immigration, of war. Although Tony Abbott presents the current situation in terms of war, the war is not really between Indonesia and Australia. Needless to say, Australia's assertion of sovereignty has implications for Indonesia's sovereignty, but Indonesia is less concerned than Australia. Moreover, it is not in fact surprising that Indonesia is not preparing to confront Australia head-on, since there exists a strong and murky history of alliance and complicity between the two countries, stretching from the past century into this.

During the Cold War the Western powers fighting a war in Vietnam viewed Indonesia, with the largest Communist Party outside of the Soviet Union and China, as the last domino. On which side of the divide would it fall? In 1965 the country witnessed a coup that toppled Sukarno, the figurehead of revolution and independence, and installed Suharto. This "coup" turned into one of the largest mass atrocities of the twentieth century. Up to two million people were massacred in this purging of supporters and thousands of alleged supporters of the PKI (the Indonesia Communist Party). It was not a highly publicized genocide; in fact, it was passed off as a civil war by those Western powers that had knowledge of the events and, indeed, that were actively complicit in them. Suharto's dictatorship lasted until 1998, during which time he enjoyed the support of various Australian governments, including Labour. Since then the genocide has been unacknowledged not only in Australia, the U.S., and the West but also within Indonesia, where "forgetting" has been institutionalized.

A small boat in an ocean of impunity.

There is in Indonesia now a growing civil society movement, with survivors playing a key role, to "fight forgetting." In the absence of an official truth commission the Coalition for Justice and Truth is conducting its own truth-seeking process, organizing public hearings across Indonesia, gathering testimonies into one database, and producing a final report—"A small boat in an ocean of impunity," writes Galuh Wandita.

Just as both the Labour and Liberal governments in Australia today have contributed to the construction of islands of inhumanity between "our" island nation and Indonesia and Papua New Guinea, so too in the past both parties/governments supported the Suharto regime. Paul Keating, as treasurer and prime minister, did much to open Australia up to the world in terms of trade and finance, to a recognition of its place in the region, to save it from the imminent fate of becoming a banana republic. But his 1994 assertion that "no country is more important to Australia than Indonesia" was underwritten by his exoneration of Suharto from blame for the genocide. Liberal prime minister Malcolm Fraser met Suharto in October 1976, offering de facto recognition of the Indonesian invasion and annexation of East Timor (the eastern side of an island in the Indonesian archipelago).

Just as the history of relations between Australia and Indonesia prior to European settlement cannot be encapsulated in histories which only use the proper names of countries as we now know them, so too the postcolonial unraveling is more complex than that summoned purely by diplomatic accounts; government policies do not always represent all of the people all of the time, and even within the diplomatic corps there are surprising incongruities and paradoxes. Such as the fact that Australia, while supporting Indonesia's invasion and occupation of East Timor (1975 to 1999), provided sanctuary to East Timorese independence advocates like José Ramos-Horta.

Between Australia and Indonesia boats come and go. Yet, once, there were ships that did not sail.

The year is 1945. On the Melbourne docks Indonesian crews walk off Dutch ships and members of the Australian Waterside Workers Federation, supported by Indian and Chinese workers, artists, and activists, mount a rousing and effective blockade. Dutch ships loaded with arms and ammunition (to be used against the independence struggle in what was then the Dutch East Indies) are prevented from leaving the port. "The ships that didn't sail": This is a refrain that structures Joris Ivens's 1947 film, *Indonesia Calling* (revisited and contextualized in John Hughes's 2009 film, *Indonesia Calling: Joris Ivens in Australia*), made in support of the Indonesian struggle for independence, after three hundred years of colonization. The film was shot largely in Australia with a predominantly Australian crew and researchers. In fact, there were many Indonesian nationalists living in Australia during the Second World War (following the Japanese invasion there was a massive evacuation, a Dutch East Indies government in exile was set up in Australia, and political prisoners were transferred to Australian prison camps but subsequently released. Their number included a who's who of nationalist leaders).

The ships that didn't sail.

Mick Counihan told me about this film, and John Hughes sent me a DVD. It arrived as I was struggling to write about the Yirrkala drawings. At first I made no connection between *Indonesia Calling* and the Yirrkala drawings. . . .

One man who was a young teenager in Garut in West Java in 1947, linguist Rabin Hardjadibrata, remembers seeing *Indonesia Calling* on a couple of occasions and speaks about it in Hughes's film:

> They showed it preceding *Gone with the Wind* [Victor Fleming, 1939] . . . it was indeed a surprise to see that here is a country well known for being "white Australia," and yet they are supporting us! And of course a second time I went to make sure whether it was the same thing that I saw, and it was, of course. We always have a soft heart for the Australians because of that, of the support for Indonesian independence.

Surprising indeed. Even more so, the fact that in 1949 the Menzies government was one of the first to recognize the new Republic of Indonesia. In subsequent years, however, Australia certainly did its bit to contribute to the destabilization of the Sukarno government by covert trafficking of arms to support anti-Sukarno uprisings. Many of the young activists seen in *Indonesia Calling* were murdered or "disappeared" during the coup of 1965.

Between *Indonesia Calling* and the Yirrkala drawings . . . a sea of difference. A sea of difference in which echoes and similarities skim the surface, leaving a trail like surf breaking. Like a heron.

A heron zips across the blueness of Whiteley's painting, leaving a trace, a flurry of whiteness. The streak of white is here now, but only just, at any moment it will disappear, out of the painting, out of the world.

Between Australia and Indonesia stretches ocean. Boats come and go.

I have never visited Indonesia or Arnhem Land. I have never been on a leaky boat or in a detention center. I can only imagine what it must be like to have escaped persecution and torture only to be trapped on a boat between Australia and Indonesia, refused landing here or there, restrained in a detention camp on some small unspeakably hot god-forsaken island in the middle of nowhere. Visiting Australia this time, in the summer, the first thing I had to do was take a dip at Bondi. To be on Bondi Beach is to be at home in the world. It is as though the world begins here—with the bodily sensation of diving into and through cold salty waves—and stretches out forever, through time and space. But back in San Diego, as the Yirrkala drawings reverberate, as I don my frock for a party, the blackness of Sydney Blue seeps slowly to the surface, and spreads. It spreads way beyond Whiteley's Lavender Bay, Preston's harbor views, "my" Bondi. Between the memories of the Yirrkala drawings and the reading, here at home, of newspapers online and books borrowed through interlibrary loan and DVDs that come as gifts through the post, I begin to imagine . . . an other Australia, opened to exchange with the world beyond, through sea cucumbers and words. Their language is in ours, but what of our language? How can it imagine?

Imagine standing on Whiteley's balcony, looking out over Lavender Bay: You effectively turn your back on the rest of Australia. Such a tiny part of the country, that southeast corner. You turn your back on a history—long and benign, short and brutal—that has linked two regions, at the shortest point only one hundred and twenty-five miles apart, where the sea and the land segue into one another.

Now when I wear my Von Troska frock I hear all these stories, their language in the dress, in the blueness. I love the blueness of Sydney, but now the frock speaks other languages, underneath the blue there is the black that Whiteley used as a base, and there are murmurings of other shores, of an other Australia. Next time I return to Australia it will be to the Northern Territory, to Arnhem Land, perhaps even to Yolngu country, where the land and the sea are continuous, where boats come and go.

Missed Connection

30

I am on a tram from the city, heading out to Northcote. Behind me, two academics are discussing grants, who gets them and who doesn't, how to pitch a project. One of them is disgruntled, kvetching about a colleague who suddenly has started embracing their Jewishness, excavating family history and writing about the Holocaust. He says, "I'm a good Jew as Jews go, not religious mind you but gotta track record, been doing this stuff for years, and they knocked me back. Again." "Suck it up, sunshine," says the other bloke. During this exchange a man shuffles into the seat next to me, talking as he comes, talking as he goes. Torture, he says, on the other hand what about torture, in and out of the hospital, that's me in and out, schizophrenic they say, they say it's a diagnosis, well maybe who's to say but that's no excuse to torture a person, they'll use any excuse the government, any excuse, on the other hand who's to say I'm not Australian, whose business is it, don't have to tell the world where you come from, they'll get it out of you in the end, what about the camps, detention camps they call them, well what's legal if it comes to that, what's a Holocaust, tell me about diagnosis me mum they diagnosed her as leukemia they got into her bones they said things in her bones, on the other hand how can you save a person when it's in the bones, and there's no flesh there's no fat skin and bones, they say I'm a bob short you can say a slice short of a sandwich but that's no reason to torture a person the government they want to get into yer head, want to put everyone in camps so they can say things in peoples' heads but on the other hand where are you going to find food skin and bones it's a good day today sun shining well I hope you have a nice evening and look out for yerself, yeh it's a nice evening.

I have turned my head to look at him during some of the speech, he is addressing a point in space, seemingly unaware of my presence. I turn back. We sit next to each other, each looking straight ahead. "Nice evening," I assume, is simply part of a stream of consciousness, which will last the entire tram ride. But as it turns out, "Look out for yerself" is in fact the termination of a speech at once public and private. Yerself is me. I turn to look at him, to reciprocate, but a fraction too late, just as he turns away, gets up, and lopes off the tram.

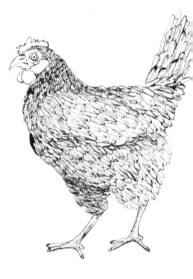

Blown through the Air

Falling asleep in the air, surfacing in San Diego, creepily hot in this midwinter, January 2014. The garden is confused: fruit trees blooming, lettuces wilting, chickens discombobulated, facing with befuddlement the question: To lay or not to lay today? Today is it winter or is today not winter not today?

Leaving Australia as temperatures climbed over one hundred degrees. On the East Coast of the U.S. in grubby, smoldering cities where only sometimes snow flitters fitfully across the landscape, there are four inches today.

Wild fires are breaking out in Australia and in California. How wild I wonder? Raging yes, but unrelated to the domestic?

"Breakfast in bed," says J. "It's a bit like sex in the grass, it *sounds* like a splendid idea." Nevertheless he brings me a tray with coddled eggs (Holly's eggs: creamy saffron yolks), demure in pastoral china, and a slice of toast festooned with two thick slices of Fat Dave's bacon: succulent, salty. Lula Mae stopped laying this week, the day that Holly started. They coordinate the rationing of human pleasure.

I have been a trifle chookless while traveling, though in Hawaii at Hanauma Bay, where I went snorkeling, there were feral chickens on the beach, not exactly cuddling up but certainly making do quite well with peckings and pickings from human picnics. Polynesian voyagers about a thousand years ago brought the first chickens to Hawaii. Those birds were less like today's chickens and more like the red jungle fowl (*Gallus gallus*) thought to be the ancestor of all chickens. You'd think these feral birds would be reverting to a red and jungly look. Feralization looks, on its surface, like domestication in reverse. But genetic analysis suggests that these chickens are evolving into something quite different from their wild predecessors, gaining some traits that reflect that past but maintaining others that have been selected by humans. In this way, they are similar to other populations of animals that have broken free of captivity and flourished, bearing a mixture of traits from both modern and ancient species.

In Austinmer, south of Sydney, on our way down to the beach for an early morning swim, Sarah took me by some chickens to whom she ritually throws her apple core, broken into pieces. In Melbourne each morning I would let Helen's chickens, making an almighty ruckus as soon as light filtered into the world, out of their coop. After I left and temperatures soared, she put ice cubes in their water and posted photos of them sheltering under the shade of the lime trees. And an image of the dog standing, just standing motionless, in the heat in the fish pond. Dazzle the water nymph, wrote Rosa.

So much to do. Pruning in particular—fruit trees, roses, grapevines—and searching for missing library books, buried under dust and piles of other books and mountains of accumulated fines. There is one I cannot find, Notes of a Native Son. I had begun to think of this book as mine, I've had it so long, renewing it each year. Perhaps someone nicked it, or I left it somewhere, or perhaps it has gotten mixed up with gardening books, I'll check again today. Or perhaps not. When a book goes missing this is usually what I do: buy a replacement cheap and take it into the library, mock-mournful, shamefaced, and the nice librarian Jimmy always says, You know we don't do this, you have to pay the fine online. And then he takes the book I offer and looks it over, quizzical, as though it's a novelty for him and a vaguely wondrous event, to hold a book in his hands. And then he says, OK, this time, but it's the last time. But this time I feel in my bones that eventually James Baldwin will turn up at home, and I shall keep him, or it, that library book that has spent so many hours in my hands, made grubby with breakfast stains. After traveling with a Kindle, its lightness—while in motion—has now become unbearable, hence this compulsion to pay the fine, as though then the book will materialize. Partly through superstition (as though paying the fine will magic the book into the world again, but also via an irrational though tenacious inkling that my heroic fine will keep the doors of the library open) I bow to institutional punishment, but I also bow down in homage to the world of books, of solid three-dimensional sticky objects that sometimes carry you away on a fluid flowing stream, a river into which you can dangle a foot and, despite what the philosopher says, you can return and do it again and again, it is the same river, you can find yourself again, albeit differently.

In homage too to Baldwin. How he manages words and how they correlate or not with feelings and how feelings infiltrate and stoke the fire of politics. The fire. "Stranger in the Village" is, at any time and in any place, even though of course time and place are specific and matter, an extraordinary essay, in its evocation rather than description, of what today is endlessly in so many contexts called "otherness." A fire that burns through thickets of sentiment. Exile: What does it feel like, where does it feel, how to think it?

In Australia there is much provocation to think of exile and asylum. Thousands of asylum seekers confined in detention camps, on and offshore. One government after another, Labour included, passing the buck. A sticky sensation of shame adhering to my Australian passport.

But this sensation was not everything. The Australian sojourn was simply marvelous: a passport to pleasure. It came at the right time: Bondi Beach in summer, Fitzroy street, friendships renewed, gardens—native and otherwise—to walk in, long conversations, spicy Asian food, the bats the black bats swooping through an indigo sky, all this worked better than any drugs and as well as all my quotidian rituals and obsessions. If obsession is potentially curative so too is travel. Obsession narrows the gaze and travel expands it, though they are not as antonymous as it might at first appear. Travel—good if you can get it—is a way of interrupting and shaking the quotidian. Recharging and reshaping.

I got better and better. But was blindsided by others getting iller and iller. I guess this happens when you are away and return and see we are not quite as young as we all once were. I felt a niggling sense of guilt that I—who make such a habitual hue and cry about this thing called *illness* (yes, I call it thus even though there are therapeutic regimes that advise rethinking it as a "wellness opportunity")—should be so well when others all around me were teetering like skittles, battling with demons of pain and separation, incomprehensible medical diagnoses and imminent death. I remind myself: There is no hierarchy of suffering.

I take heart from Pamela Brown, ironically wry and curiously lyrical. In her latest book of poems, *Home by Dark*, which she gave me over cups of tea in a café at Edgecliff station, she writes,

Like Michael said,
Now we'll spend
The rest of our lives
Watching our friends die.

But, and elsewhere, she also writes,

This is my quotidian
But it's not everything.

Don't Think about It (For the Moment)

32

JANUARY 2014

I had an immunoglobulin infusion the day after returning, blood tests still looking good, feeling fine, but of course it's a just a matter of time before the symptoms return. Dr. K asked me if I'd finished the book. I think he does not know what a holiday is. Lucky for me he works so hard. As expected the ball is in my court, but the choice is more clear-cut than often: Continue without drugs for as long as six months, if this good run lasts that long, or start back on a low dose of Revlimid with or without the Ritoxumab. Certainly I would opt not to do the combination. Too many infusions and all the stuff that goes with that. But Sheila, wonderful Nurse Sheila, said it would be possible to do the Revlimid off-protocol so I wouldn't be tied down by endless testing and could arrange labs with her and be able to travel. It'll cost something but not a lot. The simple truth is this: I don't want to think about it now. Am going to put it off for a month but then will probably opt for what Dr. K sees as a proactive move and the possibility of staving off the next big treatment for longer.

Spheres of Glass

33

I wandered, lonely, escaping from the Seattle Sheraton, from the giddiness of social encounters and a plethora of conference talk, escaping Chihuly. Chihuly orna-
ments and glass sculptures are nested in every niche of the Sheraton, commanding
attention from every shiny polished vantage point. Almost every hotel in Seattle
(and many other hotels around the world) exhibit Dale Chihuly glassworks, but
his great popularity is centered on the garden installations.

I saw "Gardens of Glass: Chihuly at Kew" in 2005 but was neither charmed
nor seduced. As a tourist and gardener and sometimes critic, like others of my
ilk I would always rather be seduced than not. On the other hand, I'd rather be
intrigued than charmed (but of course you cannot always choose the things that
move you, you cannot orchestrate those moments when the air turns cold and you
shiver or when a hot feverish breeze gets under your skin or when perplexity renders you speechless; for all that a certain kind of taste is trained into your body,
you cannot always predict how you will react). So now, visiting Seattle for the first
time, Chihuly Garden and Glass is on my bucket list. I'm intrigued to see how
these glassworks work in their native setting, hoping my mind can be changed.

After all, the conceit of these garden installations is potentially intriguing: the
insinuation of fantastical glass sculptures in among real plants. They are mostly,
though not entirely, gigantic, these sculptures, bearing names like garden grass,
reeds, blue herons, sun, French blue ikebana with orange and scarlet frog feet,
green trumpets, red orange reeds. They imitate and mimic. As you wander through
the garden you encounter vegetative landscapes, living matter, interspersed with
signs of the synthetic, squishy materials juxtaposed with brittle surfaces, warm
and fleshy with glassy coolness. Of course no garden is entirely natural, but if all

gardens are to some degree designed, then grand public gardens like Kew are meticulously curated (and so, too, one imagines, the "original" Chihuly Garden). As a viewer ambling through a series of interconnected gardens or galleries, one's curiosity could be tickled, one's sense of assurance about which goes with what. Mimesis in this mise-en-scène possesses the potential to provoke the irreality of the garden itself.

But the garden and museum fell short of conceit.

So here I am, escaping the extravaganza, walking back to the downtown conference along Fifth Avenue. Walking segues into trudging. It seems as though I have been hiking for days through rough terrain. A sliver of anxiety worms its way up, up from heavy footsteps into my stomach and buzzes there, a caged mosquito, looking for blood. An old familiar feeling, a feeling that hasn't visited for months. Perhaps, I tell myself, it is not somatic at all, just disgruntlement, the massive gaudy Chihuly glassworks—luridly pretty, drained of affect—weighing heavily upon my fragile psyche. Suddenly a wave of homesickness ripples through me, a yearning—to be home, curled up in bed with Elvis and Roxy, or in the garden picking fava beans, or in with the chickens, cooing, stroking their silkiness.

Lonely as a cloud.

When all at once I see a crowd, a host, of spectral chickens. Dead, plucked and headless chickens, impaled, fluttering and dancing in a shop window. Two washing lines slice the window vertically. Meat hooks hang from the cord lines, piercing the elongated yet rather fat necks, all skinniness concentrated in the legs, which dangle in the air, feet splayed open like hands stretching, feeling for solid ground. In between the legs and the necks plump appurtenances, rounded if rather lumpy breasts. Is it a shop, a restaurant, an office? There is no lettering, no description, no invitation.

My dragging footsteps freeze.

Behind the chooks hangs a large Chinese paper lantern, once scarlet now faded to puce, and in the right foreground, on a dusty cluttered desk, a jar of bright lively daffodils. Golden. In contrast the chickens are pasty and pale, a grimy faded yellow. The sickly yellow of Bird's custard, dished up in my childhood at the end of every vile boarding school meal, smothered over every horrible pudding, the horribleness only exacerbated by this fraudulent cover-up. Or is it whiteness turned old and musty and tinged with the ochre of decay? I step closer, nose against the glass. There is something odd about these chickens, they are too smooth, too drained of blood, too dusty, their necks—inauthentically fat—are hollow. There is something about them that makes me want to reach out through the glass to feel their textural duplicity. I realize: These are imitation carcasses, synthetic chickens, plasticity. Relief and hilarity. The sense of laughter, however, isn't just provoked by the discovery of the hoax; rather, it's to do with the uncanny persistence of irreality, an undecidability that persists in the scene before and after discovery, for now I'm part of this scene that I stumbled upon.

The sense of unease, shadowed by the intimation of disease returning, the horror provoked by this exhibition of dead and naked chickens, the unasked-for juxtaposition of my silky girls and these synthetic mute corpses is somewhat alleviated by the certainty that they are merely imitations. I'm off the hook, "my chickens," whose heads I would never chop off, who I would never pluck and hang and eat, are OK, they remain in the realm of the real while these phantoms are merely incarnations of a spectral brutality. But then the scene I witness—as though in a museum, as though this is an exhibit, as if it were a still frame from a movie—insists on including me in its mise-en-scène, on incorporating the dissociation from which I suffer. Cognitive dissonance shot through with strains of the uncanny. When I see ducks hanging in Chinese butcher shops, gleaming and velvety in their soy basting, I can't wait to taste and to experience in the mouth the crunch of their crispy skin. Even chickens, I never hesitate to eat chicken, I enjoy the cooking of chickens and chicken parts. Chickens in general. Not particular chickens. Not my chickens.

I was sitting alone in my wagon-lit compartment when a more than usually violent jolt of the train swung back the door of the adjoining washing-cabinet, and an elderly gentleman in a dressing-gown and a traveling cap came in. I assumed that in leaving the washing-cabinet, which lay between the two compartments, he had taken the wrong direction and come into my compartment by mistake. Jumping up with the intention of putting him right, I at once realized to my dismay that the intruder was nothing but my own reflection in the looking-glass on the open door.

Freud, writing here about the uncanny, presents us with a scene conceptualized as a frame within a frame. He is jolted, subjected to a shock. We might almost say that the movement involves transference, it is a movement between—between the viewer and the image. Enter the chickens as a third term, a mediating twist.

How bizarre to come upon this apparition on an ordinary street, while ambling along, to encounter thus the uncanny echoing or correlation of living and dead, natural and artificial, self and other, chickens and daffodils. Somehow this view into another world (office, butcher's shop, Chinese restaurant?) wakes me up, looks back, interpolates. The austerity of the frame, string strung across the window asymmetrically, the sickly color coordination, the insinuation of springtime and gardens, of a host of golden daffodils, into this macabre composition is provocative in a way the Chihuly is not.

It would be wrong to say that on glimpsing those daffodils my heart with pleasure danced. But a lightness did indeed enter into my leaden feet, as I imagined
a dance macabre between those denuded plastic chickens and my feathery cooing girls.

You have to walk through the Chihuly museum in order to reach the garden.
Which means your experience of the garden is overdetermined by the sense of
aesthetic homogeneity indoors. Actually the transition between the two realms is
striking. It is called the glasshouse, and though modeled on the great glasshouses
of the nineteenth century, such as the Crystal Palace, it is a very simple structure,
bare and austere. In contrast to the nakedness and transparency in which you find
yourself, a huge sprawling floral abundance hangs from the ceiling: glass flowers,
larger than life, fashioned in red, gold, and orange, drip lusciously, suspended in
space, suspended forever. As you stand under them it is almost impossible not to
imagine the whole gigantic structure crashing, splintering, dispersing into a thousand pieces. It's a gloriously extravagant composition, this mixing of glass textures,
this invocation of an aesthetic of timelessness through an allusion to practices of
preservation, to ways of keeping things alive in artificial environments. Like glasshouses, like museums, like tombs.

In the glasshouse a space opens up in which to meditate upon scale and materiality.

But after the glasshouse is the garden and before the glasshouse there are galleries, endless iterations of frilly floraliciousness. The psychedelic underwater
worlds are interchangeable with the flowery abstractions. The garden is just another gallery, a medium of display, a staging for the performance of anxiety: to
elevate glass blowing from a craft to a grandiose art. Such production requires
factory conditions and many workers. Nothing new in this, but the process of ef-
facement in the name of a single genius artist serves to efface process in general.
I so wanted the installation to yield a tension, a gesturing to something outside
itself, to the multiple imbrications of nature and art, to the materiality created out
of breath and fire. What I found was an abundance of precious cheerfulness but
little sense of the uncanny, or of the fragility of glass, how close it is to splintering. Nor much sense of how the social is inscribed in the material world. *Wonder*
is a word often used to describe the Chihuly effect, but for me, wonder served to
efface the complexities of process.

Wonder is also the predominant response elicited by another famous and popular display, the "Ware Collection of Glass Models of Plants," in the Harvard Museum of Natural History (often acknowledged by Chihuly as an influence). This
collection is composed of three thousand models of glass flowers constructed by
father and son Leopold and Rudolf Blaschka over five decades, from 1886 through
1936. In fact all kinds of plants, not just flowers, make up the collection, which was

commissioned in order to teach students of botany. The models are disturbingly life-size (too large to be miniatures, too small to be sculptures) and remarkably accurate in anatomical detail and color.

The wonder that these flowers elicit is complicated by a range of emotions and epistemological speculations, as evidenced in the richness of critical writing that circulates around them. Much of this writing hovers between description and defiance of description. How unlikely that these scientific models should be made of glass rather than other substances so much more amenable to modeling (they are constructed primarily though not exclusively of glass) like wax or papier-mâché. Their materiality, in practical and imaginative terms, is of the utmost importance. While extremely thingy, they are also chimerical. Wonder is generated in the play between seeing and not seeing, knowing and not knowing: You know they are made of glass, and yet . . . "They look real enough but as if the real is from another realm," says Jamaica Kincaid. It is she who captures the uncanniness of the artificial perfection and nails the relation of these objects wrought in glass to the garden.

The glass flowers and their many stages of being are in a state of perfection stilled. It is always a gardener's wish to have perfection and then to have it forever. It is also within the gardener's temperament to first desire forever and then to do everything possible to dismantle and smash forever. If the flowers encased in cabinets stored in the museum make up a garden, they are not the exception to this latter sentiment. Though it seems as if they will last forever, every cabinet bears a legend warning of their fragility. The people taking care of them give assurance that they will last forever. But as every gardener knows, forever is as long as a day.

Glass matters here, but other materials matter elsewhere. Plastic and yarn, for instance, can be exploited for their mimetic potential. What matters is scale and texture and the way that the materiality of the sculptural object is able to gesture outside its own perfection (its mimetic perfection or formal coherence) to chisel a crack in the cognitive dissonance that glues everything together.

Think of Ian Hamilton Finlay's glass poem, "Wave/Rock." The poem is constructed not on the page, but on a thick sheet of glass onto which the words *Wave* and *Rock*, many times over, are sandblasted. The letters of the word *wave* break on the rock constructed not on the page, but in glass. The form of the words mimics their meaning, enacts their materiality. Waves break, and simultaneously the process of waves breaking is frozen, the cycle of nature is eternal, and at the same time fragile, vulnerable to destruction, particularly in and by human hands: the one who sculpts, composes, the one who reads and sees and knows and does not know. "Wave/Rock" dislodges a habitual cognitive dissonance. We might almost say that the movement involves transference, it is a movement between—between the viewer, looking at and through the glass, and the image.

Enter the chickens, proposing a third term, a mediating twist. For me the chickens in this instance represent an ecological dimension that Hamilton Finlay most likely did not intend but through which the work now speaks.

Glass in the end is not the most important thing (though glass contains a particular potential). It is the materiality of the process incorporated into the sculptural object, the "work" in the "work" which gestures toward something playful and also potentially destructive. The wave, this one wave which is also many waves, all waves, breaks over and over again but is itself vulnerable, and perhaps after all not so eternal.

Take "Hyperbolic Crochet Coral Reefs." This is a project initiated by the Institute for Figuring, run by Christine and Margaret Wertheim. The Wertheim sisters, inspired by a type of mathematical modeling called hyperbolic geometry, put out a web call to invite women to join them in crocheting a coral reef, following some simple mathematical rules for generating a certain kind of spatial configuration and dimensionality (interestingly embodied by reefs and reef creatures). Women from all over the world responded to the invitation, contributing individual items and elements. The Institute for Figuring initiated workshops, crocheting workshops which incorporated an ecological component, learning about reefs, about the threats posed to their existence particularly from the onslaught of plastic detritus. The artists, as well as using more familiar materials such as wool and yarn, incorporated into the sculptures recycled materials, such as plastics. Leslie Dick, from whose fabulous essay I learned of this project, writes of a "mental shift in scale (from individual item to larger combination)," which is "mirrored by the relation of the Hyperbolic Crochet Coral Reefs to their real-world counterparts, particularly the Great Barrier Reef in the Pacific." Leslie Dick contends that the project, drawing on so many practitioners, produces a new kind of artist (and thus artwork), one immersed in reverie, in a project that enables a rich variety and combination of imaginative explorations. She invokes this kind of artist:

> While she may have confidence in her expertise, her work avoids grandiosity, remaining at a manageable scale (until it joins the larger combination). This artist particularly enjoys the invitation to sink below the ocean, to enter its dreamlike darkness, an alternate reality of color and shape. She enjoys making phallic shapes, using her hook and yarn to build leaning towers, star shaped fortresses, a landscape drawn in lumps of color. She en-

joys making vaginal shapes, fuzzy, curly edged openings, soft to the touch, fronded and weird.

I have only seen images on screen, but these marvelously thingy things look so incredibly lifelike, so reefish, it's uncanny. And dissonant too, the way seemingly alien materials are almost seamlessly crocheted into the sculptures. There is a cognitive dissonance at large in our world now: We revel in the beauty of underwater worlds, of forests and canyons, of places like the Great Barrier Reef, and we are filled with wonder at art that mimics that beauty and preserves for eternity a platonic perfection. Peeking into the world of "Hyperbolic Crochet Coral Reefs" jars that perfection, chisels into the glue of cognitive dissonance, invites reverie and wonder and playful engagement but also a cognitive recalibration, a reimagining and re-spinning of a conceit that intertwines the natural and synthetic worlds.

Speaking of cognitive dissonance—as we were making our way back from the spectacular San Juan Islands where we spent a night on Orcas island, a catastrophic event occurred in beautiful Washington State: one of the deadliest landslides in U.S. history. As we hiked around Cascade Lake and climbed to the top of the tower on the top of Mount Constitution, marveling in this world seemingly so pristine, a community in Stillaguamish Valley in the foothills of the North Cascades was suddenly, without warning, buried under mud. A natural disaster? Unforeseen, said the emergency manager of the area. Timothy Egan wrote a week after the event that in fact there had been warnings, most notably a report in 1999 that outlined "the potential for a large catastrophic failure" on the very hillside that just suffered a large catastrophic failure (though it seems the inhabitants of the endangered community were never told of these official reports). Egan reports visiting the area twenty-five years ago and being shown a mudslide occurring on a hillside above the river, a hillside in which old-growth forest had been clear felled, leaving nothing to hold the hillside in torrential rain. Just like the hillside above the small, disappeared community of Oso.

Egan says, "The 'taming' of this continent, in five centuries and change, required a mighty mustering of cognitive dissonance. . . . A legacy of settlement is the delusion that large-scale manipulation of the natural world can be done without consequence."

Scale and texture. A continent, an ocean, a garden, a shop window, forests, mud, glass, yarn, plastic, plants, the real and the imitative, the beautiful and the catastrophic.

I return to San Diego where rather than rain there is a drought and the river, if it can be seen at all, is skinny. I make a routine visit to the hospital on the UCSD campus and am astounded by the number of new buildings, massive grandiose medical buildings mostly, being developed on the very edge of canyons. Mesas have been sliced into and rearranged. Glass and concrete structures teeter on air. We have no old-growth forests here, just coastal scrub and chaparral. But they too hold the earth down. What, I wonder, is the cognitive dissonance we suffer from here? I imagine a performance art project enacted by chickens let loose on the medical campus or even an installation of dead, plucked, and headless chickens, hanging from the canyon walls, dangling over freeways, reaching for the daffodils.

Purple Haze   34

We return from Seattle craving food from the garden, home cooking. I make chard cakes, roast beets, and a fern green sorrel sauce, tart and raw on the tongue. We are glad to be home, in familiar territory, but the garden emanates an unfamiliar sadness. Perhaps it is a sadness we have brought with us.

J and I were at the Seattle Public Library designed by Rem Koolhaas, when a figure in a long purple coat swept into view. It was Maureen Turim, who was also escaping the conference and being given a personal tour of the library by her cousin who works there. We were fortunate to glom on to the tour. We took photos of each other, as we have done over the many years of meeting up at the screen studies conference, even though we do not keep in touch in between conferences. I recall how Scott, her husband, had taken a photo of us with Connie Penley three or four years ago. Ask Scott to find the photo, I said. As Maureen and I walked back to the conference she told me of how Scott had been diagnosed in the past year with leukemia. She told me what type of leukemia, a much more acute form than CLL. He had a bone marrow transfer, and the recovery had been tough. Still, she said, I'll tell him how well you are doing. We talked of retirement. Yesterday Facebook tells me of his sudden death.

The tiny tomatoes I planted just before leaving, acquired at Tomatomania, have expanded, forming flowers, looking like plants. I have to start clearing the beds for the summer crops. Tuesday: pole beans where the peas were planted; Wednesday: bush beans; Friday: summer squash seeds. In the process of clearing I've pulled up masses of New Zealand spinach. Tonight I will mix it in with beets and beet greens and make a casserole of sorts. Usually this transition between seasons imparts a joyfulness, generating expectations. But today I feel a little like an interloper in my garden, as though I'm here by proxy, allowed a moment of pleasure just so long as others pay the price.

There is a sadness settling as a purple haze over the garden. I am so sorry, Maureen.

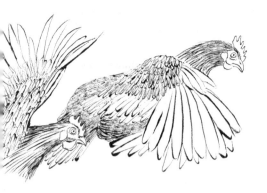

Cantankerous Rooster

35

Marathon, Texas. It is early morning, and light is creeping into the motel room. Last night we walked back to the motel under a huge black sky, so black the stars shone like the burnished feathers of a silver rooster, burros brayed, flights of angels winging us to our rest. I remember living in San Agustín Etla near Oaxaca, being kept awake and woken and harassed all day and night by the sound of braying burros, turkeys, a rooster, dogs, people. *Gracias a los burros* my rooster does not have to crow. He stands on the dressing table in front of a mirror, so there are two of him. Sculptural. Silent. He is double and a doubler. I open the door and step out into the dusty parking lot. The sky is now a soft donkey grey, fringed to the east with vermilion, redness seeps out of the earth, filtering into the sky.

I can stretch my arm in any direction and reach the edge of solidity and then my fingers will close around the sky.

I take the rooster outside and photograph him. He is immobile. His coxcomb is scarlet, his body painted in swathes of yellow, green, and blue. His tail is feathery, the featheriness of sliced tin, a shiny indigo blue. He is perfectly proportioned. His toes are splayed, giving him a firm purchase on the ground, or the dressing table, or wherever he alights. Always out of place, he will be my register of place as we travel through desert regions toward Marfa.

The rooster joined us before the desert. In Johnson City, home of LBJ, we find somewhere to pee: a tiny coffee shop in a large yard filled with ironware. Flying pigs and alligators and cows. All painted. On the counter a faded photo of a Starbucks van, the side door slid open so that "tarb" is eliminated. What you see then is the Starbucks icon and the word *sucks*.

While he fixed me an excellent espresso, John and I swapped a few minimally anecdotal details—he'd lived in San Francisco, he could tell I wasn't from Texas.

Probably not from San Francisco either. The old guy he's swapping yarns with, toothless, dusty, feels like he's roamed the local block for years, and probably drunk every bottle in town, but who knows? Who knows peoples' stories unless you drive with them for days and days through the desert and can talk of this and that and failed relationships and swap another hilarious story of another disastrous episode in the life of love. I asked John who made the rooster and the other creatures, where they came from. He looked at me quizzically as if to say, Which leg can I pull? Which story will she buy? Or, as if he were asking himself, Is this a trick question? What's she after, this foreigner? Who on this wide earth wants to know about the provenance of painted tin tchotchkes? Who gives a flying fuck where the rooster comes from? Then he laughs and says, Juan, Carlos, Roberto, Ricardo, Miguel . . . an army of anonymous Mexicans. I realize then it was indeed a sneaky question, the sort of question that a snooty gardener asks, either to elevate her purchase, raise it out of the realm of tourist art and into the realm of artisanal individuality, or simply to trip up a pretentious vendor.

I could go back to Old Town in San Diego and buy this rooster, closer to the source of its production. Or just nip across the border and buy it by the side of the road. Probably I could even nip back to Zimbabwe and buy the same rooster. And yet not exactly the same.

There was a bigger rooster, grander. But as soon as my eyes alit upon this one I knew he was the one for me. He is life-sized, perfectly proportioned, he has stepped out from a child's picture book, from meticulously illustrated Mexican playing cards. R for rooster. G for *el gallo*. Watch out, says the old guy, he's a cantankerous rooster, that one.

Molly, who has turned up at the coffee shop with Allen and Lynsey, says, We will photograph the rooster everywhere we stop on our journey toward Marfa. He will be our sign, our register of place. The problem is, Molly drives off with her lovely camera, and I only have a phone. Luckily the rooster responds well to iPhone attention: preens, holds still while I teeter and shake.

In Harper, where we get gas, he stands beneath a wall on which is painted a much larger than life U.S. flag and under it a large star of David and the slogan STAND BY ISRAEL. Over the doorway on the same wall it says BUILDING FOR SALE. Somehow my focus is screwy, and the rooster is cut out of the picture.

He does appear, albeit tinily, at the bottom of the frame, under two bucking broncos, at Lowe's, a local market in Fort Stockton. We had a cup of tea at a restaurant here, and the young Mexican American who served us wouldn't take any payment. It's just water he said. I bought a bar of fancy dark chocolate with sea salt, an anomalous foreign import, and Katie bought a local newspaper. We ate the chocolate at the Rock House by the Rio Grande, it was musty.

In Marathon we have breakfast at Nancy's Coffee Shop. Under the large sign is scrawled, faintly, barely legible, FOILED AGAIN. The rooster stands in the large expanse of the dirt parking lot in front of our rooms. The horizon is so low it just peeks over his head.

We drive down into Big Bend National Park. The rooster sits silently in the backseat of the car, but the air around him is volatile, and even though the car appears and feels to us like an airtight razor-sharp capsule slicing through space, something escapes, the rooster's colors vibrate, charging the landscape, inviting reciprocal attention. A doubler, he is an attraction and he attracts, he elicits color, winkling out of desert hues streaks and swathes and seas of vivid primary color.

Eventually we arrive at Terlingua Ghost Town. There is a row of seats along the veranda of the saloon, which is also a gift shop and also the hotel, next door to the Starlight Theatre and Bar, which only opens at five so we will not get there, but it looks enticing, the ceiling is painted midnight blue. On the veranda everyone has a bottle in hand, slow gossip fuels the atmosphere. New people in town, everyone is alert but pretends to notice nothing, though they all noticed Nora. Someone has already picked up the keys to the Rock House, and when I ask who, she says a boy and a girl with tattoos. Nora later tells us that on her way out a woman grabs her arm to comment on her tattoos and confides loudly that she has her ex-boyfriend's name tattooed on her butt.

At the Rock House the rooster sits on a table, the Rio Grande behind him. And then I bring him in for the night to sit safely at the foot of my bed. There are rooster thieves abroad, and vigilance is required.

Now we are here, in Marfa, the rooster and I. You would not exactly call him Judd-esque, my rooster. Picturesque, yes definitely. Ex-situ incarnate.

I shall take him home this rooster, a Texan I guess, home to California where he will be charged to remember all the fantastical details of this journey that I shall forget slowly, memory by memory.

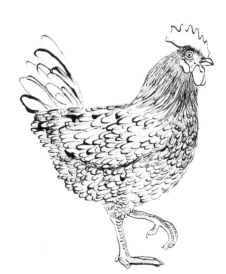

Dead and Alive

A TENUOUS CONTINUUM

It was the aroma that lured us. Sometimes smells are attached to memories and desires and can then manifest as pungently as though the source is inches from your nose. We were in fact hundreds of miles away when the distinctive aroma of bread began to tickle our nostrils. Actually we were not consciously aware of this prickling desire as we set out in the morning. We left our B&B on the edge of Point Reyes National Park in Northern California, anxious about catching our plane home from San Francisco. But it turned out we had a smooth run and arrived in the city with hours to spare, musing about a flying visit to the De Young Museum. Somehow we missed the exit to the museum. Mysteriously, the rental car, propelled by unconscious aromatic tickling, detoured and found its own way to 18th Street, half a block away from Tartine Bakery.

So there we were, along with half of San Francisco, standing in line, succulating in the scents that oozed out of the bakery into the street. Then we were inside, sitting at a long wooden table slowly guzzling the best *pain au chocolat* in all the world. We left with two sandwiches for the plane (for me, the pecorino panini filled with almonds crushed with olive oil, lemon, and sage) and two loaves of sourdough bread.

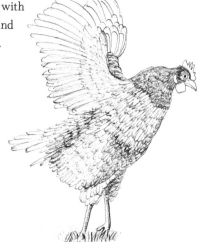

I was seduced, like many people, into regular bread making by Jim Lahey of Sullivan Street Bakery, who popularized the no-knead method. You might call it the lazy way, but Lahey figured out two important things: that a lot of kneading is not necessary if the dough is started with a minimum of dry yeast and allowed to ferment for a long time (eight to eighteen hours); and secondly, that the conditions of a very hot wood-fired oven could be reproduced or mimicked in a home kitchen by baking in a preheated sealed cast-iron pot in a very hot oven. All Lahey's recipes are wonderful, guaranteed to produce rich dark brown crusts; I regularly made the pan integral (whole grain) but also rye, walnut, olive, *stecca*, coconut-chocolate bread, Jim's Irish brown bread, almond-apricot bread, fennel-raisin loaf, as well as pizza and focaccia.

The main thing Lahey did (and Mark Bittman, who popularized this method in a widely read *New York Times* piece) was tickle my appetite for good bread. On the farm as a kid bread was baked daily; I don't remember it being very tasty, though I do remember the seductive smell, always braided in my mind and therefore body with the smell of the dogs' soup on the woodstove—the large pot of bones into which all the vegetable leftovers were chucked—that simmered very slowly all day and was fed to the dogs with *sadza* each evening. On the farm in Toora, Australia, where again I had a woodstove, I also baked bread, immersed in *Elizabeth David's Bread Book* that Jeannie Frankel gave me for my thirtieth birthday. Whenever I open up this book the sizzling smell of bacon and eggs, embedded in its pages, escapes. We partied that night, the night I turned thirty, through the night and then went to Waratah Bay and watched the sun come up, on a new day and a new year, trundled back to the farm, collected eggs from the Toora Holiday Flats hens, and cooked bacon and eggs.

Apart from the aroma, there are many advantages to baking your own bread. There is the tactility of dealing with flour and water, feeling sludge turn to silk. There is the gratification as you pull your bread out of the oven, put your cheek against the warm loaf, and feel the warmth spread into your face and through

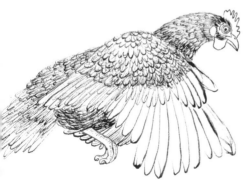

your body and you hear the singing. Like burying your face in the fat furriness of a cat like Elvis, the warmth and the vibrations of his purring spreading through you. One of the most obvious advantages, however, is knowing what goes into it. Most store-bought bread is steeped in sugar and salt and other preservatives, and the quality of the flour

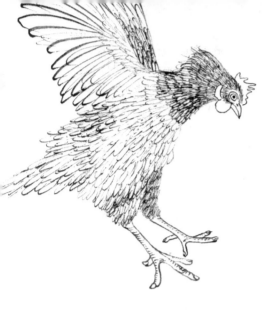

is often dubious. Though not as dubious as in nineteenth-century London where, in eating your daily bread, you would also consume "a certain quantity of human perspiration mixed with the discharge of abscesses, cobwebs, dead black-beetles, and putrid German yeast, without counting alum, sand, and other agreeable mineral ingredients."

A few years after I was diagnosed with CLL, when the lymph nodes were growing and my energy was sapped and treatment loomed on the horizon, I started thinking about sourdough bread, about the ingredient missing from the bread I was making: live yeast. Hours and hours would pass as I read my way—in bed, unable to make it into the garden—through a huge pile of bread books. Bread, the mystery of bread, the elusive formula for the perfect loaf, this can preoccupy a person for hours and days and years on end, a perfect mechanism for exclusion (pain, discomfort, anxiety, not knowing—all such sensations dissipate as one reads and kneads and plots new loaves). But it was really only after that particular visit to Tartine, after I had finished the second treatment and was, for a while, drug-free, that I became preoccupied by the health benefits of fermented food, including sourdough bread.

I had been using dried yeast—small granules encasing a speck of live yeast. The production of this form of yeast is standardized and therefore predictable. It enables a quick rise of the dough, but since it is a monoculture the bread lacks the complex flavors and nutrients derived from a slow sourdough ferment using natural, live, unpredictable yeast.

To make sourdough bread you need a starter or levain or mother. My first starter came from Jill Giraud, who left it for me in the sangha with my name taped to it (and email messages—Good luck and have fun! There's always more if you blow it). I brought it home. Imagine the scene:

It sits on the kitchen counter in a glass jar. "It" is like a fragment from the tar pits, captured and bottled but instead of black it is a yellowish-brown, pukey-looking substance. It grows, it bubbles and splutters. The kitchen smells like a back alley the morning after, awash in stale wine. It is undoubtedly alive. It is yeast. "It" is not a singular thing, but many, a myriad in fact of tiny single-celled creatures, *Saccharomyces cerevisiae*, the microbes we call yeast.

Magic. This glass jar heralds two transformative magical acts.

First: something out of nothing. Out of thin air the yeast appears. Yeast microbes are all around us, on our skin, on the surfaces of the kitchen and the utensils that hang from the ceiling, in the air. When you make a mix of flour and water and let it sit there in the jar, exposed to the air (covered with cheesecloth or a fine metal grille), the yeast moves in, starts gobbling and multiplying. You have to keep feeding it, every day a few tablespoons of flour and the same of water. And there you have it: the starter for your sourdough bread. The gobbling and bubbling is the beginning of fermentation, the process of turning starch into glucose, a simple sugar. This process ferments the sugar, which converts to alcohol and carbon dioxide that leavens or lifts the loaf.

Second: when you add a small quantity of this mixture to a larger mix of flour and water, and then add a little salt and let it sit for a while, expanding, and then fold and fondle it and then eventually place it in a large hot pot and place that large hot pot in a very hot oven, well then a magical act of olfactory transformation occurs. The stinkiness of fermentation mutates into the smell of baking bread. That smell spreads throughout the house, inhaling that aroma your body involuntarily mimics the process of the baking bread and you feel yourself lifting, levitating. Before long that wet shaggy mess of flour and water and salt will have turned into the most delectable bread: nutty, a little sour, soft and airy inside and crunchy outside.

Theoretically. In fact I managed to kill my mother. I put her in the fridge when I went away, and when I returned she was as hard as a rock and a horrible color, so I gave up, though Jill told me it would have been easy to revive her.

Later I tried again, this time to make my own starter. It was after I was back on the Revlimid as a maintenance measure (also boosting the immune system). Mostly doing well, good blood and platelet counts, feeling fine but experiencing intermittent gastro problems. One night I was woken by severe constipation that after a few days provoked diverticulitis: gut-wrenching pain, nausea, feverish, your body a feeble cinder box. Of course you are given antibiotics but yearn for something less virulent to restore harmony in your gut. You start thinking about microbes.

As distraction from the dizziness and nausea and because the thought of food was repulsive, and because I couldn't garden, as a substitute I started avariciously reading about yeast and soon found my way to Louis Pasteur. Nowadays, especially in fanatical fermenting circles, Pasteur is the bad guy, the anal disciplinarian who warned us about bad bacteria and encouraged obsessive antiseptic cleanliness. The injunctions of the sterilization brigade are numerous: no playing in the dirt, always wash hands, swab down countertops, use bleach, kill all visible and invisible creepy crawlies. And in the process, kill all the good bacteria. But there is another Pasteur or another way of looking at him, imagining his legacy. This Pasteur is on the side of life.

. . .

Pasteur's work was enabled by the invention of the microscope in the mid-nineteenth century; it was the microscope that revealed the presence of a previously invisible entity called yeast. Pasteur was a chemist, working within a discipline that saw yeast as inert and fermentation as a purely chemical process. The incredible contribution of Pasteur is that he identified yeast as a *living* organism, the agent responsible for alcoholic fermentation and dough leavening. He did this by weighing the ingredients before and after fermentation, thus showing that during this process yeast takes something from the sugar and produces something new (alcohol and carbonic acid). Fermentation, he declared, is "correlative to life and to the organization of globules, and not to their death and putrefaction."

While demonstrating a strong connection between bread and alcohol production Pasteur also showed that there are different kinds of yeast involved in each process and also that there are two types of fermentation: alcoholic and lactic acid. Alcoholic fermentation occurs by the action of yeast; lactic acid fermentation, by the action of bacteria. All the other fermentations that grab my fancy and take my time—yogurt, cheese, kimchi, sauerkraut—occur through lactic acid fermentation, through the action of types of *lactobacilli* microbes. Pasteur described the relation of the different yeasts and bacteria involved in fermentation as similar to the relation of plant families. Thus he ignited the ecological imagination that enabled later writers, such as Michael Pollan, to think about gardening and fermenting as similar activities, both involving different organisms that form their own ecosystems through coevolution and symbiosis. And he paved the way for us to think about the place of people in these ecosystems and the kinds of interactions that occur there between humans and nonhumans.

But how did Pasteur make an impact? What sort of dramas did he stage to bring yeast into public awareness? How did he orchestrate scenarios in which the relationship between people and microbes appears as a life-changing scientific event? Bruno Latour, in a series of fascinating studies of Pasteur, argues that it was an epistemological drama he was staging through a series of questions and demonstrations: How can a new entity emerge out of an old one? How can the yeast extracted from nothingness become everything? How can a nonentity become an entity? How can it become a full-blown actor? In the process the relation between human and nonhuman is elaborated. Latour talks about the way Pasteur modifies the relationship between human and nonhuman in a story that "converts a nonentity [yeast], the Cinderella of chemical theory, into a glorious and heroic character." In the process yeast and lactic acid become actants. They modify; they enable him to win medals. In reflecting not only on Pasteur's practice but also on his own, Latour suggests that we need to abandon the division between speaking humans and a mute world, to acknowledge that *we are allowed to speak interestingly by what we allow to speak interestingly.*

. . .

That canonic Buddhist text *The Tassajara Bread Book* begins with a dedication:

with respect and appreciation
to all my teachers
past, present and future:
gods, men and demons;
beings, animate and inanimate
living and dead, alive and dying.

So you start thinking about microbes, about the imbalance in your gut, about the relationship of your body to the myriad of minuscule bodies within it, about how these minuscule bodies—microbes and bacteria—play a part, perform as actants in changing the composition of your gut. And how you can modify your gut through what you eat. Pondering the conundrum of dead and alive, that tenuous continuum, you also realize that it is braided into some other entangled distinctions—that between fast and slow, for instance, or between you-yourself and you-not-entirely-you.

Reading about bread can be very absorbing, but there comes a time when you have to put your body on the line. I began with Chad Robertson's book. Buying bread from the Tartine Bakery is one thing, trying to make your own bread following the recipes in the book *Tartine*, well that is another thing. Alluring images, seductive writing, recipes that unfold like a dancer's fan, a sensuous falling series, one instruction opening out into another and then another, never-ending. I soon gave up. But then I found what promised to be a kind of Tartine super-healthy fast-track—Michael Pollan's adaptation of Tartine's bread to a whole-grain recipe.

Disaster. Then I was captivated by the poetic minimalism of a new title: *Flour Water Salt Yeast*, by Ken Forkish. Such simplicity, I felt, would surely be transferred osmotically into the baking process. Wrong. Then I was wooed by Nancy Silverton on YouTube enthusing about squishy black grapes and the yeasty microbes conveyed on their skins. All I got from that encounter was squish.

The problem is that yeast, being a living thing, needs feeding. As the flour-and-water starter brings the yeast to life, so the yeast starts eating the flour and water, demanding more more more. I'm quite happy to consider yeast an actant, just like myself, but this microbe is revealing itself to be willful and combative. You have to feed the little monster. However, you can't just throw in some more flour and water and hope the avaricious yeast will be happy. No, the operation is a lot more complex. You have, each day, to throw most of the starter away, retaining a small but very specific amount, to which you add fresh and very specific amounts of flour and water. Not only are you keeping the yeast alive, you are nurturing it, refreshing its environment. It is a very messy operation.

Flour flour everywhere.

My beautiful magenta slippers are coated with flour. The whole kitchen is coated with flour, everything is shrouded in a dusty pale patina. Flour wafts into the air and settles like snow on the butter dish that sits uncovered on the kitchen bench. You pick up a salt cellar and your hand comes away floury, you pick up the olive oil bottle and your hand comes away curdled and sticky. Worse than this, worse than the flour that billows into the air, worse than the feathery pillows of flour that nestle in every crevice, in every minute crack, on every surface of the kitchen, worse than all this is the gluey mess of flour and water that sticks not only to you, to every exposed surface of your skin, but also to the floor and the ceiling and the benches and the sink. You try to scrape it off and it either clings tenaciously or flies off in fury, globules landing on high shelves—and low footwear. You tread in the mess and spread it throughout the house.

And it only gets worse. Not better as you might expect once the well-fed starter has been added to your dough mix, once the dough has been shaped and fondled and turned and proofed and put in the oven. That is when you face true disaster, failure and despair. Loaf after loaf fails to rise sufficiently, fails to cook sufficiently, overcooks, drops in a puddle, or crouches malevolently like a disenfranchised frog.

. . .

One day J brings home a loaf of bread he has bought at the Sunday farmers' market. It is unlike any other bread we have eaten in San Diego: light, chewy, nutty, very slightly tangy but with a whiff of caramel. It is bread that you can eat unadorned and feel you are in heaven. Though it doesn't hurt to dip it in oil or smear on some butter and fig jam. And toasted its crunchiness is delectable. The loaves are made by a company called Prager Brothers. I run to the market the next week and find that they are two young brothers, Clinton and Louie, one trained as a musician and the other as a plant biologist, who decided to combine their talents and turn their hobby of dabbling in dough, making pizzas, and experimenting with bread into a business. There is a quiet fanaticism to their demeanor, a zeal about bread that is infectious and inspiring. I become a groupie, following them around at markets and tracking them down at their bakery and at the Fermenters Fair where Louie gives a talk.

What's wrong with gluten?, he asks. Gluten is what makes bread, it's that gorgeous stringiness that develops as the dough leavens, it's what gives bread its shape and strength and goodness. But an anti-gluten hysteria has swept the nation. Convinced that gluten is causing all kinds of diseases and upsets of the body people are swearing off bread and embracing gluten-free as the new panacea. "What has been the staff of life is now perceived as the spirit of disease," says Stephen Jones, the director of Bread Lab. Gluten is indeed a serious issue for people with celiac disease and some other conditions who really can't process the gluten in wheat. Most people actually can, though the reactions to commercial bread are not all hysterical or imaginary. The problem is that most industrial bakeries only allow bread to rise for a very short time—not nearly long enough to let the yeast and bacteria digest all the gluten in the flour, let alone the extra dose in the additives. Moreover, wheat, like corn and other commercial crops, has been developed to enhance what—for the producers—are seen as advantageous or desirable qualities, such as increased yield, fast growth, resistance to disease. But all of this means a loss of flavor and nutrients and a higher gluten content. As a result, all sorts of problems can arise in the gut. Long fermentation, as well as partially breaking down the gluten, also slows the body's absorption of starch. Freshly milled organic flours are the best; not only are they more flavorful, but fresh flours also tend to be more active and ferment at a higher rate than store-bought flours.

Later, the Prager brothers, following in the tradition of other artisan bakers, would buy their own mill and churn out all sorts of organic flours, including California-grown Yecora Rojo red wheat, Tibetan purple barley, and organic cornmeal.

Having discovered the Pragers I submitted to a higher truth. When you can buy such perfect loaves why make your own bread? Peace, order, and cleanliness returned to the kitchen. J was relieved. But more recently I've been experiencing an itch, the imp of the perverse has started dancing, luring me back to the precipice, inviting me to rise to the challenge. How to approximate such perfection? I peruse the books the Pragers recommend, read the list of ingredients on each

Prager loaf, I taste, sniff, and compare. I start dreaming of spelt, rye, buckwheat, millet, teff—ancient grains that give to bread a complex taste. I start gathering and hoarding seeds and nuts in preparation for a long siege.

. . .

This past summer in a town in Tuscany called San Gimignano I was meandering when something caught my eye—a lush, deep-green shininess. It was a leather shoulder bag, shimmering in a small shop crowded with bags of all shapes and colors. Almost forest green, reminiscent indeed of the dank darkness of trees, but when you turned into the sunlight it glimmered with an emerald sheen. I stroked it, smelled it, tried it out for size, slinging it over a shoulder, feeling it settle against my body. And then I left it. J went in search of gelato, and I wandered with Therese and Patty. Later when we returned to the bus, there was no J. We waited, the driver becoming impatient. And then, at the eleventh hour, he appeared bearing in his arms a gift: the green bag. At that moment, in the moment of the gift, the name San Gimignano started pealing, ringing a bell. I remembered: This is the town where Jim Lahey learned to make bread. The gift of the bag was also an invitation, or perhaps a provocation, sent from the gods of the forest, the gods of ancient grains. This new gift was a reminder of an old love, my first love in the sourdough adventure: the nonchalant Jim Lahey.

As it turns out, I will find myself in hospital in the city of Prato in the early hours of the next morning. The ambulance is very old and creaky, and the ambulance assistants are alarmingly young. By the time we get to the hospital I'm a bit out of it, but Therese and J assure me that the hospital is modern and efficient. A sense of relief as the painkillers trickling into my veins begin to take effect and the excruciating pain starts to diminish. All around a veritable cacophony of sound, not just what I know as the normal hospital noise, but people yelling, laughing, calling out orders I suppose. The best thing of all: no hospital gowns. So much more congenial and comforting to lie there in your own clothes, to see other people's holey socks peeking out from under a blanket. Despite the apparent chaos things roll along, and the doctors and nurses display a reassuring nonchalance. The next day I'm sent home with painkillers and antibiotics. Not Flagyl, please, I beg. The doctor laughs and says, No no, we want you to feel better, not worse. But I do have some bad news, he says, a little anxiously, his nonchalance slipping for a moment. You will have to pay something, at least for the ultrasound. We find the tiny payment booth and get the bill. It's 156 euros! A viable health-care system available to all. In the U.S. this would have been many thousands of dollars, double-digit thousands.

Back in San Diego I return to Jim Lahey. Inspired by his nonchalance I will start anew, I will aspire to an easygoing grace under pressure, to a conviction that things will turn out OK. And I will slow down, enter into the spirit of the long slow-fermentation waltz. I order his new book on sourdough. That very day I get an email from Katrin: Tim has made a new starter, we can drop some round for you if you'd like. I do like. Tim tells me to store the starter in the fridge when not in regular use; don't be fooled, he says, it plays dead, but it will soon come alive. I begin again. And so far it is all going fairly well. Adriene visits and tells me she is embracing imperfection. I can't go as far as an embrace, but my grip on the fantasy of perfection seems to be relaxing—not a lot, it's true, but a little. A little is OK. My dough skills are improving, though some days there is a regression to loaves that look like cow patties, flat and dark and curious smelling as though aliens have landed and left their turds in my kitchen. But mostly I am tossing off loaves with all the nonchalance of an old baker, feeling more comfortable and less harassed by Lahey's biga method, which doesn't require constant refreshing of the levain. I'm beginning to enjoy the feel of the dough, the patting and turning, and am thrilled when it responds, seems to curl into the shape my palms make. Perhaps I am becoming more attuned to the life of the yeast as it burbles, quietly transforming an inert mass into something alive.

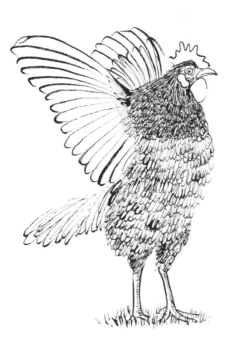

Breakfast Anecdotes

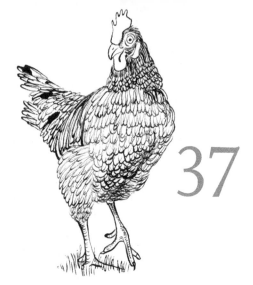

37

The worst thing about B&Bs is the enforced conviviality at the breakfast table. At a charming B&B where we spend a night on gorgeous Whidbey Island we are treated to a range of hair-raising stories, all of which provoke communal hilarity. A woman who makes Christian-themed dinosaurs narrates her enlightenment journey. A couple tells about their friend who owns properties all around the globe, particularly in "third world" countries, places like Mexico. First thing he does when he gets off the plane is go and buy some old clothes from a homeless person (or a thrift store) so he doesn't get harassed.

I want immediately to distance myself from this version of tourism. This story of grotesque mimesis provokes disgust and distaste. I would prefer not to see myself as part of the crowd, more like a cloud, or a single daffodil, wandering lonely and enlightened, benighted by the miasma of tourist mores, an exceptional tourist.

Tough shit, says J.

Landscape

Giant (1956) and *Paris, Texas* (1984): two movies filmed in and around Marfa and Big Bend National Park. Stretched out in the living room, J and Elvis and I watch both movies, me hoping to summon again the bodily sensation of being in that landscape.

Katie and I stayed in the Hotel Paisano in Marfa, headquarters for the filming of *Giant*. It is a lovely old Spanish-style hotel built in 1926, and there are large signed photographs of Elizabeth Taylor, Rock Hudson, James Dean, Mercedes McCambridge, Dennis Hopper, Sal Mineo, Carroll Baker, all beckoning you into the hotel. There was a very long happy hour on the day we stayed, lasting all afternoon; the courtyard was thronged with a mix of vacationing Texans and art tourists from New York. I negotiated my way through the crowds and meandered down the main street to the bookshop where our "ex-situ" workshop was taking place. On the way I spotted the Bearded Ones and Joey and Nora, small figures in the vast deserted landscape of the outdoor covered market, an oasis of shade. They had paper cups of tequila spirited away from the happy hour. They shared some with me. Then Katie ambled along and joined us, and then Derek and Yoke-Sum. Sipping tequila out of the noonday sun I thought of James Dean, teetering drunkenly at the end of *Giant*.

Somehow I had remembered *Giant* as presenting fabulous widescreen shots of the landscape. As we drive into West Texas to Marfa, via Big Bend, I recall *Giant*, but what I see imprinted in the landscape is James Dean. And something more elusive, a shady black-and-white memory that smells. Turns out my memory of the film's rendition of landscape is unreliable, but the insistence of Dean, his embodiment, is accurate. The smell continues to simmer, not quite rising to the surface, not graspable.

As regards landscape, I discover in my living room that *Giant* is far less scenic than *Paris, Texas*, in which the desert images are infused by Ry Cooder's melancholic slide guitar. Wenders's film is much more geared to contemporary artistic sensibilities: achingly beautiful, suffused by remorse and regret and undecidability. But between *Paris, Texas* and its intense sentimental machismo and *Giant*, give me *Giant* any day. For all its lumbering epicness, there is an aberrant intriguing air of desolation in *Giant*, clinging to and exhaled by James Dean.

Giant clutters up the landscape with stuff, first with cattle and then with oil. James Dean (Jett Rink), working day and night alone on his tiny parcel of land, finds oil. A gush of black liquid, transforming into a torrent until black sticky goo covers him and fills the screen. It's tactile: rich and dirty.

Giant is an old-fashioned movie. A classic Hollywood story, it delivers a liberal message in a language a trifle too labored, too explicit for today's sensibilities: Elizabeth Taylor's spirited feminist speeches (I do love it when she lets fly), Rock Hudson's eventual stand against Texan racism when he gets into a fistfight (which he doesn't win) in a diner along the highway. The good values win out in the end.

But along the way it is James Dean who commands attention. He is the magnetic charge of *Giant*, you can't take your eyes off him. His bodily presence displaces the landscape. The way—as a young man—he lounges and slouches and glides and leaps like a cat. His way of looking up, head downcast. Shy, insolent, inarticulate, edgy, gestural. The way—as an older man—rich and powerful, miming sobriety in a pathetic pantomime, he struggles to walk a straight line, to read his speech, to wave to his adorers as though he were king. And yet even here—burnt out, a drunken wreck—he performs a gesture that is definitive, sharp and clear, a gesture of cutting, slicing his hand through the air. It is a repetition of the gesture he performs when he resigns, preempting the sacking. Thematically, Dean represents the corruption of wealth, the corrosive effects of being a loner, living outside the community, of "not sharing"—through language or material goods. But it is not just thematic; Dean embodies a different universe, his mannerist, campy yet somatically charged acting style—it is said that he liked to listen to opera, especially Renata Tebaldi, before going onto the Warner Brothers set of *Giant*—is at odds with the dominant and more naturalistic acting register of the movie. As a figure, he is also at odds with its sentimental trajectory.

If we view the film through a queer lens, as today we cannot help doing, we might ask what if anything it means that the two male leads, playing heterosexual men in a straight story, were gay. Acting of course is about performing a role; it isn't generally, or at least in the Hollywood narrative tradition, about an expression of self-identity. But Dean's performance disturbs the equilibrium. Just as he is covered in black sticky goo when the oil spurts forth, so he in turn is a big fly in the ointment that is *Giant*.

In its closure the film makes good on the exclusion of Mexicans from a state that was stolen from Mexico; it ends with the blonde baby and the mestizo baby sharing the screen. In that move the film welds together liberal notions about race with a discourse about the family, triumphant in its capacity to assimilate and expand. But this expansiveness is secured at the expense of exclusion. In an interesting paradox, Dean's performance, so sexualized, so riveting, contradicts the meaning assigned to his figure by the narrative. The narrative consigns him to the margins, renders Jett Rink a self-elected outsider, redundant to the plot. His performance, however, places him at the center. We might say that he represents all that the straight family and the state (the family standing in for the state) exclude. But this would be to imply something more overt and graspable and representable than the actual experience of watching the film yields.

So I went looking for landscape and found something else. Or perhaps landscape is always chimeric. Perhaps I was superimposing onto my distant memory of *Giant* other Hollywood images—westerns in particular—of Texas. Or, in the process of driving through Big Bend, down to the Rio Grande and up to Marfa, perhaps I was trying to catch and frame my sensation of the space by projecting it onto the film. Or perhaps it was a haunting. Those black-and-white images exuding a stench, infiltrating *Giant*.

George Stevens, who made *Giant*, had been an official war cinematographer a decade earlier. He had filmed at Dachau when the allies went in at liberation. A fragment of this footage is shown in Godard's *Histoire du Cinema*. He gives a shocking juxtaposition—of Elizabeth Taylor (in *A Place in the Sun*) and Holocaust corpses. How, Godard wonders, did Stevens go back to Hollywood and carry on as though nothing out of the ordinary had occurred? Business as usual, he says, with the utmost disdain. And he extrapolates from Stevens to an indictment of Hollywood in general. When I went to the Bauhaus university in Weimar a few years ago, J and I planned to take a detour and do the day trip to Dachau. When we woke that morning J said, I just can't do it. I was driven by a quest—to see this footage in its entirety, having written in some detail about the Godard fragment, so I went on the bus alone. To the outskirts of the city of Weimar, to where Dachau is. It was better to be alone. To not be touched, to not share. It rained. You have to walk and walk and walk. I had no idea how immense the camps were. I had never thought about them in terms of landscape. I found the film on a loop in a black room within a large warehouse-like building filled with evidence. What was most striking was the footage of the good citizens of Weimar who were forced by the allies to visit Dachau, to witness the evidence of atrocity on their doorstep. They begin as though embarking on a picnic, there is an air of bonhomie, laughter, sharing. Good middle-class folk, well dressed. This changes when they see, are forced to look at, the piles of cremated bodies, the skeletons. They shriek, cover their eyes, some faint. Simply, they are shocked. This is a revelation—of horror.

But how could they not have known? They must have seen the trains, they must surely have smelled the smoke, the smell of burning bodies. This is the question so often asked by those who come later, by those of us who are enlightened.

Faced with this footage in this environment I too am overwhelmed by the stench, I almost pass out, even though it is not a revelation. I too see what I do not want to see, what I know and do not know.

And Stevens? He (like others—John Ford, Frank Capra . . .) returned to a culture that was victorious, to a people who saw themselves as liberators. He returned to a country entering the Cold War, as though there were no hot wars, genocides, exterminations of large populations, mostly written off as distant and minor civil wars. Yes, Stevens went back to making Hollywood movies. He is not like Sirk, he is not a self-conscious subversive, he is a good burgher. Yet there is something that troubles his films.

Godard is not wrong. I would not want to counter him by arguing that *Giant* is simply an expression of repression, a surfacing of Stevens's bodily apprehension of the Holocaust, nor that the burning of the Jews equates to the exclusion of gays. What is fascinating to me is rather the failure of equivalence, the something out of kilter, the filming of a landscape that smolders with something inexpressible and painful. I went looking for landscape in *Giant* and found what I thought was its absence: no wide-open spaces, no Texas sky. But I found a different kind of landscape, one in which the human body sculpted a space, one in which a memory of the landscape of Dachau imprinted its affective resonance, one in which memories of a road trip edged their way into a film made sixty years earlier.

Tootin Pootin

39

The doctor pulls gloves on as though donning a wig in the high court, sticks a finger up the patient's ass, and declares—with a curious mix of bravado and contempt— "No blood!" The patient is in the ER again, feels as though she has been caught out in a lie detector test, attempting once again to con the system (the next day, when the lab results come back showing that there is indeed blood in her stool, she wants to run back to the hospital, find that particular doctor and say "told you so"). Forty minutes later a bouncy junior nurse prances in and looks at the computer, reels off a list of drugs, saying, This is what the doctor has ordered for you. Excuse me, says the patient. What are the drugs for? The doctor hasn't even given me a diagnosis. The nurse is nonplussed. Maybe, says the patient, you could ask the doctor to come and tell me what he has found. Forty more minutes pass. The doctor looks in as though it is a huge imposition to be asked to explain his diagnosis, especially when it amounts to nothing much. Tests have been done, and more results will arrive over the next few days, but at this stage it looks like a routine infection, and so he's prescribed the standard drug: Flagyl (metronidazole). I'd rather not take Flagyl, she says, is there something else you could prescribe? The doctor replies: You'd *rather* not! Why not? And no, there's no alternative. She explains that Flagyl makes her pretty ill (Dr. K has agreed that it could be the case that it reacts adversely with the cancer drug she's on, has said that there are alternatives but they work more slowly and can't be guaranteed to work as effectively). The doctor holds his ground. Would he have to lose face if he changed his initial mind and came up with an alternative? She asks to see the physician in charge, who eventually comes and reiterates that there are no alternatives to Flagyl. She reiterates her reluctance, though she does not mention the fact that in addition to ten days of nausea there is the issue of how many courses of Flagyl she has taken and the issue of antibiotic resistance. Flagyl is well known to women with vaginal infections and also to those who have suffered from Montezuma's revenge while traveling in Latin America, where it targets the anaerobic protozoan called giardia. But as a broad-spectrum antibiotic it also broadly affects the resident bacteria of the gut and, in some cases, loses effectivity against whatever it is treating. She sticks to her guns, trying not to sound adversarial, trying to reassure everyone that it is only small guns she's playing with, and only one, the kind of toy a lady carries around in her purse. Eventually he says, OK, but be aware of the risks. Probably, she thinks, but does not say: no riskier than being here in a hospital where people commonly pick up deadly superbugs that have become resistant to antibiotics, like staph and C. difficile.

In "El Niagara en Bicicleta" the Dominican musician Juan Luis Guerra describes, hilariously, the ER experience as akin to crossing Niagara Falls on a bicycle:

Don't tell me they lost the forceps,
that the stethoscope is out partying,
that the X-rays melted,
that the serum was already used
To sweeten the coffee

She goes home and takes the alternative antibiotic, does not feel nauseous, the cramps begin to subside but the pain takes longer. She is able to function normally, but each day asks herself if it is working. Eventually, though it takes a while, she recovers. Despite the antibiotic or because of it? Who can say?

It is a risky business, this she knows, and this is why she is in the ER. She is scared of a repeat of the episode that occurred almost two years ago to the day. She knows how quickly your body can move from a-little-bit-out-of-the-ordinary into near death. That episode, in retrospect, began with a couple of weeks of low-grade intermittent diarrhea. One day she drives them home from a day trip to LA, and since J is tired and she is feeling sprightly, she cooks dinner at home, J goes to bed early but she stays up and watches a movie. The next day she wakes feeling fairly awful and knows she should get to a doctor. But she can't get through on the phone and eventually realizes it's Saturday. This hasn't occurred to J either, who goes off to yoga. By the time he returns (an hour and a half later) she is very ill and shivering severely. Arctic winds are blowing into the house. He can't feel the wind on his skin and can't grasp that she is very sick. She instructs him to make her a hot water bottle, get blankets, help her to the car so she can lie down in the back, she can barely keep herself upright. They get to the ER, and the system kicks in remarkably fast and efficiently. The whole day she lies there in a high fever, shitting, being cleaned up, shitting, being wheeled here and there for one test and then another. J stays by her side. Her nurse is extraordinary: patient, swift, unpatronizing, the doctors and technicians likewise. At the end of the day she has been stabilized but is admitted, and the admitting physician explains, We have to keep an eye on you and be sure it is not *Clostridium difficile* (C. diff), and those results will take several days. Four days later, on Christmas Eve, the ward doctor lets her go home. Turns out it's not the dreaded C. diff, just colitis, an ordinary infection which began in the region where she had prior surgery. An ordinary infection that flared dangerously because of the CLL. She is so relieved to be freed that she exudes energy and well-being, and at their annual Boxing Day party on December 26, most people have no idea that she has been in hospital the prior week.

. . .

Albutt Einstein, Dumpledore, Vladimir Pootin, and Winnie the Poo. They fill up the space in her cubicle, dance jovially at the end of her bed while she waits for the chief, for the next round in the antibiotic war. They dance at the end of her bed, cheerful and chanting, offering a temptation, a way around antibiotics, a quick and painless cure. Who are they, and where can they be found? Are they real or characters conjured by her fevered brain, or by some comedically inflected scatological imagination, by precocious poo-obsessed children, perhaps, or by a modern-day writer of coprophiliac fun?

. . .

A couple of weeks of low-grade diarrhea, sometimes bouts of severe cramping—this is how it goes. You are never quite sure if you can dodge drugs and hospital through diet, resting up, or if you need labs or even to get straight to the ER. The regular monthly intravenous infusions of immunoglobulin (IvIg) have been a godsend (if there are gods in the medi–sky mall up there); being on IvIg means that in fact I have had no such similarly severe infections in the past two years (but lots of low-grade and unpleasantly disruptive episodes). You never know whether it is something you ate, a flare-up of diverticulitis, gallbladder, stomach cancer, the drug you are on to treat the cancer, or if these are the first symptoms of something like C. diff.

. . .

Albutt Einstein, Dumpledore, Vladimir Pootin, and Winnie the Poo are and are not real. The names are pseudonymous labels for real people who generously donate their feces samples to OpenBiome, a nonprofit storehouse collecting stools from healthy donors, which are safely checked before being sent out to hospitals.

. . .

And what will happen with these stools once they reach their destination? Why indeed are they needed? Do we not have drugs to treat these conditions? The answer is yes and no. The drugs (antibiotics) exist, but often, particularly after repeat usage, they become ineffective. The crisis is particularly acute in the case of C. diff, where often nothing seems to work and people waste away and die. But then, not long ago, a cure was found, very widely publicized because it seemed so outlandish and gross. If the diluted feces from a healthy body were somehow (using an enema, turkey baster, nasogastric tubes . . .) inserted into the bowels of someone suffering from C. diff, the condition seemed to very quickly disappear. The procedure became known officially as fecal microbiota transplantation (FMT). Many people afflicted by a range of severe and debilitating gastrointestinal conditions have had their symptoms relieved or cured by FMT, though so far it has only been proven to actually *cure* C. diff. But here the evidence is strong. A 2013 Dutch study comparing the use of drugs to FMT found a 31 percent cure for those taking the drugs and 94 percent for those receiving FMT.

"It's the closest thing to a miracle I've seen in medicine," says Zain Kassam, a gastroenterologist who is OpenBiome's chief medical officer. Terms like *miracle* and *magical* circulate a lot around discussions of FMT. And indeed there does seem to be something magical about it all. The fairy-tale aura of Albutt Einstein and his merry troupe invokes such associations. In fact, however, there are perfectly good scientific explanations for why FMT works.

People often say, "I" have become resistant to such and such a drug, as though it were the cells and tissues and organs of their body that have become resistant. Because this is what it feels like, especially if you are sick. But in fact it is not "my body" that has acquired resistance but, rather, other bodies, ones invisible to the human eye, that live within my body: microbes. Nevertheless, although human bodies and the microbes that live within them are distinct and behave in distinct ways, they are symbiotic and interrelate in complex ways. So when people say— groaning in pain, wracked by fever, shitting uncontrollably—My body has become resistant to antibiotics, there is a material basis for their sense of bodily upset, even if caused by microbial action.

One of these microbes is C. diff, a microscopic creature that resides in all healthy guts (as does *E. coli*). Sometimes, however, the population goes rogue and multiplies, causing severe upset to the balance of the ecosystem that is the gut (or perhaps it's the other way around—imbalance, caused by some other factor, precipitates a derangement of the C. diff population). This is when those ghastly symptoms appear. This is because the microbes, when deranged, do indeed start to affect the very substance of the body, that is, human cells, to spread and produce toxins that penetrate the epithelial cells lining the colon. The colon then becomes porous, and fecal matter oozes out of the bowel into areas that are usually bacteria-free.

Antibiotics are likely to be prescribed, until recently most probably Vancomycin. However, this drug and others have become virtually ineffective against drug-resistant hypervirulent new strains of the C. diff microbe. Antibiotics seem not only to be useless but also to exacerbate the condition. According to some theories, this is because antibiotics, especially broad-spectrum ones, are themselves the major culprit: they destroy indiscriminately, and in wiping out the "good" bacteria as well as the "bad" they severely upset the ecological balance of the gut.

It was only in the late seventies that C. diff was identified as a major cause of antibiotic-related diarrhea. Most cases occurred in hospitals, hot beds for contamination. It was not uncommon to go into the ER or hospital with a knife wound or broken ankle, say, and come out (or stay in or never come out) with C. diff or MRSA, the infection due to antibiotic-resistant staph. You are still at risk of picking up these infections in hospitals (though basic hygiene, most notably hand washing, has been improved), but the offending microbes are also now at-large. "Like a lion escaped from the zoo," Martin Blaser, in *Missing Microbes: How the Overuse of Antibiotics Is Fueling Our Modern Plagues*, announces dramatically, "C. diff has escaped the confines of the hospital and is now loose in the community."

What the fecal transplant does is simply this: restore microbial balance to the intestine. It appears magical because it is so simple. What imbues it with an aura of magic in this day and age is that, by all accounts, it is frequently able to cure a virulent, often deadly, disease very quickly and without chemicals or synthetic medicines.

Needless to say we are not the first people to have discovered the benefits of FMT. Emily Eakin reports that the first known account dates to a fourth-century Chinese handbook by the physician Ge Hong, who prescribed "yellow soup"—a fecal suspension—as a remedy for severe diarrhea. We surely can assume that versions of FMT have been used in a variety of what we, in industrialized medicinal cultures, refer to as folk remedies. In the U.S., the first description of FMT appeared in 1958, but from the eighties well into this century virtually the only known proponent of FMT was Thomas Borody, a gastroenterologist in Sydney, Australia. Then, suddenly, around about 2012, the idea was in the air, all sorts of experiences were being reported.

The inspired figures (at the time grad students at MIT, one of whom had a friend with C. diff) who founded OpenBiome in 2013 recognized that many people who are suffering from chronic or severe gastritis conditions do not have ready access to healthy stools or to ways of ascertaining that the stools are healthy. By providing clinical conditions for testing and through a strict screening process for donors, they became a clearinghouse for doctors, hospitals, and individuals (though they only ship to hospitals) interested in trying this treatment. It is, as one of the founders describes it, a kind of Red Cross for poop.

Poop is now a medical commodity, and many biomedical companies are in the race to develop and patent poop pills, which will probably become available at considerable expense. But OpenBiome is already offering a capsule (in addition to two kinds of liquid treatment)—and at an affordable price. Moreover, they offer a pro bono option.

But, while it is relatively straightforward to buy treatments from OpenBiome for C. diff infections, it is more complicated for other conditions. This is because stool is classified as an Investigational New Drug (IND) by the FDA, approved for C. diff but requiring special application for other infections. Those who contract C. diff infections are really in danger, and FMT has surely appeared for them as a potentially miraculous solution. But there are a whole range of gastritis conditions for which good results from FMTs have been recorded or for which it makes some sense that they might work: Crohn's and celiac disease, for instance, as well as everything that falls under irritable bowel syndrome (IBS).

I, at the time of writing this, am remarkably well—off all drugs and with good results on all the blood fronts (though the immune markers remain wonky). Without the stress of teaching and administration I have the luxury of being able to concentrate on writing and being healthy. In particular, I can take the time to be attentive to diet and make sure that I eat probiotic and prebiotic foods to feed those microbes in the hope of thus contributing to the ecological balance of my gut. But to be realistic this fantastic streak of well-being won't last, the CLL symptoms will return and with that all the other upsets like gastritis issues that have so often landed me in the doctor's office or the ER. I am all for giving FMT a go before embarking on more antibiotics, and I would certainly rather do it through clinically safe and regulated channels than by DIY.

But Dr. K is not so enthusiastic. When I raise the issue with him he looks sardonic and says the human body is like an elephant (depends from which end you look at it whether you see a trunk or a tail). I like this inversion—normally everything else, especially microbes, are anthropomorphized; it tickles me to have the human body elephantized. I guess what he means is that, as Rob Knight puts it, although we know that the microbes in patients with IBS are not behaving normally, "we don't yet know if this altered behavior is caused by the body's immune response or if microbes are at fault." And because CLL is a disease of the immune system it is doubly complicated.

Still, there is no need to throw in the towel. Things are looking up for many who need help more than I do, and I believe that I too might benefit at some future stage by the kind of research that is being undertaken (prompted by the success of FMT in treating C. diff infections) into other diseases. OpenBiome's own research is particularly encouraging in this respect. They report on their website that early clinical evidence suggests that, for other diseases, some healthy donors may be more effective than others. Each of their donors has been characterized by a broad range of molecular biomarkers, and it is anticipated that this data can be used, along with other data and statistical tools, to predict donors who are likely to be especially well-suited for a given disease.

. . .

Albutt Einstein, Dumpledore, Vladimir Pootin, and Winnie the Poo are avatars of the future, magical beings or presences who exist in the everyday, charging the field with new energy, new ways of thinking, and bringing with them the capacity to transform despair and less savory emotions, such as revulsion, into hope.

Dragon Inn

40

A dagger flies, so fast you register its movement in your gut rather than sight. And then it is caught. Caught, amazingly, between a pair of chopsticks. A bowl of noodles is flung across a room, whirls in the air, lands on a table, spinning. Spins and then settles, settles perfectly intact, ready to be eaten. An arrow slices the air, gaining velocity it moves at the speed of light, a speed that cinema can hardly register let alone the naked eye. Suddenly, a hand reaches out, closes over the arrow, stops its flight. Such an elegant gesture, it hardly seems to be a move of war, it is as though someone has been there all the time, waiting for the arrow to arrive, waiting to receive it. There is nothing predictable in this scenario, in this battle where everyone is on their toes, called on to respond in a flash, in the beat of a heart, in a leap across the room. Where there is a breathtaking orchestration of cinematic technology and kung fu techniques.

Imagine you are in a green ferny valley cocooned in a mossy nest, greenness all around you, feathery fronds enfolding and stroking. Or walking in a cloud forest, Spanish moss draping the trees, orchids peeking through the undergrowth. In a white garden at night, the scent of roses, moon flowers, tobacco plants, jasmine. One by one you sense the smells as they infiltrate the darkness. Or you could be making bread, the process unfolding from the very beginning with flour and water and salt, and days passing by as the starter becomes yeasty, the proofing and kneading and shaping and the smell as it bakes, the singing of the bread as you hold it, warm, to your cheek and listen to it.

It is commonly called visualization, though it is not only the sense of sight that is mobilized. For me, anyway. Visualization is a mode of meditation, or you might call it a therapeutic tool. Most simply it is a way of focusing and calming the mind, of conjuring and making present a world that displaces and overwhelms this worldly world of suffering and terror. It is a way of getting through pain and anxiety. When I had the surgery for lung cancer I used visualization. Gifts came in the mail, friends made and copied tapes. Jacquie Lane recorded the sounds of water in a wild place she loves and often visits in Washington State. Lynne Tillman and Diane Serafini sent tapes that had worked for them during surgery. Later, I started attending Shambhala, where the meditative process—at least in the early stages of training—is more focused on being in the here and now, focusing on the breath, though some of the teachings and some of the teachers are particularly attuned to the sensory world, of awakening our senses. Being awake, a basic precept of Buddhism, is partly registered through the aliveness of the sense perceptions. Even though Shambhala has shifted some of my homegrown, cobbled-together practices, nevertheless sometimes still, when in a hospital and particularly when the sense of panic and anticipation arises, I draw on visualization. The scenarios I conjure up are mostly very simple, calm and quiet, but they are also sensory, the sensations they awaken transport me to an elsewhere. The scenarios are not, however, always saturated by calmness. Sometimes I conjure up vignettes from kung fu movies, in particular, from the movies of the great director King Hu.

Recently I was lucky enough to see again his *Dragon Inn*, a 1967 Taiwanese Wuxia film—this time a 35mm print, in glorious wide angle, and with all the imperfections, the scratchings and dust smears, of the original print. So exhilarating. A startling shift from extreme close-ups to extreme wide shots, an exciting sense of improvisation, ingenuity in both the cinematic skill and the dancerly moves of the fighters. Every attacking move is a surprise, elicits ingenious countermoves, moves that take your breath away and leave you gasping, laughing. Sometimes the landscape is immense and sparse, stretching across the known world, other times the screen is crowded with people and action. There is a theatricality of gesture and pose and action in this version of Chinese opera. The performers in this film were mostly not martial artists, all the action was performed by Chinese Opera people, who were the stuntmen. As the big confrontation at the end closes in, there are sudden cuts to frames filled with scarlet, associated with the eunuch emperor, his robes, his parasol opening out and filling the frame with redness.

To be caught up in this cinematic world is exhilarating but hardly calming. One might point out that there is a Buddhist element to *Dragon Inn*—the composure under duress, the moments of stillness. The heroes in and of themselves do not convey much interiority or display psychological characteristics; there is a sense that these dramatic episodes are part of a procession of events in which the individual lives are specks in an ocean, in the stormy waves of birth, old age, sickness, and death. But there is also the extraordinary rhythm and timing: of bodies and things, poised or hurtling through space—the cutting, the length of shots, the movement of the camera in relation to the movement of bodies. This is indeed, overall, exhilarating rather than calming, but it is also a way of recalibrating the breath and channeling it into a kind of distillation. Seeing *Dragon Inn* on the big screen has inspired me anew, feeds my hospital fantasies, not fantasies *of* hospital, but fantastic scenarios that enable me to breeze through episodes that otherwise would be hard to endure.

All along the Highway

41

As we leave the desert behind the radio crackles into coherence. A deep male voice exhorts us to dig into our pockets and contribute to the Leukemia and Lymphoma Society. A lone voice crackling in the wilderness, I think.

All along the highway on the plateau before the western edge of the Texas Hill Country we listen to country music, all along the highway where wildflowers bloom: swathes of bluebonnets intermingled with red and yellow.

We stop for lunch in Ozona, a small big town in the Edwards Plateau region. Hunters come to Ozona in search of white-tailed deer, javelinas (pig-like hoofed mammals), and game birds. Ozona is the county seat of Crockett County, named for Colonel Davy Crockett, a hero of the Alamo. We drive through the town looking for a steak house Katie once ate at and remembers hungrily, but it is nowhere to be found. The streets of the town are deserted on this Sunday, faded tatty shuttered shops are strung along the main street fanning out from the civic center—gracious and impressive buildings, solidly built of stone. The Café Next Door is the only non–fast food place we can find off the freeway. We expect it to be full of travelers like ourselves, but it is chockablock with families out for Sunday lunch, dressed up a little, probably coming here after church. The little girls have bows in their hair, some of the men wear clean bright shirts, mostly red, with their black jeans and skinny black ties and polished boots and Texan hats. People are eating big, but we delicate and discerning city girls order toasted cheese and salad. The sandwich has been heated, but the cheese resists melting, its plasticity and psychedelic orange hue pronounced by heat. We don't say anything to one another, we are hungry and wolf the sandwiches down. But later, as we drive through an expanse of nowhere, Katie says, "That cheese was scary."

Outside the town of Harper we pass a ranch where an extraordinary sight hurtles me out of Texas and back to Africa. The grass is brownish, the landscape savanna-like; as though on a safari we cruise past African gemsbok, eland, gazelle, kudu, springbok. Later I discover that there is a price on each exotic animal's head, and if you are prepared to pay the price you can come in and kill it. It will cost you, for instance, upward of twelve thousand dollars to bag a kudu, though you can get a springbok for half of that.

In the town of Fredericksburg, with its lovely stone buildings that seem to have been eerily transported from an earlier European era, we are again craving tea and so return to the Old German Bakery and Restaurant. On the way out to Big Bend and Marfa we had delicious bratwurst and sauerkraut and a pork cutlet that was even better cold the next morning in the motel at Marathon watching the sun come up. The bakery is closed this Sunday, so we wander around a backstreet and Katie shows me the Sunday houses and tells of how she stayed there with her mother and father when they were both still alive. These are small weekend houses that the ranchers and farmers built in the late 1800s so that they could spend a night or two when they came into town for church and perhaps to party. They are small craft houses meticulously constructed out of local materials, now mostly rented out to tourists. Katie's voice softens as she tells me about these houses.

We find a cup of tea at a biergarten where two young girls in their sparkling twenties are taking their grandparents out for dinner or lunch on this Sunday midafternoon and have to shout a lot; and at the table next to us, a party of retirees, just off the coach, are checking out the town on their iPhones, comparing maps and statistics.

North of Fredericksburg we pull into a wildflower nursery and walk through fields of blue, fields of red, whole fields like oceans, like we are swimming through a diaphanous red sea, light as air. Yoke-Sum, in Marfa, had shown us the seed packets she and Derek had purchased here. She is going to take them back to England to plant in her garden, where, if the bluebonnets grow, they will become exotic rather than native. Here, though native, they did not sprout spontaneously along the highway. It was Lady Bird Johnson who was largely responsible for getting rid of the junkyards and billboards that graced the highway system, replacing them with native plantings, through her support for the Beautification Act of 1965. Before this road trip if you had tossed to me the words *Johnson* and *1965* and asked me to say whatever came into my mind I would have said Vietnam, napalm, and the Civil Rights Act (of the previous year). That word, *beautification*, it slightly churns the stomach and curls the lip. Botox and pansies, landscaping and real estate, Sunday best, veneering.

Yet Lady Bird's legacy is substantial, her campaign for national beautification was linked to environmental concerns, to improving urban decay and pollution as well as to preservation of natural wonders. As we swim through the crimson air of the poppy meadows in the flower fields I remember hiking through the Lady Bird Johnson Grove, one of the most spectacular stands of old redwoods in Northern California. And as we hit the highway again, pondering the shiftiness of terms like *foreign* and *domestic*, *native* and *exotic*, I feel grateful for the way her legacy lives on in, for instance, the infelicitously named Surface Transportation and Uniform Relocation Assistance Act of 1987, which requires that at least 0.25 of one percent of funds expended for landscaping projects in the highway system be used to plant native flowers, plants, and trees. As we swim through the crimson air I ponder the trickiness of that word *beautification*, the slipperiness of terms like *native* and *exotic*, the chimerical propensity of color and how it can be strangely conjured into being through political process and the enactment of policy but also, strangely, through the agency of objects charged with magical propensity.

. . .

As we hit the highway again, on the home run to Austin, the deep male voice greets us again on the radio, still pitching persuasively for the Leukemia and Lymphoma Society. Although it induces a degree of squeamishness, this exhortation to charitable giving, I nevertheless feel grateful; not only does this society fund a great deal of research, it also is generous with information and support. Still, I think, probably a lone voice crackling in the wilderness. Then the voice segues smoothly from leukemia to climate change, actually to the fiction of climate change, to a rant about how our president, his voice sneers on this word, *president*, how our president, Obama, is hobbling and dictating to the EPA, preaching an alarmist philosophy that bears absolutely no relation to reality. He claims that the planet is heating up, says the voice, And where does he get this information? I ask you where does he get this information? I can tell you where he gets this so-called information; he reaches into the air and pulls statistics from nowhere, out of the air, that's where, out of the air. We realize we are listening to Rush Limbaugh, the most listened-to talk show host in the country. I guess, with all those listeners, he might raise some money for research that will come my way. Oy vey.

A Lion's Roar 42

I board the plane in Austin, buckle up, and with eyes closed hear again the country music that accompanied us, driving across the vast expanse of a small part of
Texas. All of a sudden lightning streaks across the darkening sky and hail stones
start falling. The wing of the airplane is soon covered in whiteness. A shiver shoots
through the plane, there is a quivering in the air. We prepare to disembark but
then the crisis subsides as quickly as it erupted, the sky clears, the mood shifts.
Sparks of electricity remain in the atmosphere, however, people start talking,
there's an expansiveness that wasn't there before. I am sitting next to a young
woman who endears herself to me by showing concern for the rooster, who, in
his overhead bin, has been jostled by a bag stuffed in haphazardly by a rough and
rude young man. She tells me that her mum collects roosters and even has some
from Soviet-era Russia. I'm not really a collector, I demur. I can understand that,
she says, he is clearly the one and only.

My surly hermetism is instantly vanquished, the conviviality of airplane small
talk sucks me into its orbit. Maria tells me that she volunteers as an animal res-
cuer, fostering creatures from the wild so that they can eventually be returned
to something like a natural state. As a student she worked at the Austin Zoo and
Animal Sanctuary. Occupying a large acreage in the hill country, this zoo is home
to many domestic and exotic animals that were either rescued from, or unwanted
by, their owners. Toads are rescued, goats, donkeys and snakes, but also coyotes,
cougars, lions, tigers. All the big cats are endangered in their native habitats, and
in quasi-legal captivation too, and so zoos often see themselves as places of preservation and restoration. A mode of domestic rewilding. Maria tells me a story
about a lion.

The story she tells goes like this: A lion was rescued from a church where he had been used in religious theater. Drugged out of his mind, overfed and malnourished, confined to a small cage in a trailer, never exercised, he would be wheeled onto the stage with a lamb. When he was released and stepped onto the ground for the first time he buckled under his own weight. All the bones in his feet shattered.

Later I will find on the internet a photo of a blond man, a pastor as it turns out, in a pink jacket, open-necked shirt, and khakis, clutching in his arms a lamb. He stands on a stage and you can see, behind him, a caged lion. Ed Young is a megachurch pastor, best-selling author, and televangelist. The lion and the lamb were brought onto the stage as part of his Wild sermon series. He is often described as creative, is a flamboyant performer, in his services he deploys props, gimmicks, visual theater. He is prone to putting into play everyday sayings and of dramatizing biblical metaphors through literalization and embodiment.

In "How to move from whining about the economy to whoopee!" Ed Young paced on stage in front of a large bed, now and then flopping down and flipping through the pages of a Bible. This was an enactment or embodiment of the metaphoric: Time for the church to put God back into the bed. The lion, you might say, like the bed and the Bible, was simply a prop, a visual aid, an illustration of language.

Maria told me that there is a happy end to the story, they eventually managed to rehabilitate the lion, and in the Animal Sanctuary he can roam, as though in the wild. I cannot say with certainty that Maria's lion is the same lion that Ed Young brought onto the stage. There was a flurry of media exposé, but a spokesman for the Fellowship Church says the lion was back "at home" in his California preservation where he has thousands of acres on which to roam. No permits were requested for the theatrical sermon because none were needed. No prosecutions ensued.

. . .

All the way home, and for days afterward, the stifled roar of that lion is trapped in my body. Back home Elvis springs onto the bed, looks me intently in the eyes, and says: Tell me a story. A growl ripples through him, just below the skin, as he stretches danger flashes and then he retracts his claws, his paws curl inward and there's a deep rumble, the echo of a roar, a vibration.

I write this story but do not read it aloud to Elvis, as is my wont. This is a story I cannot tell out loud.

The Ecology of Cancer, and
What Do Ants Have to Do with It?

43

Ants are like cancer cells. Conversely, we might say that cancer cells are like ants. Even though they sometimes feel more mammoth-like and slothful, lumberingly prehistoric rather than tiny and socially frenzied. "They feel." Of course cancer cells do not have feelings so far as I know. What I mean is that they feel to me—these colonies of CLL cells that circulate through, and clog up, the bone marrow and the blood and the lymphatic system—they feel to me massive and heavy and slow. More accurately, I should say that they make *me feel* like a sloth, I imagine myself as one of those creatures I saw a few weeks ago in the Tar Pits in Los Angeles: slowly dragging my massive body over the never-ending earth.

When I heard Deborah Gordon declare that ants are like cancer colonies I experienced a rush of resistance. I did not welcome the idea of analogizing my condition to a common-and-garden insect that lives in colonies, rather than to the singularity of an exotic species of megafauna now extinct. I was alarmed not charmed by the image of colonies of ants scurrying around in my body. But also in some peculiar way I did not yet quite understand, this analogy—of cancer cells to an ant colony—struck a chord. Suddenly a new image, one not immediately accessible to my habits of thinking and feeling, began to reverberate.

Ants, the ants that I know, live in my garden, not in my body. It has always been mysterious to me the way ant colonies would spring up in the garden, how they would know where the aphids were congregated, how they would march and scurry from their nests to my favorite rose bush, devastated by a colony of aphids. Aphids are small insects that suck the life out of plants and then secrete a sugar-rich sticky honeydew that ants love. In fact they "farm" the aphids, protect them from predators and parasites and nurture their eggs. In the face of this alliance—a mutualistic relationship or type of symbiosis—I would feel very small and ineffectual. All I could do would be to hope for an invasion of ladybugs (to eat the aphids and thus deflect the ants), or I could spend hours every day hosing off the aphids with jets of water. Sometimes you would sink a pitchfork into the compost pile and as if from nowhere a black mass of moving matter would crawl up your arm. After initial panic—rushing around dementedly shaking arms, trying in a frenzied manner to brush the ants off—I figured out that in the process of pursuing their own ends, foraging for fabulous stuff to take back to their nests, they were doing me a favor. Like worms, they were doing their bit to toss and turn and hasten the process of decomposition in the compost. In the end by leaving things be—as much as is possible for a neurotic controlling gardener—the garden settled into its own ecology. Or, rather, it became more possible to observe the interaction of plants and creatures: to see, for instance, which plants attracted bees, and when. African blue basil and rosemary are bee magnets. The weedy fennel, when it's younger, is a host for the swallowtail caterpillar that turns into a spectacular butterfly, flits around the garden, and then sashays off to Mexico. Later, when the garden is festooned with the fennel's yellow umbels, the bees come swarming in.

But the story is not so simple, not such a paean to natural balance and harmony. Enter the chickens.

Nowadays there are no infestations of ants, no plagues in the garden. The beak of a chicken and a squirrely squirming ant—these things exist together in a powerful force field of attraction. Heaven if you are a chicken, pretty dismal, I guess, if you are an ant. Though maybe the ants have just changed their habits, become invisible to chicken and human eyes, or moved on over to my neighbor Mrs. Tam's garden. Chickens also love worms, but since the birds are surface scratchers and since the vegetable beds and the compost are barricaded the worms survive there, in fact they survive everywhere deep in the soil, doing their work, sifting and turning.

Ants are like cancer cells, says Deborah Gordon, insofar as they are regulated but without central control.

An ant colony is regulated; its survival depends on the distribution and coordination of tasks and roles. Communication, or an exchange of cues, exists between the ants. The tasks and roles themselves are not fixed, but shift and change as the environment shifts and shapes. The ants exist in a dynamical social network. A hub may form, for instance, simply by ants moving into a space where there are lots of interactions. Gordon calls it the anternet. Ants do not always behave the same way. Foraging behavior, for instance, changes in times of drought. If one element changes (e.g., the availability of water) then the behavior of the colony changes. These changes, in turn, shape social and reproductive patterns. By observing these changes in patterns of behavior or modes of regulation, scientists can observe how natural selection is working on this colony.

There are many biological systems, apart from ants, that function without hierarchy. Bird flocks, without a leader, turn in the sky; fish schools swerve to avoid predators; tropical forests develop patterns of diversity . . . and cancer cells mutate and metastasize. For all of these systems, we still don't fully understand how the parts work together to produce the dynamics, the history, and the development of the whole system.

It has often felt to me as though the garden is a battlefield. The march to the rose bushes and the swarming in the compost bin seem to be ant maneuvers carried out with all the efficiency of military campaigns, masterminded by some center of control (and sometimes the body too feels like and is popularly conceived of as a battle zone where the war against cancer is waged). Indeed, this is how the great and pioneering ant scholar E. O. Wilson described ant society—in terms of hierarchy, conflict, and regimental organization. So why should we relinquish this view (or feeling) in favor of the model proposed by younger scientists, including Deborah Gordon? Most significant for me, in terms of the efficacy of the analogy, is that Gordon and others tell a different sort of system story, emphasizing situated (therefore variable) processes of recognition and response. They understand the ant colony as composed of flexible units (whose functions change according to situation) and propose a system characterized by different architecture and components. Nodes of interaction are at the heart of Gordon's model, and frequencies of interactions at nodes are what shape material social orders. Ants, she argues, don't provide moral lessons or insight into behavior or feelings, but they do provide insight about the dynamics of networks, systems without central control.

It's a tricky business, this maneuvering (is it a dance or a battle?) between feelings and conceptual models, between the garden and the body, ants and cancer cells. Sometimes new images, just as much as new data, can interfere with feelings and reorient one's thinking.

What matters in networks is the ecology of the system.

So, taking our cue from ant colonies, how might we think about the ecology of cancer? What are some of the ways that cancers diversify and spread? How is organization regulated? How, with answers to some of these questions, might we approach intervention in ways less dramatically belligerent?

Cells in the body act collectively—for example, as networks of neurons to produce sensations or as patrolling T cells that mobilize other immune cells to respond to pathogens. It seems they communicate with one another. In the process of metastasis, the cancer cells may use signals from healthy tissue to recruit other cancer cells to a new location, where certain areas of tissue constitute an attractive resource. If researchers can figure out how cancer cells are recruiting then maybe they can set traps to prevent them from doing this.

This makes clear sense in the case of solid tumors, but how can we understand the behavior of malignant B cells in CLL, given that CLL is a cancer of the blood not manifested in tissue areas or solid tumors? What happens in a "normal" body is that the B cells are recruited to fight infection; they regularly die off and new ones grow. In CLL, because of some genetic glitch, they don't die off but in fact relentlessly proliferate, course through the marrow, and travel through the blood and lymphatic system, interfering with and crowding out the production of healthy white cells, red cells, and platelets.

Although the cancer is in the blood and not localized in tumors, the cells do cluster, they form hubs, just like ants. They cluster in lymphoid tissue. Research has identified a form of regulation in this lymphoid tissue, or microenvironment, whereby malignant B cells communicate with other healthy cells. Curious about the relation of the cancer cells to certain healthy cells, Dr. K and his colleagues looked at this relationship in the lab. They found that when the CLL cells were removed from the "suspicious" healthy cells, the CLL B cells began to die, whereas the same cells, when replated back onto the healthy cells, perked up immediately. Because they supported the survival of CLL cells and because CLL B cells became attached to them, the researcher group called them "nurse-like cells" or NLC. They concluded that one of the ways CLL cells survive is by recruiting these protector cells.

Dr. K describes CLL as a very social beast. By this he means that the survival of the cells depends on a network of relations, which indeed amounts to a form of regulation without central control. The relation between the NLC and the CLL B cells is symbiotic, just like that between ants and aphids. In a dynamical system like an ant colony, it is possible to observe how when one element changes (e.g., the introduction of drought) the behavior of the colony changes. So, similarly, by focusing on the microenvironment of another dynamical system—a colony of cancer cells—it becomes possible to envisage forms of intervention more akin to the strategic introduction of drought rather than war. Rather than therapies which are the equivalent of carpet bombing, indiscriminately destroying good blood cells along with the bad (which, anyway, doesn't generally work with CLL, which is notably resistant to stand-alone chemotherapy), the solution might be to try and intervene in the signaling system to change the behavior of the cancer colony. Or, as Dr. K puts it: to foster therapies that isolate the CLL cells so that they die of social neglect.

To observe how cancer colonies evolve, how cellular activity is regulated, how selections are made: this chimes with other ideas vibrating in the air in this second decade of the twenty-first century when the Darwinian inheritance is being reconfigured. We humans have made such a mess of the planet that perhaps our only hope lies in attending more closely to other forms of organization, to looking more closely at ants and fungi and chickens (with whom we share about 60 percent DNA) and extinct species like the sloth from the Paleolithic era to species like bees that are disappearing by the day as we poison the environment and our own bodies. By looking outside the human body to other "bodies" or clusters of living cells in the natural world it seems to me that we have more chance of figuring out solutions, or ways of being in the world, perhaps even ways of living with cancer rather than definitively conquering it, just as in certain approaches to invasive species in habitat studies. It's a reversal of the gaze or perspective. Rather than trying to understand the natural world through the lens of human society, we reverse the perspective so that a description of a natural society—an ant colony in this instance—can illuminate how we think about modes of organization in the human body.

I doubt that Dr. K and company are preoccupied by such analogies. They are in the laboratory, separating the malignant B cells from their nurse-like protectors, replating them and trying to figure out how to intercept the signals. They are running algorithms. In defining the various cells, structures, and molecules that protect the CLL cells they are working on the development of novel anti-leukemia agents, such as monoclonal antibodies and immune-based treatment strategies and genetically engineered T cells. No, they are not looking at ants; but for me, as a gardener and a nonscientist and someone with cancer, bells start chiming.

In writing this I have become less alarmed by the ant analogy, more attuned to the reverberations sparked by hearing Deborah Gordon speak. At some point analogy clicks and opens up a different link. A link to the ecological.

Even though he places emphasis on the environment, Dr. K is cautious: We still don't fully understand how the parts work together to produce the dynamics, the history, and the development of the system, he says. There isn't a single explanation for how CLL happens, let alone how it evolves, adapts, transforms. Unpredictable things happen. Needless to say, there also isn't a single solution.

Nevertheless, this perspective gives me hope. Not that a cure for CLL will be produced tomorrow, but certainly that more efficacious and less damaging possibilities are opening up that might prolong the life expectancy of people with CLL (so far this has not been possible). The outlook is considerably brighter than when I was first diagnosed six years ago.

It fills me with energy and hope: that this research can be understood in terms of a larger project, within an ecological matrix encompassing micro and macro environments, timescales ranging from the big bang to now, symbiotic relations as apparently diverse as the relation between ants and aphids in a garden and malignant B cells and nurse-like cells in a CLL environment.

It gives hope when things are going well (like now, when treatment is resting in a sweet spot). But in the dark times it is the sloth that imaginatively materializes rather than a colony of ants. Although the ant analogy has greater scientific resonance, the sloth connects affectively to my bodily experience. But in the process of writing this piece I have relinquished the idea of ants scurrying around inside my body, am more able to situate ants and cancer cells in an analogous relation, within the framework of dynamical systems. This I realize: It is not necessary to *feel* ant-like in order to grasp the import of the analogy. You might say my cognitive apprehension has marginally improved. On the other hand, it is only through sensation, through ways that the body experiences being in the world, being in the garden as well as in the hospital and the lab, that understanding grows. Figures of speech, often fantastical, may seem to be at odds with scientific data, but the human sensorium involves a rich patterning of signaling networks.

What Does It Matter? 44

The saltwater for the Pesach eggs is presented in beautiful tiny hand-painted bowls that Parastou's brother brought from Turkey. Elana has brought chopped liver and a fennel and orange salad sprinkled with mint leaves. The liver enlivens considerably the matzoh. Parastou has made Persian rice with lima beans, crispy on the bottom; and the lamb, it melts and dances in the mouth. Brian's chicken broth is light and clear, the kreplach fluffy, saffron scent infiltrating the broth, rising steamily out of the soup, enveloping us all. J also makes a delicious chicken soup, and so did my first husband, NS. Both the Jewish men I married were/are creative cooks. NS's mother prayed that her son would shed the shiksa. Not likely, when the shiksa, who had for years been resisting her own mother's admonitions to learn to cook if she wanted to find a husband, found a man most handy in the kitchen. If you marry my son, NS's mother told me, he will never become a doctor, and anyway you will get divorced. She was right on both counts. But something good came out of it: After the divorce I had to learn to cook.

It was an infusion day, and afterward, as often happens, I'm done in and only want to be horizontal. But I cannot miss the feast, tastes curling up and around and into every bodily crease and crevice. The food, but not only the food, also the ritual, the kerfuffling over protocol. This night, as so often, we muddled our way through the service, arguing about interpretation. Why do we have to wait to start drinking before the candles are lit and the first part of the service performed? What do the bitter greens signify? Why do we have to eat them rather than just look at them? Why are we eating lamb? The young ones were impatient—What does it matter? they asked insistently, all this ritual; but us old secular Jews and/or fellow travelers like myself, we want to remember, get it right, immerse ourselves together for an evening in the theatricality of the symbolic dimension.

But the next day I suffered, felt like I'd run into a truck. Elvis was ecstatic, a day in bed. Every so often he would lope out into the garden, roll around in the dirt, and then slouch back into the house and spring onto the bed. Such softness, the pad on his paw, despite the clambering up trees and stalking of *enemigos* in the bamboo thicket. I love to stroke his pads, so soft, and the tufty fur on his feet.

As he settles next to me, chin leaning on the Mac Air, I ask him: What does it matter? He has no answer. I tell him that even though there is no answer, it is not an empty question.

So Unctuous and So Tender   45

"Filthy creature! Filthy creature!" she screams at the chicken. The chicken resists attack, she grapples with it, trying to split its neck. After it is dead and she has collected its blood, her resentment persists. She looks down at the carcass and addresses it one last time: "Filthy creature!"

The narrator witnesses this scene, bloody and brutish, as a child when he goes to the kitchen anticipating the golden succulent roast chicken that always appears on the table for Sunday lunch, prepared by the family cook Françoise. The smell of the chicken turning on the spit—this is a Sunday smell, associated with Françoise, summoning her virtues, and of all her virtues this "aroma of that flesh which she knew how to render so unctuous and so tender" summons most specifically her quality of gentleness. However, on this particular Sunday when she serves the chicken, "its skin embroidered with gold like a chasuble and its precious juice drained from a ciborium," the witnessed scene of carnage puts her saintly unction a little less in evidence.

Leading up to the chicken scene is an anticipatory description of the asparagus that will be served with the Sunday chicken. It is a description primarily of colors—seductive, voluptuous—but it ends with the sense of smell, how after dinner the asparagus changes the chamber pot into a "jar of perfume."

The narrator, describing this incident from his childhood, tells of how he fantasizes about getting his family to dismiss Françoise immediately. But a cowardliness creeps in to mar his resolution. "Who would have prepared me such cozy hot-water bottles, such fragrant coffee, and even . . . those chickens?" As it turns out, and later he will come to realize, he is not alone in his compact with cowardliness. His great aunt and other adults in the family are wise to the fact that Françoise's kindness is shadowed by cruelty and sentimentality. Although she likes to weep she also likes to hate. She is particularly cruel to the frail pregnant kitchen maid. While Françoise loves inordinately her own family and the family she serves, she has little empathy for others. When the kitchen maid is shrieking in pain, Françoise is sent to fetch the medical book that the doctor has marked up with instructions for what to do in such an emergency. Françoise doesn't return and is eventually discovered reading the book and weeping over the description of the symptoms from which the maid is suffering. Meanwhile, the pregnant sick girl waits. Just as she weeps torrents for unknown persons when reading the newspaper Françoise weeps for the idea, not the person. For those she dislikes malice is her mode. The chicken incident alerts the narrator to the reason that they have been having so much delicious asparagus this season—because it causes allergies for the detested maid.

I am reading this Lydia Davis translation of Proust's first volume of *In Search of Lost Time* in Mexico, in a village called Xilitla where we are visiting Las Pozas, a surrealist garden of fantastical concrete structures built in the jungle. I don't know why I am reading this particular book, here of all places, perhaps it was there on my Kindle, lying in wait. What I do know is that irritation and impatience have been slowly smoldering as the wretched hawthorns, even more insistent than the soggy madeleine, provoke endlessly attenuated passages of tremulous sensitivity.

Why are you reading about hawthorns in the jungle? I ask myself. Surely this voluntary immersion in excruciating European sensitivity is a kind of perversity. Then I reach the chicken incident. And suddenly I'm reconciled to Proust, the hawthorns fade out of the frame, and everything else falls into place. Or, rather, I feel more attuned to resting in this place we might call Proust. This is the Proust I prefer, the clarity about cruelty, for instance, the way in which detail can be made to count, a single detail, or an accumulation of details, delineating over many pages qualities or characteristics. The way he has of unfolding a person, of teasing out how people accommodate to living with things, even the things they despise, often because they have no idea of their own worst aspects (vanity, snobbishness, greed, hypocrisy, jealousy, envy, to name just the familiar vices). These characteristics, or maybe even "essences," migrate between characters, across the pages. What hooks me back into the Proustian fabric is something other than an existential dimension, it is a more primal engagement with storytelling, with the spinning of a fictional web in which characters are unfolded ever so slowly, so slowly that they change over time. And so, slowly, almost imperceptibly, you feel yourself changed.

Slow immersion, infinitesimal change, the possibility of not being incarcerated forever in a decidedly fixed character description—this is perhaps the lure of the long and sprawling novel and television saga in an age of the sound bite, of flickering attention, of the instantaneity and ephemerality of social media. Think of the Patrick Melrose novels in which Edward St. Aubyn manages to sustain interest in a small cluster of characters over five novels. Or think of television sagas, such as *The Sopranos* and *Breaking Bad* and *The Wire*. Think especially of *Wentworth*, a remake of the incandescently trashy Australian soap *Prisoner*, which ran from 1979 to 1986.

From the first episode I was hooked into *Prisoner*—the unerring sense of drama, the virtuoso enactment of cliffhangers, the tension between gritty realism and flamboyant melodrama, the flimsiness of the cardboard sets, the grandiosity of plot ambition. And yet and yet, despite the display of artificiality, *Prisoner* lured us fans into a complicit but also delicious compact: an engagement with the characters of this fictional world. No matter that the only consistent thing about these characters was that they consistently acted out of character. In fact this was the lure. *Prisoner* was a machine for generating signs; it distributed qualities or essences across a network of characters and simultaneously generated an affective charge that caused us to fall in love (and into addiction) and to imagine these characters, affects, essences as part of our world. If *Prisoner* played on the paradox of a closed world, of incarceration, in which anything was possible, change was axiomatic, then by entering into the charged ambience of this world, we enlivened our own immersion in mundanity.

The flesh of *Prisoner*, and *Wentworth* too, is neither unctuous nor tender. The only chickens in *Prisoner* are the kind that come home to roost. And they roost uncommonly fast.

. . .

Back in San Diego, when I return to Proust I am back in the jungle. Now Proust summons the smell of tropical rain and the burning of copal. In the mornings and the evenings a man would walk through and around the house where we were staying, gently swinging a crucible in which copal, a kind of frankincense, was burning. Smoke wafted up and around, through doors and windows. After a day in the jungle garden, climbing and slithering on wet slippery stone paths, after heat and sweat and revelations one after another, what bliss to lie at last under a ceiling fan. Outside a thunderstorm dying down, the scent of rain and lushness and copal smoke. Sweet, dense, spicy.

Dorland 46

Mountains, bare Californian mountains stretching away into the east, where the sun rises around five in the morning. I get up, open the door, breathe in the high desert country air. Usually take my pot of tea and Mac Air back to bed, but this morning I have been sitting at the small desk, listening to the birds, feeling the wind come up. There are two cabins for writers or artists or musicians—a piano sits in this room—perched right on top of the mountain as though in the wilderness, but they are next to a grove of live oaks where Robert and Janice, artists and gracious custodians of this very special place, live in one trailer and paint in another since Robert's cabin burnt to the ground when a devastating fire ripped through, destroying everything in 2004. He stood at the bottom of the mountain and watched it burn.

I have a week here, a precious week carved out of a jumbled, somewhat pressured time crammed with classes (in which I am a student—tai chi, Feldenkrais, qigong, Spanish, Shambhala), seeing the grad students I still work with, keeping up with friends, medical and acupuncture appointments, visits to the vet, arranging flowers and hosting and sitting at the sangha, dealing endlessly with insurance and Social Security and email, reading, keeping up with films, politics, the garden, meditating, walking, preserving lemons before they all fall off the tree and rot. Trying to write every morning a little and not always succeeding. Retirement supposedly opens up space and expands time. It is true that the stress of a daily job evaporates, but details, a myriad of details, edge their way in, scurry around and multiply, migrating from one pocket of time into another, where they colonize, congeal, ooze, spread like Indian ink seeping into and staining a new manuscript.

Here I talk to no one. No internet. The phone works and I have used it to look up a few things, but since I'm not skilled at reading on the phone it mostly serves as a time machine. Talking to no one has its virtues. It might not be the way to live, except for Trappists and hermits and Buddhist monks on long retreats in caves, but for a while, for a defined period of stolen time, it means your focus is sharpened, your ideas crystallize, images materialize out of the fog with extraordinary clarity. Without distractions and interruptions and choosing your own ideal rhythm you find you are charged with energy. I am working mainly on reworking and polishing sketchy and rough parts of the book. Somehow these are pieces that I knew not to gnaw on (often I gnaw to the bone, bury the bones, dig them up, suck the encrusted soil away, then hammer and splinter the now dry and brittle words), I put them aside only slightly reluctantly, aware that in some instances they might never work, but in other instances they just might—when the time is right—be amenable to shaping.

The two cabins that were built after the fire are built to code, they are the prototype of post-Katrina housing—a single main room which includes a kitchen and a wood heater for winter, with a porch out front, a small bedroom, and a bathroom. Since I first came here there are a few plantings around the cabin—rosemary outside the bedroom window, a few Mexican salvias growing in among the cactus, attracting hummingbirds, and a wisteria over the porch. I did not know Dorland before the fire. Earlier residents speak of the enchanting adobe main house, filled with books and antiques which were also distributed through the eight cottages. The arts colony was founded in 1979 by concert pianist Ellen Dorland (who had owned the property since the 1930s) and environmentalist Barbara Horton; the three-hundred-acre wilderness area was transferred to the Nature Conservancy, with the colony retaining rights over ten acres. Dorland is part of the easement plan that is designed to allow mountain lions movement through different areas of Riverside and San Diego counties. I would love to see a mountain lion—perhaps not, however, on a mountain with only the lion and myself in sight.

This is not one of the well-endowed artists' residencies, you pay a token amount and provide your own meals. I like this. Even if there is minimal preparation I enjoy letting the food possibilities ripple through my mind during the day. This morning I boiled an egg, a Sabrina egg. Of the three hens she is the one whose eggs vary most: Sometimes they are a deep-chocolate color, other times densely freckled, and today's egg (not gathered today but brought with me) was a pale buff color with just a few spreckles of reddish brown. I ate the egg with the Prager Brother's walnut bread. Then a bowl of my own yogurt, creamy and slightly tart, with peaches and blackberries from the farmers' market. Dark rich roasted coffee from Caffè Calabria down the road in North Park that I had to hastily grind before leaving home so that I could use it in my small French press. I brought with me greens from the garden, cucumbers and tomatoes (brave Stupice, always the first of the season, small and juicy, each bite a taste explosion after the long months of no tomatoes or cardboard-flavored imitations), shishito peppers, frozen cubes of green curry made when I pulled out the last of the cilantro and had all those roots to use, frozen chicken, a dressing for the kale—anchovies and garlic and olive oil and parmesan—too complicated to make here. Have to keep up eating the same quantity of leafy greens each day because of the new drug regime. Such a pain trying to keep track.

As I left the house I saw in the front garden a bud of the odorous rose Secret just beginning to open. Snipped it and put the stem in my water bottle in the car. It's been slowly opening and changing color. When I'm stuck, when the words turn leaden or all freeze up, I lean over and sniff. Sniffing doesn't actually liberate the words, but it does enliven the soul. At night I breathe in the rosemary.

It might seem as though I might as well have stayed home. Haven't roamed far, food-wise anyway. It's true that Dorland is only about sixty miles from San Diego. I can load the car up, drive, and be here in an hour. But it seems another world. And I'm cautious about staying healthy because last time I was here I came down with some bug and J had to come and fetch me. My immune system is stronger this time, the Revlimid has afforded me overall energy and resistance. Although, I had a fright last night. J, as requested, made his marvelous ragu and froze a container for me to bring. Still at home last week, just after he had made the sauce—it sits on the stove for ages, just a bubble breaking the surface occasionally—as we were about to dig in, he remarked that he had included some liver. Oh no! I shrieked. Liver! Liver! It will kill me, liver is a killer! I have been warned since starting the Coumadin that there are two forbidden substances: liver and mango. Do not even taste these, they react dangerously with Coumadin. Oh, well, luckily I cut them into little bits rather than grinding, says J. So I picked out the disgusting chewed-and-leathery-looking morsels and promised to do the same when at Dorland. Well here I am, and guess what? I forgot. Suddenly I remembered. Halfway through a portion. Oy vey, here I am in the wilderness, I don't even know what will happen but it could be dire. Should I warn Janice and Robert that they might have to drive me to a hospital? I decide against panic performance. I had not eaten a lot and once I realized, picked out all the bits from what remained and finished my dinner. And then decided to do something very distracting while I waited to see what would eventuate, so I watched *Topsy-Turvy*, about Gilbert and Sullivan, on the Mac Air.

Oh what a marvelous film, a brilliant evocation of performance, of the exchange between cinema and theater, of the onstage-offstage dynamic. And as always with Mike Leigh and his ensemble group of actors, the delineation of characters and the small gestures and intimations that make up the relationships between people are great. The sense of rhythm and timing is impeccable. I do not know how he does it. What I love is the way in which he is able to chart both the stubborn persistence of character traits, the pernicious hold of habit and dependence, and also the little chinks of hope—in those moments when something almost imperceptible occurs in an exchange, something that might lead to something. This happens too in *Mr. Turner*, where the characterization, especially of the women, is superbly nuanced, and Timothy Spall's performance is riveting. The dense texture of Victorian interiors, of things, things, things, is tangibly thingy. But the attempt to render one medium through another, painting through film, produces a horrible mess. It seems to me a misplaced ambition to render Turner-esque views cinematically. It's not that I'm against the project, but here it is too literal, it aims at an equivalence rather than at a palette that exposes and explores differences, fissures, and particularities. And it ends up being a bit of a cheesy mess. Leigh and Pope, his cinematographer, have made a mark by using and crafting tableaus in the past, but usually they are integrated into an intimate drama or more expansively into an edited sequence, intercut brilliantly with close-ups, as in *Topsy-Turvy*. Here we get cinematic chocolate box tableaus.

At night when not watching *Topsy-Turvy* and when eating, I've been reading *How to Live, or A Life of Montaigne in One Question and Twenty Attempts at an Answer* and rereading—or rather, scanning—a few books on microbes and our endangered microbiota. When, with much effort, I pull the two-volume *Complete Edition of the English Oxford Dictionary* off the bookshelf, a tiny pocket edition of *The Tibetan Book of the Dead*, with a commentary by Chögyam Trungpa, previously hidden, falls to the floor.

Once or twice a day I meditate, sitting on the porch. Yesterday a lizard clambered up the wicker work table, blending into the aged weaving. Once he realized I was there he held still, and so I was able to contemplate him, his coloring: many shades of gold and brown and burnt umber. I wonder if he was contemplating me, and if so, what did he see? Drawn into lizardness, my mind kept veering off to rattlesnakes. The wretched snakes will not keep out of my head, they writhe their way in, occupying emptiness, emanating fear. Janice warned me when I arrived that they have so far seen five, quite a few more than is usual so early in the season. Robert lent me a long stick, so when I walk I use it to tap in front of me, warning them that I am coming so that neither of us will be taken by surprise. But this morning I walked around the upper pond. It used to be choked by reeds but now has been cleared by friends of Dorland, including the Boy Scouts, and is beautiful, you come upon it as an oasis in this desert region. There are water lilies—large, waxy, pink and white—and reeds around the edges, huge old oaks and a massive if spindly palm tree, dating back to the original homestead I imagine. Now and then an almighty splash and rippling of the surface as an invisible frog plops into the water. The wind in the reeds and trees, croaking, though hard to tell from where. I became obsessed with spying a frog so had to walk very quietly around the banks, but this meant I couldn't tap with my big stick. Frogs or snakes? Which will it be? I saw neither. But this is what I think I will do next time a rattlesnake slithers and rattles into my meditating mind: I will invite him (why do I think of it as a him?) to sit there, preferably coiled rather than rearing up, ready to strike. I will contemplate him, and maybe this way I will tame my fear.

Touched by a Whale 47

We are on a small boat in a lagoon. All around: blue water and gray whales. *Eschrichtius robustus*, also called a California gray. Now and then and here and there you can spot whales spouting, spy hopping, flipping their tails into the air. Sometimes there are single whales, but mostly you will see a mother whale accompanied by her baby, they surface side by side, glide gracefully and then slowly descend again under water. We all wait with baited breath for the pair to resurface, the mothers can go a long time under water but the babies only for about a minute and a half. Sometimes there appears to be a rhythm, a dance almost, to the way in which they appear and glide and descend and reappear. But mostly it's surprising—they pop up unexpectedly, far away, or on the other side of the boat. We have learned to look for signs: footprint, which is a clear pool of water in the sea where the whales have been, or you can see their shapes moving underwater by the boat. You have to peer because the water is murky, shallow, and the whales stir up the bottom.

Sometimes they come close to the boat, or panga. You can see mother and baby rolling over one another, playing, the mother carrying her baby on her back or nudging it seemingly toward us. And occasionally, just occasionally, a baby (a fourteen-or-so-foot baby weighing a thousand pounds) lifts its nose up right by the boat, and you lean down and touch its face, a rubbery hairy face, and it looks you in the eye and then sinks down below the water. When it looks you in the eye you feel a wildness entering into you.

Or is it quite the opposite: the instinct for domestication and for reassurance of our own human capacity for empathy and compassion?

I arrive, in San Ignacio, a lagoon in Baja, Mexico, with a thundering headache. My whole skull, including the face, seems like a powder keg, ready to explode.

The day before coming to San Ignacio, along with a monthly infusion of immuno-globulin, I had a shot of Neulasta. This was to top up my neutrophil supply, which has run dangerously low, putting me into the neutropenic range. Simply: very vulnerable to infection. Neutrophils are a particular kind of white blood cell that protect against infection. Among other things, they form pus, so if your count is low you don't want to get any cuts. I didn't feel or look neutropenic, but the doctors were not prepared to take any risks on the verge of travel. I was warned that bone pain could be a "side" effect of the shot, that the skull is particularly targeted or frequently a locus of pain. It happens because suddenly a torrent of white blood cells are pumping through the bone marrow, causing pressure. It is like having a migraine. Pain migrating all over your face and head to which ordinary painkill-ers don't respond.

In San Ignacio, on the lagoon, the pain seemed to disappear. It was there but my being was elsewhere: out on the boat, in the wind, the water, with the whales. Be-ing visited by these whales is indeed like a visitation, they appear to us as though from another universe, though it is they in fact who are in their element and it is we who are the visitors. These mighty creatures from the wild ocean appear and swim around our boat, playfully nudging it now and then, swimming underneath, but never tipping it over. On the last day we saw a young baby, less than a week old, still with its fetal folds.

We feel honored and privileged to be visited by the whales. They have traveled nearly six thousand miles from Alaska's Bering Sea to the Baja lagoons, the lon-gest mammal migration on earth. We are in awe. Also, rather smug. Pleased at our human capacity for reform and betterment, for appreciating nature, for learn-ing to leave a small footprint. And we are well disposed to think that the whales approach us because they are so relieved and happy to know they are safe, that they come to us in love. In *Seven Tenths: The Sea and Its Thresholds*, a magisteri-ally quirky book written in 1992 that savagely describes and poetically mourns the devastation of the ocean by the fishing industry, James Hamilton-Paterson also lobs a few missiles in the direction of the enlightened eco traveler: The loss of creatures, the changing environment "mobilizes in him a tenderness akin to vulnerability, to a point where a large part of his wistful concern for the whales and the environment generally is displaced fear for himself."

. . .

Here we are on a small island, Punta Piedra, deserted except for this eco camp. Deserted and a desert. Sand stretches in all directions, except for the mangroves that ring part of the circumference and through which we kayak. Helen B and I are here with a tour group from San Diego. The footprint of the camp is small—

solar energy, simple tents, six chairs along the shore. Helen and I sit here after the morning boat trip with a cup of tea and, after the afternoon trip, with a glass of wine and converse, sometimes with others in the group, though we warm most to the pair from Australia as we can more easily exchange deadpan jokes with them. You can watch the whales and dolphins and sea lions and cormorants and pelicans and other birds appear and move across the view within a hundred feet of the shoreline.

An island epitomizes the fantasy of a return to originality, and at the same time it evokes territory, ownership. "Our" island. "Our lagoon." You can walk in the early morning along the Mexican seashore, see no people, just creatures, assured nevertheless that you can return to safety, far from urbanity. This is my first real exposure to ecotourism, to professional travelers, to people who have been to almost every country in the world and are able to trade country stories like other people trade Jewish jokes. Perhaps I am entering into that realm so bitingly satirized by the Australian writer Murray Bail in *Homesickness*, a novel that describes the global travels of a group of tourists to diverse museums, real and imaginary, around the world.

. . .

We are told by the naturalists that splashing brings the whales to the boats—they like the sound—and that if they come close enough, you should try and encourage them to come even closer by splashing more. We do this with great energy. Six people in this small boat splashing like crazy, screeching with joy, a spectacle of ecstasy. Do whales have a sense of curiosity and humor? This is a question often asked (of whales, not tourists). One whale seemed certainly to be playing with us. In answer to our splashing she raised a fin and thwacked the water resoundingly, creating an almighty splash that engulfed the boat, soaking Helen, who was closest and had been splashing most vociferously, but spraying us all. She then went under but almost immediately rose up out of the water, a perpendicular dive into the air, did what appeared to be a 360-degree turn, then subsided into the water and buggered off, out of our lives forever.

You imagine the whale is playing, performing, entering into a jokey exchange with us, but you do not really know. You feel in the presence of something unfathomable, a mammal like ourselves, but a mighty being, a wild creature that in our consciousness for so long has been threatening. And threatened.

These gray whales have twice been brought back from the verge of extinction. This lagoon was once a killing field. When the mothers came in here to have their babies they were prime targets for hunters after blubber, and in 1857 Scammon's whaling fleet left few survivors. The second severe depletion occurred during modern whaling, when factory ships used to process the entire whale while still at sea. Now the gray whales are an Endangered Species Act success story. Now San Ignacio is a refuge. Not, any longer, from hunters, but from other whales—from those toothed beauties, orcas, and hunchbacks. The gray whales, while birthing, find a refuge here from these mammalian killers.

The island and lagoon are a refuge for us too. For many who are ecologically disposed, the natural environment, whether wilderness or an environment like this, seemingly restored to what it once was, provides salvation from the toxicity and pollution of urban living. I am less inclined to consider nature as redemptive in this way, more cynical about the tourist slot I fill, but I too have experienced the curiously transportive sense of being touched by a whale. And for an exhilarating hallucinatory moment I believed or, rather, sensed this experience as curative, imagined that the whales might redeem us, cleanse us of cancer and the sins of the Anthropocene. The moment, or moments, for there were more than one, passed, subsided into mere mortal happiness and joyous fun. It does, however, make sense to me that when we touch the whales we are in turn touched, by the whales themselves, but also by the way they summon all those other creatures of the sea that have disappeared. As well as joy they open a path to melancholy and grieving and anger for every living being that is threatened today by landscapes and seascapes that are changed in ways that can never be reversed. But if the whales are good at channeling other creatures, they, along with those other cetaceans and large mammals (whales, dolphins, elephants, pandas), are so much more televisual, so much better equipped to channel human love than those crabby crustaceans and ugly insects and invisible microbes that too are threatened by disappearance.

This lagoon will never be restored to what it once was, the wild creatures will probably never have the lagoon to themselves again. But a new ecology is evolving. This refuge has been created through long years of environmental activism, negotiations between local and national and international interests, compromises between wilderness advocates and tourism, slow bureaucratic enactment of legislation. Once, the gray whales visited the bays in San Diego, but in the 1880s the entire herd was destroyed and they never returned. When they were on the point of disappearing in Baja the International Whaling Commission finally protected gray whales from hunting in 1946. They were given additional protection in 1973 by being placed on the Endangered Species Act. In 1988 the Mexican government established the El Vizcaíno Biosphere Reserve, of which San Ignacio is a part. It is the largest wildlife refuge or sanctuary in Latin America. San Ignacio is now a UNESCO World Heritage Site, declared so in 1993.

A new ecology. The fact that there is no fishing or swimming allowed in the lagoon during the whale season (nor in the two other areas in Baja where the whales come, Ojo de Liebre Lagoon, formerly Scammon's Lagoon, and Magdalena Bay) means that the local fishermen lose their income. But in the new environment, shaped to a large degree by ecotourism, they become boat drivers and custodians (and are skilled at cutting free the occasional whales that still get entangled in fishing nets). There is only one fisherwoman at San Ignacio, Lupita, and she is a naturalist at the camp during the whale season.

. . .

It is a place where species meet. It is the new wild.

. . .

Today there are about three hundred whales in this lagoon alone (about 10 percent of which are estimated to be friendly; it is thought that these are ones that were here themselves as babies and so have learned that the humans here are friendly too). The most recent population estimate of "our" gray whales was about nineteen thousand, with a high probability that it is close to the carrying capacity of the ecosystem of these animals. Our group constitutes one—the eastern—of two groups that exist in the Northern Pacific. One species, two populations. The other group—the western—has not been so lucky. It hovers on the brink of extinction with a population of around a hundred and fifty. They face threats from seismic oil exploration, entanglement in fishing gear in Japan and China, and ship traffic in their feeding and migration routes.

These migration routes might be changing. Although they once lived there, gray whales are no longer in the Atlantic, except on two recent occasions: In 2010 a gray whale was sighted off the coast of Israel, it was then seen off the coast of Spain and then disappeared. It is believed to have swum through a warm channel created by climate change. In 2013 one was spotted in the southern Atlantic off the coast of Namibia. This was the first sighting of a gray whale in the Southern Hemisphere *ever*. Two of seven satellite-tagged western gray whales, instead of heading down Asia's Pacific shoreline to the South China Sea, traveled across the Bering Sea to North America. In 2011 one made it all the way to Baja.

This is both marvelous and alarming. Gray whales may be about to move back into the Atlantic because we are opening a path for them through the Arctic. Climate scientists estimate that the passage will be ice-free year-round by 2030. It seems that there have been other similar migrations in the past. The whales appear to have moved into the Atlantic whenever it was warm enough for them to get through the Bering Strait. One migration took place seventy-nine thousand years ago, and then three others happened more recently, between about ten thousand and five thousand years ago. This time is different, the climate change has been produced by humans, by greenhouse gases; the whales will have to contend with shipping lanes, oil drilling, and industrial fishing operations. But they will also likely have lots of good habitat to live in, more shallow shelves (as sea levels rise), where they can scoop up food. Gray whales are great explorers, and they will go where there is food. The ocean is changing, and the species that can thrive there will change with it.

. . .

As we splash the whales and they splash us in San Ignacio Lagoon I wonder what they think, if they even conceive of us as humans, or if they comprehend us as part of a composite thing which we call a boat but which they might understand as something else, perhaps another sea creature. I wonder what a whale would say if it could speak. They, like other creatures that live in the ocean, have a much more complex sense of space than we do—gradations of light and shadow—and an acute and complex hearing range. They communicate in ways we do not understand. They seem to respond to the sound of the outboard motor. When whales approach the motor is turned to idling, a low thrumming. To me it seems undoubtedly the case that the whales who approach the boats are curious and fun-loving. But when people say, and this is a truism, that they bring their babies to you, I am prone to wondering. Maybe they just bring their babies to the boat, most probably showing them that it is safe, that the boat has many sounds: a fairly complex sonic communicative system which includes a thrumming motor and screeching sounds— wows and oohs and ahs, and you beauty, and look look it's a baby, as well as tactile extensions that ripple the water, that touch and sometimes stroke.

Wittgenstein famously remarked, "If a Lion could talk we could not understand him." There is a paradox contained within this aphorism. For the lion will not use language as we know it, she will use a system of signs unfamiliar to us and to which we do not have ready access. If she did talk she would not be a lion but a human projection, as in *The Wizard of Oz*. Of course we have learned to live with and communicate with some species whom we have domesticated and who have in their turn animalized us to some degree. Dogs and cats. And then of course there is the peculiarity of chickens.

In Pasolini's film *The Hawks and the Sparrows* birds talk. "I come from far away. My country is ideology. I live in the capital, the city of the future, on Karl Marx Street," announces the Hawk in this allegorical, caustically comic enactment of a debate between Marxism and the Church. It is also a bitter representation of a devastated landscape following the Italian boom, and it is also a delightful homage to silent cinema. Between the loquacity of the hawk and the silence of cinema: poetry.

I imagine the whales may say to us, "We come from far away," but I do not think they live in the country of ideology. And yet, like us, not outside it. Between the visible and the invisible, loquacity and silence, the reemergence of "lost" species is moving in ways that are hard to express. The way hope jumps and catches in your throat as you see a forty-ton whale rising up out of the water, slicing the air with precision and grace, and sinking down again into the deep. If poetry were at my fingertips I would tap out the words of an unknown language, but all I can do is try to negotiate the reefy shores where inexpressible awe hits the sponginess of sentimentality and cheesiness of anthropomorphism.

. . .

Back home Elvis jumps onto the bed, uttering a few guttural laconicities. I reply in human talk, a mix of English words and phatic noises. I believe he has a pretty large English vocabulary. My knowledge of "cat talk," on the other hand, is very basic. Sometimes I think he simply pretends or refuses to understand what I am saying. *Quien sabe?* Who knows?

Chickens. Well chickens are a more difficult proposition when considering this question of the talking lion. They are less loquacious and bombastically intellectual than the crow, but they do seem to communicate through sound which resonates in some way that I feel a part of. Not invariably and not all the time. They do not understand reprimands; I do not understand why suddenly, out of the blue, Sabrina has started pecking my leg quite viciously whenever I venture into the yard. She has also taken to bullying and pecking the other two, so perhaps she considers me another chicken. Yet there is what I take to be a kind of communication when I go out before bed to make sure the door to their inner house is locked. I speak and let them know it's me and not a predator approaching, and they coo and chirrup very softly, the three of them forming a song line. It is a sound that moves into my chest, calming the spluttering old heart.

Travel

48

"I hate traveling and explorers."

These words, the opening words of Lévi-Strauss's *Tristes Tropiques*, have been lying in wait; now they leap out and ambush me, mockingly, as I think about journeys, travel, detours, and interruptions.

In the past I went places generally because of work, or work was a way to visit places for pleasure. I guess, rather reluctantly and shame-facedly, I am becoming a different sort of traveler, one who simply goes to look and who sometimes takes tours. First there was the whale tour, and now a few tours here and there inserted into idiosyncratic and self-organized travel.

CLL has turned me into a traveler. Or tourist.

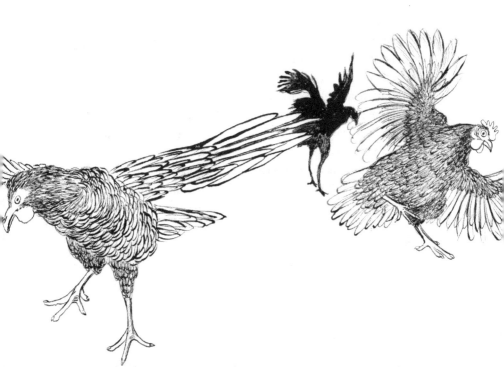

The Answer Is Not Coming

49

She waits in the freezing snow at the bottom of a huge mountain, an icy mountain lying between one country and another. It's the end of the day, light is failing. Perhaps he has ditched her, or had an accident, or fallen into a crevasse. Doubt. Waiting. "The answer is not coming." So writes Rachel Kushner at the end of *The Flamethrowers*. Though these are not quite the last words of the novel.

Two things are going on, as I see it. There's a familiar quotidian experience: hanging about waiting for someone who doesn't show. You're in that place or moment when anxiety and boredom collide, anticipation runs headlong into despair. And there's a larger metaphysical or perhaps structural thing going on: how to be in that experience, how to move through this waiting or to let the waiting materialize as a nonconclusive ending.

The answer to the question of whether he is coming or not is simple, it becomes clear as night falls: He is not coming. But there is another question not answered, though what exactly this question is you can't say and actually it doesn't matter what the question itself is. It is not a man who will not come, it is an answer. For Kushner, I believe, it's enmeshed in how to bring the novel to an end. This is a novel that is dense and intriguing in its cutting between times and places, places in the U.S. and Italy, in the 1970s and around the First World War. The threads of connection that link people to political and art movements are rendered through scenarios in which characters experience speed and slowness, talking, listening, waiting. Guns and motorbikes, riding fast and waiting about slowly not doing much. Techniques and technologies. Kushner, within the fabric of the daily, writes about a variety of technologies, mobilizing characters and ideas that attempt, variously, to forge a way out of the routine of the everyday. Her novel, too, shapes up—disintegrates, realigns—through a virtuoso enactment of technique. She herself is a flamethrower, filling the sky with colors and patterns, materializing through technique a range of possibilities, some lethal. Reading, immersed in the rhythms and the cutting between locales, alerted through technique rather than through authorial direction, to the present, you don't expect a conclusion, particularly one that embodies a triumph over adversity. It isn't simply that we are left with a question at the end, some plot thread that is left loose, given to us as a throwaway scrap from the table of literary delights. No, it's that the whole practice or technique of the novel works against triumphalism with all its moral underpinnings.

Because I'm pretty well right now I'm greedy to grab every moment to write or read scraps from lots of different books, and so I've read this novel slowly, in some senses against the grain. In the last third I speed up, glad to immerse myself in the novel during Cancer Survivors Week, thus saving myself from getting hot under the collar about all the triumphalist rhetoric in the air. Saving myself, perhaps, from insinuations of guilt solicited by sentiment-drenched exhortations to give money to defeat cancer. I want to live longer, I want them (that great big *them* in the sky) to find a better form of treatment than the ghastly chemo people with tumors have to endure (and, indeed, there are people with blood cancers who endure these too). And being implicated, a receiver or beneficiary of the bounty, I know I should give more than I do so that people not as lucky as me in terms of time and place can get a better deal. But it makes me mad that so much of cancer, medicine in general, actually everything in general in this country, is so dependent on charity, on private institutions, on individual gifts. Matters of public concern rendered as a balancing act between the fortunate and the unfortunate, where individuals can be empowered by charitable acts, acts of giving.

The objective correlative of this is the celebration of survivors, the hullaballoo about the battle won by strong individuals. Empowerment through adversity. We are the strong ones, the ones who fought back and won, we are special, not like all those losers who succumbed and dropped dead without a proper struggle.

Still, we need fiction sometimes. The fiction of survival is a charged fiction, and through the charging, the living through acquires a material reality. The reality that we are fighting, that we will overcome. When Isabel wrote to me, long ago it now seems, when I had surgery for lung cancer a year after the leukemia diagnosis, *Vencerás* (you will overcome), it was inspiring, it gave me courage, I started to believe that I would survive. She gave me a gift.

So what to do? What is the answer? Me fuming silently on my soapbox with a hand hovering reluctantly over a shallow pocket chockablock with scrunched-up tissues and lists of things to do and a little cash isn't going to change the circuit of charitable and uncharitable capital.

Nightclub Bouncers

50

Imagine your body as a nightclub: raucous pulsating music, sweaty bodies gyrating, drug-fueled desires floating free from individual bodies, forbidden fireworks bursting into flame, careening through the sky. And at the doors there are bouncers, but they are slumped over, groggy, looking bemusedly at the line of eager punters hoping to get in. They can't decide, they are unable to recognize the IDs, the fashion statements, the accents. And so the punters sidle their way in and soon the party changes.

. . .

When Helen B was here over the summer of 2013 she worked every day in the vegetable garden, clearing the jungle that had developed in every bed over the past year when I had given up trying to maintain paradise. She worked methodically for a few hours every day, usually in the cool of the day, and in between took long rests, feet up, absorbed in her Kindle. This was instructive to me, a lesson in pacing. I tend to go at it (whatever it is, working in the garden, writing a lecture, making a meal) like a terrier in a field of china dragons and then take forever to recover. At the end of her stay the vegetable beds were miraculously clear of weeds and opportunistic orphans and flowering chicory (beautiful blue cornflowers) and lettuces bolting for the stable door. There was palpitation in the air as the beds panted, asking for compost and coddling and new seeds and seedlings. But Helen's work was not finished. She announced that there was seemingly no way to stop the Wandering Christians from creeping in from the back alley, under the fence, slithering into the garden, invading. Seemingly no way. Unless . . . unless we used the Roundup found in a back and murky corner of the garage. Not actually in the garden, she insisted, it's a way of protecting the garden. I know that many gardeners protect their borders by dabbing (rather than spraying) Roundup on weeds. After much debate, we decided to do this (or, rather, it was Helen who bravely donned gloves and did the deed).

Right now (December 2013) I am on a long flight to Sydney (after stopping down for two nights in Honolulu, hardly a punishment) and have treated myself to an issue of *Fine Gardening*. In it is an article entitled "Setting the Record Straight on Glyphosate," and it rehearses the many arguments about the relative safety of glyphosate (the active ingredient in Roundup) if used properly in a suburban garden (as opposed to in large-scale agricultural farming). Most interestingly, for me, what struck a new chord was the argument about active and inactive ingredients. Inactive ingredients or adjuvants are those constituents of a herbicide that enable the prime toxin to work—in the case of glyphosates those that help the spray to stick to and be absorbed by the leaves. These adjuvants, unlike the active ingredients, do not have to be listed. Some scientists now believe that they may be more toxic than the glyphosate itself. Without knowing the science of the matter I can grasp this, it makes sense. And it makes sense to me because of the CLL treatment. Because of experiencing the way that the chemicals designed to guard against side effects can sometimes produce side effects more severe than the chemo itself.

Now it is January 2016, and I return to this piece after making myself a note last year that the story is not yet over. In March 2015 an agency of the World Health Organization declared that glyphosate probably causes cancer in people. Monsanto denounced the report. Indeed the pendulum has swung back and forth with alarming indecisiveness. Thirty years ago, an Environmental Protection Agency committee determined that Roundup might cause cancer. Six years later, in 1991, the agency reversed itself after reevaluating the mouse study that had been the basis for the original conclusion. Since then the use of Roundup has soared (between 1987 and 2012, according to *National Geographic*, annual U.S. farm use grew from less than eleven million pounds to nearly three hundred million pounds), mostly because of Monsanto's GMO Roundup Ready crops, which are resistant to glyphosate, enabling the farmers to spray their fields, supposedly keeping their crops (soy, cotton, and corn primarily) safe while killing the weeds. Unfortunately, the workers who spray the crops are not resistant, nor are the animals nearby, nor are amateur gardeners, though we are exposed to far less dangerous levels than the farm workers and their families who live in the vicinity of the spraying. But now even the weeds have become resistant to Roundup. Residue on the crops is high and so is its presence in waterways.

Glyphosate is not included in the U.S. government's testing of food for pesticide residues or the monitoring of chemicals in human blood and tissues. As a result, there is no information from this source on how much people are exposed to from using it in their yards, living near farms, or eating foods from treated fields. The EPA said, after the UN Agency for Research on Cancer released their findings last year, that it would analyze these findings, but to date, as far as I can ascertain, they have made no public report. California's Environmental Protection Agency (CalEPA) does intend to list glyphosate as a carcinogenic chemical.

. . .

And soon the party changes. . . . This analogy of the body to a nightclub monitored by bouncers comes from a researcher whose aim is to tweak and make safer (rather than ban outright) industrial chemicals that are currently unsafe. Frankly, I find it hard to imagine my less youthful body as a nightclub, but I can still remember rather vividly the fabulously pulsating environments that sucked you in so lasciviously if you could make it past the gatekeepers. So I am easily persuaded. But mostly I am persuaded because of the lucid explanation in a simple video by Amro Hamdoun of how herbicides like Roundup work on the body. He explains that because many environmental chemicals have structures not commonly seen in nature, organisms have simply not had a chance to organize defense systems. We've made something like eighty thousand synthetic industrial compounds in the past century—from plastics to fire retardants to hair sprays to pesticides—and many of these are known to have endocrine-disrupting properties. Many types of diseases, such as breast cancer and blood cancers, are caused by this misregulation of hormone systems. The mechanism for regulation of what gets in and out involves proteins called drug transporters, likened to nightclub bouncers. The drug transporters are confused, they have not had time to identify the interlopers, nor to organize their defenses. They have become feeble bouncers.

Today Luis and his son, with some help from J, are going to begin the assault on the bamboo that grows all along one side of the backyard. It is lush and beautiful and towers way over our heads, but its rhizomes have spread everywhere, depriving the vegetables and other plants of food. J and Peggy and I have been waging a losing battle cutting each new shoot as it appears, trying to starve the bamboo, which can grow six inches in a day. Now we are getting serious, without the use of Roundup. Luis is going to cut back the bamboo, dig, and pull out what rhizomes he can, and from there we will keep up the day-by-day tussle, going to the root or the shoot of the problem. Perhaps in a year's time it will give up. Perhaps it will take longer. But then we will be able to plant berries and more espaliered fruit trees.

Helen and I were acting as nightclub bouncers, keeping glyphosate out of the garden, we hoped, but possibly no more efficiently than the feeble nightclub bouncers (drug transporters) meant to keep glyphosate out of our bodies.

All Natural

51

Is an "all-natural" chicken better than a "natural" chicken? And what anyway is a *natural* chicken: that package neatly vacuum-sealed and thus labeled that swims into view as you paddle around in the supermarket, yearning for dry land?

Of course no producer calls their product "unnatural." And *natural* we know anyway to be a tricky term, often invoked to summon some notion of purity totally antinomic to the synthetic. Still, I feel drawn to those packages that declare their natural credentials since the undeclared "unnatural" suggests all the unspeakable ways chickens are raised and processed. Ghastly for the chickens and ghastly for our bodies too if we ingest them. Eating the other is, in many cultures, a mode of incorporation, of becoming the other. In our culture the chicken is perhaps the most familiar domesticated other, and yet there is a degree of cognitive dissonance—we don't seem to have registered that we are becoming chicken. A particular kind of chicken, moreover: malformed, crippled, ill, and ugly.

Each person in this country, on average, consumed more than ninety pounds of chicken meat in 2015. Almost nine billion broiler chickens, weighing fifty-three billion pounds, live weight, were produced. More than forty billion pounds of chicken product were marketed.

A century ago chicken meat was something of a luxury item. It is of course factory farming that has made chickens so cost-effective to produce and cheap to buy in the supermarket. They have been carefully bred to produce ultimately edible chickens that grow very fast, develop massively disproportionate breasts (crippling their legs), and don't require too much food. The conditions in which they are raised, lay eggs, and are killed are horrendous. There are many very shocking accounts of these industrial practices—on film, on the internet, and in print—but one of the best, which is to say one that speaks the unspeakable with brutal clarity (its effect achieved, I think, because it builds slowly from a broad consideration of the chicken, including charming whimsy, to the end point in industrial farming), is *Chicken*, by Annie Potts.

If we are as a nation becoming chicken, what are we beginning to look and taste like? If we happened to land up in the jaws of another animal, would we be considered a tasty morsel?

Val Plumwood, the Australian ecophilosopher who was death rolled three times before being released from the crocodile's jaws, later wrote, in an essay called "Meeting the Predator," that it is only when we can consider ourselves as meat for other animals that we can imagine living in peace on this planet.

Making a stab in the dark we can probably say that we would taste extremely bland but that this blandness carries traces of (at the very least) antibiotics, arsenic, caffeine, and the active ingredients in Benadryl, Tylenol, and Prozac (fed to chickens to alter their moods). We might also taste feathery.

I sit in the yard and watch Sabrina, Lula Mae, and Holly flashing their feathers in the sun—the glint of myriad colors I don't have the words for. Nor do I really have the words to describe what happens to most chicken feathers; it involves venturing into the slaughter houses of the major chicken producers. But this is what I have gleaned: The broiler industry produces billions of pounds of feathers per year. In Europe these are landfilled, while in the U.S. they are autoclaved to produce material (feather meal) that goes into feed for farmed animals and pets, including chickens. It was in this feather meal that the mind-altering drugs were detected.

Cannibals, wrote Montaigne, "do not upset me so much by roasting and eating the bodies of the dead as those persecutors do who torture the bodies of the living." On top of the torture, forcing chickens to eat themselves, that really takes the cake.

Should we then just accept that all store-bought chickens are unnatural and thereby relinquish the anxiety that fills the air as you approach the meat section, anxiety that fills your lungs and bubbles out your nostrils as you try to tread water and hope for dry land soon? Attached to my anxiety, I can't quite do that, and so, cognizant of all the provisos regarding the term *natural*, I am nevertheless prepared to embark on a fairly fanatical search to rule out as many as possible unnatural traits, properties, or characteristics.

Not so easy. America's Test Kitchen has an excellent report on this question of categorization. They say that the USDA has defined the term *natural* only for fresh meat, and the only stipulation is that no synthetic substances have been added. "Producers may thus raise their chickens under the most unnatural circumstances on the most unnatural diets, inject birds with broth during processing, and still put the claim on their packaging." So you seek comfort in some of the other proudly proclaimed labels: raised without antibiotics, hormone-free, vegetarian fed and vegetarian diet, and free-range. Cold comfort it turns out. "Raised without antibiotics" is pretty meaningless, as the claim is not strictly enforced and loopholes are rife, like feeding the flock feather meal laced with residual antibiotics from treated birds. "Raised with antibiotics," which is not a claim anyone makes, is nevertheless one of the main reasons that antibiotic resistance is so rampant (most Americans have imbibed far more antibiotics than they think they have because it comes by way not of the doctor, but of meat). "Hormone-free" is a way of plumping up all the now-ubiquitous reassurances, since the USDA does not anyway allow the use of hormones or steroids in poultry production. "Vegetarian fed" and "vegetarian diet" are categories not regulated by the government. Free-range simply means outdoor access, though how much access isn't regulated.

The only label that is rigorously enforced is the USDA organic seal. This confirms that poultry must eat organic, vegetarian feed that's free of pesticides, antibiotics, and animal by-products, and they must have access to the outdoors.

When I tell some friends about my findings they are appalled that I consulted a cooking resource. Their view is that cruelty is the bottom line and there is only one ethical response to the barbaric practices of industrial farming. They are similarly (though more so) critical of Temple Grandin, the animal activist who has designed more humane methods of animal slaughter, including of chickens.

"Would you eat your own birds?" they throw in my face. The answer is no, never, no more than I would eat my own friends (though who knows, perhaps a situation might one day arise . . .). But like many others I can eat less meat, try to buy from poultry producers who practice humane (and more healthy for all) methods, and where possible contribute, through activist channels, to political change.

Perhaps, though, that is just a justification, a way of keeping my nose in the air and my principles sloshing around in the swamp of the supermarket. Some would say you should only ever eat what you are prepared to kill or, to go even further—that which you have in fact killed, artisanally, with your own hands. I can't even contemplate killing my chickens, my intimates, though my scruples become crumbly when it comes to chickens in general. Between the air and the swamp, between taste and ethics, between intimacy and ignorance there are a lot of loopholes.

Anza Borrego

52

Driving into Borrego Springs, down from the high country through jagged moon-scape mountains, Patricia, Elana, and I stopped at a lookout point. A man was peering into the valley through his binoculars: silent, rigid, focused. When he dropped his binoculars, another man standing there asked him what he was watching. We wait eagerly for his reply, perhaps he has spotted bighorns? But no. This is what he said: My house is down there, my wife's at home. I want to make sure there isn't another car there.

. . .

A few hours later, sprawling atop a cool boulder in the breezy shade of Palm Canyon, we saw a group of hikers looking up into the rocky mountains before us. They had spied two female bighorn sheep—far away, high up, small to the naked eye. A rare and exciting glimpse of these endangered creatures.

Anza Borrego: *Anza* refers to the Mexican explorer and colonizer Juan Bautista de Anza, *Borrego* to desert bighorns that have lived here for eons but are rarely glimpsed. Three Indian nations extended into this region (just a couple of hours from San Diego) when Anza, seeking an overland route from Sonora, Mexico, to Northern California, passed through this valley in 1774: the Cahuilla to the north and east, the Northern Diegueño to the west, and the Kumeyaay to the south. It would be another hundred years or so before cattlemen moved into the Borrego Valley. After a successful well was dug in 1926, irrigation farming began. The groves of citrus trees are, today, dry and brittle, some are dying from drought.

As we returned on the walk down from Palm Canyon the pair of sheep we'd seen seemed to track us, dancing from one rocky outcrop to another. They would disappear for a while, and then there they were again, a little closer. At first the path was quite crowded and included a young woman who worked for the park as an educational coordinator and who told us that these two ewes belong to a matrilineal social structure and probably left their young with a larger group of females as they went foraging, their need for water competing with their wariness about people. She pointed out the dimples in their rear haunches. After they drink, she says, you can see the dimples are gone, the space filled out. They can go four to five days without water. Sometimes the young have a disease that inhibits their energy, so it's very important if you see young to move away quietly because if you spook them and they run they'll use up all the energy they need for fighting the disease. You could see that one had a yellow collar, and so I asked how they got tagged. Using helicopters and nets, rather than drugs, she said. The sheep are netted and brought to a base where they are examined (for healthy teeth, for instance)—a hair is taken for DNA, they are given antibiotic inoculations, and radio tags are fitted. Then they are returned to the exact same spot where they were captured and subsequently monitored telemetrically from the air.

Two young men with elaborate cameras ventured beyond a sign saying DON'T CROSS BEYOND THIS POINT in order to approach the stream, get closer to the sheep, and get good shots. Elana called out, Excuse me, sir, you shouldn't be there. I cringed, hearing my own accent in her Rhodesian twang, a touch of the Borrowdale Madam, but I also admired her for taking citizen action, for acting on behalf of the sheep, the rest of us hiding cowardliness beneath a typically Californian and infuriating laissez-faire politeness. They said, Oh, sorry, we didn't realize, and came back to the path. Five minutes later they were back by the stream. We ourselves were not without technology, though our phones, at this distance, were pretty useless.

In this new wild where animals are collared and managed, cameras displace guns.

. . .

The establishment of Anza Borrego as a state park and desert sanctuary involved a very long struggle. It is interesting that a real boost to the project came as a result of a survey done in 1928 by Frederick Law Olmsted, the figure whose name is most associated with some of the great city parks of the country, including New York's Central Park. He also submitted plans for what became Balboa Park in San Diego, but disagreements meant this never eventuated. He wrote:

Certain desert areas have a distinctive and subtle charm, in part dependent on spaciousness, solitude, and escape from the evidence of human control and manipulation of the earth, a charm of constantly growing value as the rest of the earth becomes more completely dominated by man's activities. This quality is a very vulnerable one. . . . Nowhere else are casual thoughtless human changes in the landscape so irreparable, and nowhere else is it so important to control and completely protect wild areas.

Eventually it was just us three on the path. We continued down toward the camp site, the borregos reappeared, traveling in tandem with us and gradually coming closer. We stopped, sat down and looked at each other, the sheep and we. They grazed, looked up at us now and then, came closer. My heart was beating extra loud. They came within thirty feet I'd say. Not super close but closer than I ever would have imagined being to a bighorn. They were the color of creamy coffee with white on their haunches and muzzles, less than three feet high at the shoulder, delicate faces more like sheep than goats though in many ways they seemed quite goat-like; the large horns that swept back in a half curl, large in relation to their seemingly delicate bodies, were just a little frightening. Their haunches were dimpled. One of them was wearing a yellow collar. They looked sleek, strokeable.

We hold our breath and watch the borregos. They watch us. We wait for them to turn and leap, up and away, up the rock face, along needle narrow ledges, disappearing into a crack in the universe. But they do not turn and leap, they stay and graze, every so often one of them lifts a head and looks nonchalantly in our direction. We interpret the look as nonchalant, but who knows? Time slows down. Unfolds. Each gesture is experienced in slow motion, the body slows and as breath slithers away it infiltrates the world, the wind, the swaying ocotillos, languid giants, their scarlet tips licking the intense blue sky. We always paint our lips with bright red lipstick in the desert to honor the ocotillos. Now we are silent, willing ourselves into the landscape, willing ourselves to become ocotillos or rocks or cacti so that we can see without being seen. Or do we really want to catch the eye of the borrego, to lock looks, to be acknowledged?

The borregos have excellent vision and along with their climbing abilities they are vigilant. They watch for prey. They have no doubt figured out that these curious humans who hike up and down to the springs in Palm Canyon, who wander aimlessly in other parts of the desert, are not hunters or mountain lions. Nevertheless they are on the lookout. They watch us and have no doubt seen us long before we have seen them.

. . .

There is a novel set primarily in Anza Borrego that begins and ends in a museum gallery where a man standing by the wall is watching Douglas Gordon's *24 Hour Psycho*. Hitchcock's *Psycho* slowed, slowed down so that the projection lasts twenty-four hours. Soundless. No need for sound, it is in us, in our cultural memory, those violins screeching. The shower scene, each detail: the shower rail, the curtain rod, fingers clinging, clutching, pulling the curtain down. The man is transfixed, now and again though his attention wanders as he watches other spectators: what they watch how they enter the gallery how they approach the screen suspended in the center of the space how they walk around and watch the reversed image. You can't watch the entire film in one go, the museum shuts its doors and kicks you out and starts again the next day. And anyway who has the stamina?

The middle and lengthiest section of Don DeLillo's *Point Omega* takes place in Anza Borrego, where two men are staying in a ramshackle house, the younger one is planning to make a film about the older man, an unrelenting shot, a single take in which the man is against a wall talking about his experience in the war office. He was an academic, recruited—on the strength of an essay he had written on rendition—for two years to listen to secret meetings, to read classified documents, to conceptualize. A woman arrives at the desert house. She is vague, affectless, her outlines uncertain. She is a blank slate for the projection of desire. Because she's there the younger man becomes fascinated, watches her, wants her to be aware that he is watching. But she seems disinterested. Then she is gone, poof, into the vast expanse of the desert. While others search the two protagonists stay in the house and do nothing but talk and drink. Unlike in *The Searchers*, she is never found. The men eventually leave, the film will never be made. The novel returns to the museum.

The older man's name is Elster. DeLillo lures us into his antinarrative narrative through Hitchcock, and the master of suspense and terror persists, unlikely though it seems, in Anza Borrego. Elster is the name of the character in *Vertigo*—the classic film about a woman disappeared—who hires Jimmy Stewart to find his missing wife. In the end, as all the threads unravel, it becomes clear that Jimmy Stewart, Scottie the detective, has been duped; the mastermind, he who orchestrates the devious machinations, who has been controlling the stories, is Elster.

Elster is Hitchcock and we are Scottie. We: the audience of Hitchcock films, of classic Hollywood westerns, and we who read the reports of the U.S. government's acts of extraordinary rendition, of torture by proxy. Scottie is duped but also complicit. And so are we, DeLillo seems to imply. Yet in his novel, Elster, too, turns out to be ineffective.

In a world where terror, rendition, and surveillance are at the heart of the U.S. experience, DeLillo seems to be saying, there is no place for old-fashioned narratives, initiated by enigma, fueled by terror, propelled toward resolution. The only way to experience terror/Hitchcock is to slow him down, infinitesimal motion, no beginning, no end. This is what some people think. And maybe it is what DeLillo thinks. But I feel that something slightly different is unfolding in *Point Omega*. Like the work of Elster (in the novel), *24 Hour Psycho* might parse terror, slow it down so that the components emerge, so that analysis is possible. But DeLillo's Elster doesn't, in the end, use, in any politically useful way, the knowledge he acquires by being given access to secret documents and meetings. And when *Psycho* is slowed down it lands up like an art object in a museum, where viewers watch each other as much as the image.

DeLillo's gesture is to empty time of events, of things happening, of significance. *Point Omega* is no doubt set in the desert because this is where so many of the great Hollywood narratives took place, unfolding a sense of transcendental timelessness. Tableaus where time is slowed down, before the killings. But for DeLillo the desert is not redemptive, far from it. Yet does not seem to me that it is an unremitting or straightforward critique of classic Hollywood. For me *Point Omega* is also, in a curious way, an acknowledgment that it is not possible to produce an anti-Hitchcock film because the terror that is shorthand for Hitchcock persists. We will keep watching *Psycho* and *Vertigo*, over and over again, because when the threads have been unraveled they are never entirely satisfactorily tied up again, the terror put to sleep, resolution secured. In *Point Omega* the terror that is shorthand for Hitchcock, its link to looking, persists, not just in the movies and art museums but in daily and political life, and even in the desert.

. . .

It is very easy in the desert to succumb to the lure of the transcendental. The space, the immensity, the sky: everything slows down. It is thrilling (for me, though probably not DeLillo) to look into the eyes of these beasts, of this endangered species, so close to extinction. But why? Why do we hold our breath and submit to a slowed-down universe? Is it mere romanticism, a reaching for that panda moment, a moment that expunges the terror and violence that has surely shaped this landscape? And that represses what we know in our bones: the link between all technologies of surveillance and warfare.

Ovis canadensis nelsoni: the desert bighorn who live precariously in the Peninsular Ranges, spreading from the Southern California desert regions down into Baja Mexico. They are a subspecies of the desert bighorn, but because Anza Borrego is notably different from other North American deserts, the species have adapted and exhibit some differences. The population declined from approximately eleven hundred animals in the 1970s to about four hundred in 2000. This number is considerably lower than it once was, long before counting sheep began, before the coming of the white man, before Anza came in his caravan through the valley. Human disturbance—roads, rail, and tram construction, livestock grazing, diseases, hunting—all contributed to the modification and loss of habitat. Like the native humans with whom they cohabited in the southwest for thousands of years, bighorn have little resistance to the diseases of domestic European sheep and cattle. Weather, climate, and other unpredictable natural events have also played a part in reducing numbers, but once a population becomes so small it is vulnerable in a number of ways, including inbreeding (low genetic diversity) and mountain lion predation. In a healthy population of bighorn sheep this is typically not a concern. In 1998 the U.S. Fish and Wildlife Service (USFWS) listed this population segment as an endangered species, and a recovery plan was drafted in 2000. It includes tracking the sheep through such means as electronic collars and the implementation of strategies for ensuring that connectivity among all portions of habitat be established to allow sheep to move freely throughout the Peninsular Ranges (even in more remote regions, renewable energy projects and border-enforcement activities may alter, discourage, and interfere with the path of the sheep).

Since the recovery plan was implemented things are looking up. The most recent (as of this writing) CDFW range-wide survey in 2010 estimated the number of sheep as nine hundred and fifty-five. In 2014 there were a total of ninety-five radio-collared bighorn sheep. These wildlife managers and advocates who have nudged desert bighorns along through recovery and protection programs are, as Ellen Meloy writes in *Eating Stone*, contemporary "attentive shepherds."

They are hybrid creatures, these radio-collared sheep, with their tracking and sensing technologies. The relation between them and their attentive shepherds is particular to what is often called the new wild, but it reminds me of how domestic relations between people and animals might also be reconfigured.

Yellow tag, yellow collar: Victoria, my meditation instructor, and her husband David travel with their cat Scamper in a van—from Colorado down to San Diego and then back up through Colorado, New Mexico, New York City, and on further up to Halifax. He has a yellow collar and lead. Their van is kitted out mainly around the needs of the cat. We walk around a bit with him in Coronado where they are parked in a friend's driveway. I'm amazed. Collaring a cat? But he happily leads us, we all four walk and sniff and pause and meander, moving to his rhythm, his sense of time and the world.

In "Flight Paths," Helen Macdonald writes about how, today, many thousands of animals and birds carry tags, and it is not only scientists who can follow the paths. There are many websites where the public can share the tracking:

New visualizations of traveling animals make the world a more complicated and wondrous place. They reveal that great white sharks tagged in Californian coastal waters migrate over a thousand miles to spend their winters in a remote part of the Pacific Ocean now known as the White Shark Cafe and show how Amur falcons might survive on their journey over the ocean between India and Africa by following swarms of dragonflies making the same trip and feasting on them in flight.

She talks about wonder and about how these kinds of projects give us "imaginative access to the lives of wild creatures," but she also does not ignore the complex histories of technology that enable these new engagements. Early pioneers in the remote tracking of animals sought military funding for their efforts, suggesting that bird migration studies could be used to improve navigation and missile-guidance systems. And she tells a story of a bird used as a spy. The technology of cinema too as everyone knows, after Virilio, owes its origins to the military.

. . .

Is it then true that there is no escape from the "war against terror," even by going for a desert hike? Our encounter with the man using binoculars to spy on his wife certainly casts a shadow over our day trip from San Diego and reminds us of the ever-presence of Hitchcock. But it is also true that the excitement of our encounter with the bighorns gives us a glimpse into other worlds, other pasts, into all that has disappeared—often violently—from the wilder landscapes we encounter today. In the moment when we locked looks with the ewes time seemed to stop, the world closed down like the iris of a camera. And then it opened up.

Lighten Up

53

APRIL 2015

I start working in the garden at first light, building a structure for the cucumbers and pulling out the napa cabbage that has been growing so slowly for so long but now is ready to be pulled from the earth. I want to get work done in the garden before the heat hits, but in fact it turns out to be an overcast deliciously cool day. So I keep working for hours. I strip the outer leaves of the cabbage to feed to the chickens, a favorite food, but you need to kneel and hold the leaves so they have to tug, they like this resistance, I guess they like the play and the exchange. They prefer to tug on the kale and dandelion leaves growing through the netting in the vegetable garden than to peck at the same leaves tossed onto the floor of their run. Then in the kitchen I chop and soak the cabbage—out come all the creepy crawling insects, including a myriad of slugs that get added to the chickens' feast. Actually the cabbage is remarkably intact, there are very few holes from munchers on the inner leaves. Then I soak the cabbage in a brine solution. The plan is to rinse the leaves the next morning, after a decent soak, add all the other ingredients for kimchi, put them in jars, and begin the fermentation process. This is my first kimchi so I am a little apprehensive. During the day on Tuesday I have to buy a few Korean ingredients I don't have on my shelves.

. . .

But my plans are disrupted. In the early hours of Wednesday morning I'm woken by excruciating gut pain. A piercing pain, not cramps. We try a few things: walking, hot water bottle. Nothing works. J calls 911. In the ambulance the medics, who are calm and gentle, ask me which hospital I want to go to. I say Thornton.

A few minutes later they say, We think that Thornton is too far, your heart rate is going down, we need to get to a hospital as soon as possible. Would you be OK with Hillcrest?

. . .

It's a bit of a blur after that. They seem to be attaching things—lines, tubes, sticky things, a defibrillator back and front—all over her body. In the ER she gets wheeled in and out and taken off for tests, including a CT scan with contrast of the stomach. Time passes. And then, after a few hours, the pain starts to dissipate. As she feels the pain subsiding it is as though she rises again into lucidity. She asks, Did you give me a painkiller? No, they say, not yet; we've been waiting to get a better idea of what's going on. No, the pain is leaving of its own accord.

Lying there, painless, she feels relief but also she feels a fraud. She expects that they will dismiss her, tell her to get dressed and leave, never darken their doors again. We are very pissed, she hears the phantasmatic hospital voice pronounce, pissed at you for making false claims and taking up our time and causing us to squander resources. She suspects that some psychosomatic demon has seized hold of her in this dark night, a stork that has swooped in out of the sky, picked her up as though she were a baby, and dropped her, without rhyme or reason or filiation, into this hospital. An old familiar feeling: Why am I here? On the stage in the spotlight, how can I edge out, shuffle backward, merge into the shadows before they discover the hoax? Arriving in Britain, a girl hickishly educated in the colonies, excruciatingly shy, acting, always just about to be found out yet pushing the envelope: How far can I go with this masquerade? And at school in Harare, with friends whose parents were snooty white liberals, who looked down on her a farmer's daughter, convinced that all farmers were rednecks; how she feared and despised them, these people who had no idea the war had already started. But her disdain was blunted by cowardice, a retreat, she could not speak the way they spoke, with assurance and kindness.

She lies there in the ER, a spaghetti entanglement of tubes reaching in and out of her body, a sense of quiet milling around her people speaking in subdued tones, in the background shouting, machines being wheeled, banged, orders barked. J sits by her through the night as she drifts in and out of sleep. When she wakes one time he says to her, It's morning, early, and it's raining outside.

. . .

It's raining outside, outside in the world, in California, where there is a drought. Becalmed, she drifts back into sleep.

. . .

J: endless cups of coffee discovered cold in the microwave. Ideas floated, forgotten, abandoned. The cold leftovers of domestic life. The world, there is a world out there, a drought suddenly leavened by a smattering of rain. He does this, he brings her news, every day, of the world out there. He reads the news, he reads everything, poems a few lines long, fat eighteenth-century books stuffed full of philosophy, gossip and opinion pages on the internet, crime novels galore, the whole of Proust in one continuous sequence, right-wing newspapers as well as the leftist ones because he says you have to know the world you live in. He forgets the world, the coffee in the microwave, as he reads. But he also remembers, and he brings the world to her.

. . .

Eventually the medical team led by Dr. P comes and stands around my bed in the ER. They tell me the story so far, as they see it. The CT scan of the stomach has not shown anything unusual, but what they did see, at the top of the scan where a bit of the lung was included, is an embolism or clot. They will do an ultrasound of the gut area tomorrow. It is possible that somehow the clot has put pressure on the heart, causing referred pain, but they will know more when they also do a CT scan with contrast of the lungs. They will then have a better idea of whether the clot is related to the lung cancer. They don't know at this stage whether what has happened is somehow produced by the CLL or whether Revlimid, the drug to treat CLL, is responsible.

On the basis of this they admit me to the hospital for further tests, and I am wheeled up and into the trauma ward.

The next day they do ultrasounds of the gut and legs as well as a CT with contrast of the lungs. This could not be done last night, as you can't repeat the CT scan within twenty-four hours because of the strain on the kidneys. As I lie there being pumped full of contrast preparing to slide under the huge whirring machine (as I have lain so often for lung scans) I think of the kidneys. What does a kidney look like? Everyone knows—it is shaped like a midcentury swimming pool; it is like a pool in the desert pumping and circulating chlorine and microbes, disinfectant and infections. And what do kidneys sound like? Few people know this, but I do because I once saw a food program in the series *The Mind of a Cook*, featuring April Bloomfield talking about offal. She visits Fergus Henderson of the marvelous restaurant St. John, who is cooking kidneys. You can hear them sizzling on the stove, and he says, Listen! They are talking, they speak to me.

. . .

I am in a shared room, we are divided by a curtain which gives some privacy, but you can hear everything. My neighbor sounds intelligent, polite, middle class. I'm a bit miffed because she is allowed more leeway than I, a degree of freedom to unplug and reconnect herself. I am trying to drink a lot of water to get the poison from the contrast out of my system (I know to do this because of all the scans with contrast I have had in the past, you learn to be a patient if not patient), and so I have to pee a lot and every time the nurse has to come and disconnect me from all the tubes and oxygen and then reconnect me. It turns out that my neighbor lives on the street. She is battling with alcohol withdrawal, is missing front teeth, her complexion is red-tinged, sandpapery, she looks old though I think she is in her forties. She was once, not so long ago, a nurse, and I guess this is why she is allowed to unplug herself each time she goes to the toilet, and then she hooks herself back. The nurses are fine with this. Perhaps they recognize the fragility of the distance between home and hospital, rules and routine on one hand, and on the other, a universe in which nothing is stable, there is no refuge, and you are not the person you are used to being. Except for one young nurse, who insists that the rules must be obeyed, procedures followed, will not allow my neighbor any leeway. Perhaps she too, this young objectionable nurse, on some level recognizes the fragility of the distance, but for her the incipient terror of such knowledge can only be used to defend and to humiliate.

Between routine and observance: a thin line. Between the compulsive repetition of obsessive desire and the orderliness of habit, between ritual and disintegration . . .

When I get my marching orders, the relief thoughtlessly spills out, I'm so glad, can't wait to be home. My neighbor says, I hope they don't discharge me. I'm so happy to be here.

. . .

The gut imaging has shown nothing out of the normal. Diverticula are present, as I know, but not diverticulitis (inflamed diverticula). They find a few more pulmonary embolisms in the right lung but none in the left where the cancer was, so they are unlikely to have been cancerously generated. The team concentrates on the clots. P says that now imaging techniques are more sophisticated, varied and affordable, a lot more imaging is being done, and a lot more stuff is showing up. So people often find out by chance that they have, for instance, clots. It's possible that if the "thing" had not been discovered they could live perfectly happily without treatment. Thus there is a medical dilemma, one that is also partly ethical. Can you say to someone: If you don't have treatment you will probably be fine, but there is an outside chance that you will die? And then we can use your body for science.

What is the treatment? A blood thinner, Lovenox (currently a different thinner is being given through an IV), which I will have to inject myself twice a day—into stomach fat. They have figured out the correct dosage for me. It's quite possible that one dose a day would be sufficient, but the FDA has said it should be two. I will need to discuss this with Dr. K, along with the question of whether to continue with the Revlimid. They are pretty quiet on the question of the stomach pain and the falling heart rate: "We just don't know." . . . "There are medical mysteries." . . . "There are questions we just can't answer." Not so long ago it would have been unthinkable for doctors to reel off these phrases of indeterminacy, at least with such self-confidence and composure. But now it's almost become the new rhetorical orthodoxy. Of course this is infinitely preferable to the God Doctor stance, but it's disconcerting to me that now they have discovered the clot and have something quite exciting to hang onto, other questions and symptoms are brushed aside. What about that gut pain?

Embolism is a cadenced word, it falls from the tongue like a parachute from a plane. But it is also freaky, medical, foreboding. I prefer the word *clot*, which turns my attention to clotted cream. If it comes from Jersey cows clotted cream is truly cream-colored, that very pale yellow that is at once deep and light as air. The paint in our kitchen is called filtered sunlight, and indeed the walls and cupboards do convey a sense of refracted sunlight. Clotted cream, on the other hand, is dense, but they share a tonal quality. *Clotted cream* banishes the bloody redness from my mind.

The nurse shows me how to inject myself, how to grab a bit of stomach fat, plunge the needle in, pull it out, point it upward and keep pressing on the thumb until a safety guard pops out. She did not warn me that my stomach would become a prairie of bruises, a wrinkly plateau of purple sage, tinged with blue and lavender and black and pink. When Raina comes to clean I hide the glass jar where I'm keeping the used injections in case she thinks I'm a junkie. But we talk, and she tells me she injects herself twice a day for diabetes. She complained, but her sister and nieces said, You're breathing aren't you? *Vives.* You're alive, lighten up.

. . .

I had remembered to ask J to transfer the cabbage brine to the fridge. I hope it's not been sitting in salt for too long. I rinse it out and slowly—pottering—grate ginger and chop garlic, cut carrot and daikon radish into matchsticks, add light soy, salted shrimp, scallions, fish sauce, and red pepper powder (what I bought is quite coarse, is this right? What difference does the texture make?). Then the smelly mixture is packed into jars, tops are screwed on, and thingummies, like air vents, are inserted so they can breathe and burp by themselves. I put them in the dark bottom cupboard seated on a towel, next to the potatoes.

A week later ordinary screw tops replace the vented ones, and I put the two jars into the fridge. A few days later yet you open the fridge door and an almighty stink whooshes out into your face. Now one of the jars is out of the fridge, in the kitchen. The smell smells of something other than, or as well as, itself. I'm mystified, can't place the memory, though it is sensuously present, strong. Then it comes to me: *skokiaan*, a thick alcoholic drink made in Zimbabwe from fermented maize meal. It is a stinky sort of repellant smell but also enticing, you know it will be something good. And it is.

Glad to Be Here (Plaintive Knowledge)   54

He whoops, cackles with delight, the room lights up. "God, I'm glad to be here!" We are in an infusion room at Hillcrest Hospital, it's a pleasant spacious room, large windows with great views over the city. Only three of us. But we are all hooked up to tubes and I can think of other places I'd rather be. A more relaxed rhythm here than at Moores Cancer Center, time to chat with the nurses and attendants and each other. Patrick, the guy who guffaws and whoops and cackles, is in a great mood today. His appearance changes each time I see him here, but he certainly doesn't look like a well man, nor does Jerry, the man in the other chair. On the face of it, I can pass for well. We are discussing ports and white cell counts and platelets and different kinds of chemo. "This is the only place," Patrick says, "where I can rave on, without having to explain everything." His delight is infectious. My armor of reserve and skepticism crinkles, I know what he means. He knows a great deal about his disease, as does Jerry. There's so much you have to learn, and often it feels like useless knowledge, of benefit to no one, probably not even yourself, though mostly (not always) it feels better to know than to not know. So there is a kind of camaraderie generated through the exchanges made possible by this shared terrain of plaintive knowledge. Patrick was diagnosed seven years ago, when he was twenty-seven, with a rare form of leukemia. He tells us about hospital experiences he had before landing up at UCSD—pretty grizzly—and we compare the infusion center here with Moores, more like a battery chicken farm. I come here to Hillcrest for some labs and for a monthly immunoglobulin infusion but have to go to Moores for the chemo infusion. "Every time I go to the infusion center at Moores," he says, "I am humbled." Why? I wonder. "Well, I've got all my organs." But he has just had a big toe amputated because of osteoporosis, so he's wearing a brace. He says it's great because he can stand on tippy-toe, which he couldn't do before. Jerry, a year older than me, has been having chemo for years. He looks like an old man, very skinny and hunched over, but also cheerful. Says it's been a bit tough recently, not much appetite, and then the thing is, I couldn't drag myself to the kitchen to prepare anything. So he called up his ex and asked if he could stay. We love each other, are close friends, share grandchildren. She's been making sure he gets a good breakfast and leaves him a sandwich so he's packing on the weight. Then the young guy bursts out, "I love it here! It's the only place where I don't have to explain everything."

. . .

He isn't here any longer. I haven't seen him, maybe he comes another day, I am only here once a month. But there's a cold feeling in my stomach.

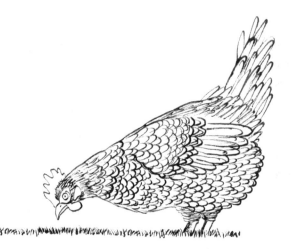

Stinging Nettles

55

Jagged red lightning flashes before my eyes, and I sense on the edges of vision an encroaching army of rats, teeth bared. It is the word *warfarin* that provokes this vision, snatches my attention away from Dr. K mildly recommending a transition from the blood thinner Lovenox to an alternative one, warfarin. Although warfarin will do nothing to get rid of the clot already formed in my lung, it will hopefully prevent further clots while we wait for the body to get rid of the embolism in its own time. When I confess my feverish overreaction to J he corroborates my hysteria: Warfarin is rat poison. We find out that, even though it is now considered a medicine, it first came into commercial use in 1948 as a rat poison. In 1954 it was approved for medical use in the U.S., and it is now on the World Health Organization's list of essential medicines.

The embolism has quite probably been caused by Revlimid (lenalidomide), the drug I have been taking for some time as a pill—first intensively, in combination with Rituximab infusions, then, after a break, on a much lower maintenance dose. It is a derivative of thalidomide. That word *thalidomide* sends me into paroxysms when I first register the connection. It is the drug that caused the thalidomide babies in the 1950s. Well it turns out that "the low level of research that continued on thalidomide, in spite of its scandalous historical toxicity, unexpectedly showed that the compound affected immune function." Revlimid belongs to a group of agents called immunomodulatory agents. It has not yet been approved for treatment of CLL, and in fact I am part of a trial, but the results and expectation are that the good results can last for a number of years after completion of a course. As I finish the book I am still in good shape (apart from chronically deficient immunoglobulin). I'm sure that Dr. K was hoping my immune system would strengthen to the point where I might no longer need that monthly infusion of immunoglobulin that keeps me going. If I had been able to continue in the trial who knows?

Who knows where to draw the line between beneficial and harmful? Doctors, perhaps. But even for them a decision relating to dangerous drugs is often a gamble. Despite all the data, all the testing, all the algorithms, it is impossible to estimate with certainty how any individual will react.

As soon as you start treatment for cancer you enter the casino and start rolling the dice. Although we could say that when you take your first medicine, as an infant, the dice starts rolling. I faced my biggest gamble fairly early on in the cancer journey.

This is how it happened: While I was still in the watch-and-wait period, a year after I received the CLL diagnosis I came down with suspected pneumonia and was treated for months with antibiotics. (Why did I submit to this regime? you ask. My now-self also asks this of my then-self and does not find an answer.) Eventually Dr. K said this is not a good idea, they need to do more thorough testing. I requested this and a non–small cell tumor was discovered in my left lung. The lower lobe was surgically removed.

All cancers weaken one, lower the immune system and prepare the body to be more welcoming to other, new cancers. Usually this is because of treatment, particularly chemo, generally a form of indiscriminate carpet bombing. Those who have CLL, because it is a disease of the immune system, are at risk from the beginning, even before treatment, because the immune system cannot easily fight off other cancers. So this should not have been a surprise. But it was.

As the surgeon predicted, the tumor seemed to have been caught and removed, leaving a clean house. The question arose, however, of postsurgical strategies. The pulmonary oncologist I saw, Dr. X, a highly regarded researcher and clinician, began to discuss the chemo regime that would be required, possibly consolidated by radiation, as follow-up therapies. This is not unusual—to follow up cancer treatment, after it looks as though success has been achieved, with further treatment to guard against the return of the cancer. But I was hesitant.

I could see the wisdom of such a course of action in most cases; however, it seemed to me debatable in the case of CLL. With an already vulnerable immune system I was wary about assaulting it further and laying myself open to new infections and possibly new cancers. Dr. X was appalled by my reticence and explained the illogicality. Without such precautions the lung cancer was likely to return, and when it did it would probably not return in the lungs so would be difficult to detect. Swings and roundabouts. Cures and damages. Poison and elixir. I stuck to my guns and told her I would not make a decision until I had talked to Dr. K. Oh, she said, dismissively, Dr. K will concur with whatever I recommend. I am treating the serious and prime cancer, was her implication. For me, this was not the case. The chronic condition I had to live with was leukemia. The lung cancer had been caught early and apparently dealt with. More chemo and radiation was tantamount to poison. I talked to Dr. K, and he was sympathetic to my position but did stress it was a gamble. But he was not about to jump into the fray and turn up at the next duel with X, as my second. Specialists, in my experience, for understandable reasons, are very reluctant to enter onto each other's turf. K, however, was soon persuaded and set up a three-way meeting at which he persuasively outlined the CLL case. X capitulated in a flash.

Although he took a little persuading, I had confidence in Dr. K. When I first saw him he told me, "There are no such things as side effects. All drugs have effects, some good, some bad, and some both." He also is much more prone to use the analogy of the sweet spot rather than the magic bullet. Where the magic bullet implies a missile that would kill only the organism targeted, it still carries suggestions of toxicity. The sweet spot is that place where a drug or treatment can do least harm and deliver most benefits. Getting there is often a matter of trial and error and a matter, too, of playing the odds.

For five years I underwent regular screening of my lung-and-a-half. And then breathed a temporary sigh of relief, though I'm now experiencing arthritis from perpetually crossed fingers. I know of course that the cancer could creep back sneakily and unexpectedly at any time. But so with anyone who has once had cancer. It would be a stretch to say I'm reconciled to the provisional and transitory, but it's the sweet spot where I rest for the moment.

After dodging the chemo bullet there was still Revlimid and then warfarin to contend with. Both are potentially effective and beneficial drugs for humans if used correctly, but both are also, under certain circumstances, poisonous and with potentially lethal effects. Such is the way of Western medicine. Although I am not about to get on my high horse about non-Western and natural products. Many plants exist on a continuum of healing and harming, delighting and destroying: the opium poppy, coca, various species of strychnine, to name just a few. And like many people, I have encountered the poisonous results of naturopathic medicine.

On the whole I tolerated the Revlimid reasonably well, but on New Year's Eve, the day before my birthday, I began itching crazily, all over, though most excruciatingly on hands and feet. It seemed an ominous harbinger: ringing out the old world and itching in the new. Tests revealed something amiss with my liver so that the elevated bilirubin levels were sending signals to the nerve endings in my skin, causing me to behave like a flea-infested dog. Day and night, night and day, unrelenting torment.

What is the cause? I ask, but no one knows. One of the medicines or supplements is probably the culprit, but it could be anything. Why has it happened now when nothing has changed, no new meds added, no dosages changed? No one knows, no one knows why the body suddenly decides it doesn't like some alien ingestion. Trial and error is the only way to find out, on this the orthodox and naturopathic doctors agree. Eliminate a suspect. Wait and see. If things don't change move on to the next elimination.

. . .

There is only one thing that delivers occasional moments of relief: to sit in a cool bath, reading a very absorbing thriller on my Kindle secured in a ziplock bag.

. . .

I try walking in the garden, examining the plants, seeing what is ripening, where the weeds are. Even this does not distract sufficiently. When, all of a sudden, my eyes alight on a bunch of stinging nettles growing in among the broccoli. These are weeds I always encourage because even though, if seized unthinkingly, they themselves can set off a terrible itching, they make a wonderful soup.

Superstitiously I imagine that eating the nettles will work as a homeopathic cure—that it will take the heat out of my body and that the emerald liquid will circulate into my veins, cleanse my liver, and devour the CLL cells.

Logic overcomes superstition momentarily as I don gloves and pull the nettles. There they sit now on the kitchen bench, two bunches: one for the chickens and one for us. For us I soften a small amount of chopped onions in butter, then (using gloves) throw in the bunch of nettles—a nondescript weedy, dull green color—add stock, and watch the liquid turn a brilliant jewel-like green. Simultaneously, in one of those marvelously alchemical moments in the kitchen, the sting goes out of the nettles.

. . .

Chickens and nettles—that is a different story.

As they devour the stinging nettles I ask them a series of questions, inspired by African divination practices. "E. E. Evans-Pritchard, in his study of the magic practices of the Azande in the Sudan, observed the use of the 'poison-chicken oracle.' In this ritual, a chicken is fed poison and then asked questions. If the chicken dies the answer is taken to be affirmative; if it lives, negative." I ask Sabrina and Lula Mae and Holly whether I am going to die soon. They ignore me, keep gobbling. They survive and so do I.

Chickens with their beaks are unaffected by the fine stinging bristles and go crazy for nettles, which turn their yolks a deep turmeric color.

Like a chicken, I feel I should eat the nettles raw. Taste the sting, swallow the sting, feel the itching dissipate, feel a feathery fluttering, watch the soft fluffy feathers grow out of my skin. So much more attractive than the angry pustules glaring at me now, interfering with touch.

Instead I start the slow process of elimination. In the end it turns out to be a naturopathic supplement. Almost as soon as I stop taking it the symptoms subside. I do not think that in and of itself the supplement was causing the itching. And it is not clear either that it is in and of itself incompatible with Revlimid (or vice versa), since for quite a time I was taking them together. But something in the fragile ecosystem of my body shifted. Two things are clear: First, when a product or substance produces a toxic effect it often has to do with context, with the relation and reactions to one another of different substances within a given environment; and, second, contexts or environments are themselves not fixed entities.

Nettles are vicious weeds in one context and delicious nutritious herbs (rich in vitamins A and C, iron, potassium, manganese, and calcium) in another. Antibiotics can save lives in one context and wreak havoc in another. With so many antibiotics becoming ineffective, though, the focus of current research is less on context and more on the acknowledgment that, as Rob Knight puts it, "antibiotics are essentially poisons that are more toxic to bacteria than they are to us." The overuse of antibiotics (not just through medicinal application but also through eating meat from animals that have been routinely dosed with antibiotics) can cause chaos in the ecosystem that is the human gut, and microbes (it is the pathogenic microbes that antibiotics are meant to target) have developed resistance. Microbes are able to absorb new genetic information extremely fast (largely because of their propensity for horizontal gene transfer), which means that the resistant microbes have multiplied and become ever more virulent.

Some scientists believe that the mistake of overprescribing antibiotics was made because of a fundamental misrecognition: that destroying the microbes that make us sick would give immunity. The immune system, in this view, is about sensing and fighting off pathogens, about securing a poison-free environment. "Alternatively, you could say the microbes are calibrating the immune system, triggering responses that create a suitable niche for themselves while pushing out their competitors." To many scientists the immune system's main function is not warding off pathogens—it is "to manage our relationships with our resident microbes. It's more about balance and good management than defense and destruction."

Indeed, but the exuberant enthusiasm currently sweeping through fans of the microbiome tends on occasion to produce a view of the microbial kingdom as an essentially benign regime. Words like *symbiosis* and *ecological balance* are invoked with incantatory relish to summon up a kind of harmonious utopian love-in. Microbes are conceived of as invariably good and beneficial or, alternatively, utterly and invariably bad.

Given my verging-on-fanatical interest in fermentation I am guilty of flapping away with the rest of the fans. But it was in the garden rather than the kitchen that I was brought up short with a shock.

As a gardener I'd rather not use poisons on pests or on plants, and so when there is an upset in the ecological balance of the vegetable garden, in the cabbage patch, say, I first try using that universally effective deterrent—a strong spray of water—and if that doesn't work I reach for an organic or natural treatment, such as Bt (*Bacillus thuringiensis*), a soil-dwelling microbe that you spray as a live toxin onto the plants. I, like other organic gardeners and farmers who have been using Bt—harmless to birds, fish, and mammals—since the 1950s, assumed it worked by starving the insects (effectively by punching holes in their guts, thereby paralyzing their digestive system, causing them to stop feeding and die). But it turns out that this is only a part of the gruesome story; it takes a week for a caterpillar to die of starvation, but Bt kills much more quickly. It seems that the caterpillars' gut bacteria, that you would assume would protect them, are actually the means through which Bt kills.

They are harmless if they stay in the gut, but they can pass through the holes created by Bt toxins and invade the bloodstream. When the caterpillar's immune system senses them, it goes berserk. A wave of inflammation spreads through the caterpillar's body, damaging its organs and interfering with its blood flow. This is sepsis. It's what kills the insect so quickly. The same thing probably happens to millions of people every year. . . . As in the caterpillars, the same microbes can be good in the gut, but dangerous in the blood.

It's all about context. But context itself is variable. And the gut's immune system is selective and reactive—not constant and standardized.

Contexts and substances are not fixed. One of the most amazing stories in modern medicine concerns the way in which the most lethal of viruses can be transformed into something like an angel of mercy. The HIV virus, for instance, turns out—once the toxic component has been disabled—to be the perfect vector for delivering information to the immune system so that it can mobilize T cells to target particular cancer cells. The very attributes that make viruses so virulent

("They live to infect and reproduce; they infect and reproduce to live," as Siddhartha Mukherjee notes) have been exploited for different and hopefully much more beneficial ends. In CAR-T therapy blood is taken from the patient, and in the lab the T cells are genetically modified by being cut with the disabled virus vector, multiplied, and reprogrammed. These cells are then infused back into the patient's body, where the modified killer cells are let loose to do what they have been retrained to do.

Are there any medicines that are free from poison? Yes (but they are not necessarily available in pill form or via infusion): therapeutic practices, such as tai chi, qigong, meditation. Those are my choices but they are not the only ones. Nor are they guaranteed to deliver you from the maws of cancer or other illnesses. There are those who believe they do possess such power, and though I don't share that belief I understand and am sympathetic to the choice made by some to reject all orthodox treatment. The over-medicalization of cancer treatments in this country propels patients into an either-or choice. I do believe that these therapeutic practices do two important things: They reduce stress considerably (and stress is very likely one of the most underestimated exacerbaters of illness) and they nurture and stimulate the immune system—in gentler ways than the killer T cells, for instance.

. . .

The nettle soup sits on the stove, ready to be consumed. To finish it off I hesitate between sour cream and yogurt. But only for a moment, there is only a small amount of yogurt left—to be saved as an offering for the chicken sphinxes. I pour the soup into bowls, scoop out a spoonful of rich thick organic cream, and swirl it into the emerald sea. It is warm, tartly sweet. I feel it entering my gut, placating the hungry microbes. I imagine the greenness spreading through my body, calming those greedy lymphocytes, those hungry ghosts that haunt my body and soul.

A Talent for Cancer

56

My relative examined you, observed a few of your normal body cells, compared them with what it had learned from other humans most like you, and said that you had not only a cancer, but a talent for cancer.

It is an alien creature—her captor/savior—who speaks these words to Lilith, the main protagonist in Octavia Butler's 1987 science fiction novel, *Dawn*. A young black woman, Lilith, is one of the few humans to have survived a nuclear apocalypse that destroys Earth.

It is not in fact only humans who get cancer; mammals, fish, reptiles, and even plants share this talent. But as far as we know it is peculiar to earthly beings. And though, at this time in the world, it seems to us that cancer has never been so bad, so close to a pandemic, and yet simultaneously never so close to defeat, in fact cancer is as old as time, the time we humans know. Cancer means crab, cancer cells were named for a reason, because they have claws. They dig in and hang on, the image is vivid and apt. But they also mutate and adapt, and perhaps this is something that contemporary biology and medicine understand better than before. In this sense cancer, far from being exceptional, is a model of evolutionary diversification.

Instead of the crab with claws, we are now encouraged to envision molecular communication and exchange. Time for a species might be long, but for an organism it is condensed (and for the creature who has a talent for cancer but not necessarily for outliving it). By the time you get through the various stages of cancer, it has often reproduced and diversified and it might not be much fun hanging on and enduring the changes. But it does seem to be quite a lot of fun for scientists interested in diversification, mutation and adaptation, and questions of how species emerge and evolve. Cancer is a dynamic ecology, and the gold standard now is about diversifying the singular crab-like entity named cancer and investigating what it is: on one level, what different cancers have in common and, concomitantly, how they can be differentiated; and, on another level, fine-tuning the treatment for individuals by understanding how their cancer is adapting and responding.

I can't say that it's exactly fun to have this talent but it is fascinating. We have a talent for it not because we have survived for so long, not because we have outlived cancer, but because we have coevolved with it. Now, with an increasing understanding of and attention to stochastic models, we can apprehend cancer not as something deviant and exceptional, but as a part of being a creature and as a model that might help us to make sense of so much evolutionary activity. To see evolution not always as a structure manifested in straight lines, in lineages of descent, but in a patterning more akin to the shape of algae or fungal webs.

Lilith is saved by the Oankali aliens. However, she has not only to learn to coexist with other species, but in order to survive, to mate with an Ooloi, the Oankali's third sex, to produce a nonhuman, genetically altered child. In the *Xenogenesis* trilogy (of which *Dawn* is the first book), Butler explores human beings faced, via hybridity, with a decentering of the human. Her story is, through the allegorical dimension of a science fiction fantasy, a survival story: of African Americans in this country and of humans in a postapocalyptic world. Perhaps it is just a story, the story about a talent for cancer, but as Donna Haraway has written in relation to Butler: "It matters which stories we tell to tell stories with; it matters what other concepts we think to think other concepts with."

Phobia

57

THE CHICKENS COME HOME TO ROOST

Now take your average brain tumor. Who gets brain tumors? Intellectuals get brain tumors, that's who. And heart attacks? Well, if you're emotionally fucked up, you'll get a heart attack for Christmas.

All my life or for as long as I can remember I have been in thrall to a phobia, a blood phobia. And then, without warning, I am diagnosed with a blood disease.

"Lesley Addison leave the room!" We are in a biology classroom at Queen Elizabeth High School for Girls in colonial Salisbury (now Harare), and Mrs. MacDonald, pretty pert popular blonde Mrs. Mac, is addressing her with a smirk, winking at the other girls and soliciting sniggers. Easier to get her out of the classroom before she faints, so predictably, when the "B" word is mentioned. Part of her is relieved, grateful to be spared the sensation of spinning nausea, the smell of the slaughter yards, the dripping of blood in the butcher's shop. There was a man, called the butcher boy, who delivered meat to neighboring farms, riding around on dirt tracks on a heavy bicycle in the sun with a huge pannier on front loaded with brown paper parcels seeping blood. Every new moon he would abandon his bike and become a raving madman. Struggling against losing consciousness in the biology classroom, she would experience herself becoming the butcher boy, spinning out of control.

It is humiliating to faint, to be carried out or to lumber groggily for the door and fresh air. But it is equally humiliating to be told to leave the room and to be laughed at. Moreover, since Mrs. Mac never called her back, the girl was destined, as the teacher well knew, to aimlessly roam for hours the deserted corridors of Queen Elizabeth High, reeking of disinfectant and urine, and thus destined to fail O-level biology. However, she calculated that she could pass with only a few marks in physiology if she did brilliantly in botany. But this wasn't enough. She also wanted Mrs. Mac to be humiliated by her public success. So, despite sarcastic discouragement, she elected to enter the National Student Science Competition, with a project on poisonous plants.

For six months she rode around the farm with a hessian bag tied to the saddle that she would soak before going out and in which she would store the wildflowers and suspicious-looking plants she gathered. Back home, with whatever books she could muster from the town library and visits to the botanical garden, she would try and identify them all, poisonous or otherwise, and then either press them or pickle them in formaldehyde. There was one book she loved above all others, it had a dark green cardboard cover with an illustration of a flame lily, or *Gloriosa superba*, in orange and yellow, the country's national flower. The book was called *Common Veld Flowers*, and all its color was condensed into this glorious lily on the front; all the other flowers were illustrated in black and white.

When she left Rhodesia before it became Zimbabwe but after the war of liberation had begun, she left this book along with so many others behind. Samuel Chigwedere took care of all their literary books, and the others went into storage or were given away to the Red Cross, where her grandmother worked and collected books donated for book sales. There were rooms there filled with books, books heaped in great piles on shelves and under tables and on top of tables and in boxes and on the floor. Unsorted, disorganized, dusty, books once loved, read over and over again or never read, rejected, spurned, tossed out the window, books that circulated in and out of the Red Cross over the years. You would enter those rooms and be engulfed by a musty enticing smell. The smell of words. The aroma of fiction.

Browsing through these books over the years, ever since she was a little girl, she acquired a different sort of education than that offered by Queen Elizabeth or the junior school where she had boarded. Here there were no divisions into subjects like biology and English and French and domestic science, no constraints shaped by notions of age and suitability of reading matter. There were hundreds of books without covers, usually a murky green or dirty brown color, but when you opened them up all sorts of worlds emerged. You might find yourself in the Soviet Union or in the classical world or in Grimm's Fairy Tales or in the Deep South of the USA. Caressing those gorgeously color-coded Penguins—orange for fiction, green for crime, and very occasionally poetry in blue—you might learn a lot about the unknown. Sex, for instance. This is where, at the age of thirteen, a few years before the poisonous plants episode, she read *Lady Chatterley's Lover*.

Fueled by malevolent ambition and righteous revenge she won a prize, that fifteen-year-old girl, and in the process learned a little about botany. Winning the science competition made absolutely no difference to her blood phobia. She would soon abandon science, and so, many years later, when diagnosed with a disease of the blood, she would be doubly overwhelmed: ignorant *and* phobic. Albeit fairly well read. And well versed in obsessive, deflective, substitutive modes of compensation.

When I left Zimbabwe and went to live in Glasgow as a graduate student and suffered terribly from the cold and the alien culture, *Common Veld Flowers* turned up one day in my letter box. A Glaswegian lover had found it in an antiquarian bookshop.

She: a girl on a farm long ago. I: a woman diagnosed in her fifties with a blood cancer. Between that girl and I vistas unfold.

She tried a lot of things. As a teenager she volunteered to work in a hospital, a foolish fantasy of heroism that lasted a day; she tried various therapies, such as writing, forcing herself to watch movies. She even wrote a book during which she had to watch a lot of bloody scenes in movies, would not turn away, would make notes, observing every cut.

Nothing cured her phobia.

In therapy images and fragments of stories would emerge: a patchwork memory in which frayed images, fragments of violence, were sewn. She imagined drunken driving through the night, on country roads, a woman in labor, a collision, something fatal. She elaborated a history—infidelity, recriminations, discord.

I imagined this as the origin of all our family unhappiness. Now I am more inclined to view it as a screen memory, a constructed coherence screening out less accessible (though also possibly more banal) troubles.

You don't have to actually see blood for a phobic reaction to kick in. It doesn't have to be real in the sense of there, visible, touchable, sticky. You can just hear the dreaded word, hear someone describe a simple incident, and like Pavlov's dog the symptoms spring to life. There is no logic to the mechanism, you do not stop and think, you are totally at the mercy of your bodily reactions. It wouldn't be so bad if you just passed out, conscious one moment, unconscious the next. But no, it's a slow dragging through a murky liminal zone where there are no borders, no edges, no center of gravity, no solidity, nothing to hold on to. You feel as though your insides are emptying out, everything blurs and spins. You can't stay upright, you go weak in all your joints, the world swims drunkenly. Sweat pours off you. Clammy.

. . .

And then one day she receives a diagnosis. She has leukemia, a disease of the blood. She almost passes out as the hematologist explains to her in simple terms what produces this condition. He tells her that if you are going to get cancer this is the best cancer to have. Chronic Lymphocytic Leukemia. It's a mouthful, hard to remember. Oh don't worry he says, there's a more friendly name, we just call it CLL. He says he cannot say exactly how long she has to live, he thinks at least six years, but who knows? maybe twenty. He is an elderly man, and kind, doing his best to break the bad news as he has been doing to so many people for so many years. He says that one of the world's top researchers in CLL and other blood diseases is here at UCSD, and he will try and refer me to him: Thomas Kipps.

Blood work. The very worst thing about having CLL turned out to be the blood work. Muffled hell and torture and high anxiety every time I had to do blood work, and I had to do blood work a lot. It got worse as the years passed and my veins became hardened and more and more incalcitrant. Anticipating and dreading needlestick. Spilt blood. Blacking out.

It was Sybil, who had been through chemo treatment and had a port installed, who told me to ask for one. It changed my life.

A port (or portacath, a portmanteau of *portal* and *catheter*) is a small medical appliance that is installed beneath the skin, usually in the upper chest just below a collar bone. A catheter connects the port, under the skin, to a vein. Ideally, the catheter (a long narrow hollow plastic tube) terminates in the superior vena cava, just upstream of the right atrium. A needle can be inserted into the portal (a small silicone bubble), and infused agents can be spread throughout the body quickly and efficiently. Blood samples can also be drawn. Contrasts can be inserted for certain scans (particularly for the lung cancer which develops after the CLL). The only evidence of a port is a slight bump and line under the skin. When not in use the port is closed and the skin is as smooth as after any needle insertion. Most commonly a port is inserted for a long chemo treatment and then removed, but it can be retained for several years.

I guess that for some people a port is a rather formidable object. It seems to make solid the fact that you are in for a long haul, a long chemo treatment or perhaps a long cancer. But for me it was an object invested with magical properties.

Why did no one on my medical team (in general responsive, knowledgeable, supportive) suggest a port years earlier, during chemo even? Perhaps there are issues about expense/insurance. Or perhaps the risks are seen to outweigh the benefits (having to have it flushed regularly, for instance). Or the fact that there is some minor pain associated with each use, perhaps they feel that this might deter people. But ultimately I think it is a case of imagination reaching its limits or, perhaps, a case of two incompatible imaginaries colliding. The doctors and nurses probably have no idea what the phobia feels like, since the phobic patient, overcome by an excess of imagination, is accustomed to subterfuge, pretense, performative nonchalance, to warding off humiliation by shrugging off their condition as though it were a minor irritation. You say, fairly casually, I'd like to lie down please when you do the draw, I get a bit woozy, not so good with blood, need to look the other way, but you cannot bring yourself to describe what a phobia is like, how frightening and humiliating too. A superstitious sensation that if you speak the symptoms they will appear. The doctors and nurses on my team are not unimaginative people. On the contrary. But here's the thing: I guess that they are either inured to blood or in thrall to it, in the sense that it is utterly fascinating to them, this is what they work with, what they think about, scrutinize, read about, and imagine. Imagine in all its complex permutations, in particular they imagine how CLL blood might be recomposed so that patients might not suffer so and one day even be cured. You can sense the excitement of the researchers when we have lectures in the support group. For them my response is probably and quite simply unimaginable.

I myself can imagine people who might not like to garden, but I can't imagine people who simply don't like gardens, who find a garden a frightening and overwhelming place to be. Or eggs. People who don't like eggs or are phobic about chickens.

And now? Now, if the port was taken out (and eventually it will have to be), I dare say I will revert, infantilism will seize hold. But I am a bit better in thinking about my body and its circulating blood. For instance, I am able to write these sentences without taking long breaks to lie down, drink water, think of other things. I can read about my disease. I can have discussions without passing out or making an excuse and deflecting the conversation. Not cured though.

Once, recently, in the infusion center, they had to use the veins for a trial, it was a long blood draw, I was scrabbling around on the edge of consciousness as tubes and tubes were filling up, panic rising. Amie, the nurse assistant, panicked sympathetically for a moment and then began to tell me how to make chicken adobo, step by step, the Filipino way. Are you paying attention? she asked sternly, you have to remember every detail, every step of the recipe. No short cuts. She described the smells, the taste. The smell of vinegar, how it overpowers everything, so sour, but when the chicken is cooked you don't taste or smell the vinegar, there's just a tanginess. Kind of magic. That's all it is, she said eventually, not complicated, you can make it yourself. And when it was over, the draw and the story of the recipe, she confessed to me that she had never made it herself. So perhaps I told it to you all wrong, my son does the cooking, before that my husband.

So this is the irony: It has taken leukemia to begin to cure me of a blood phobia. Although, the way things are going, I will probably die of leukemia before I am entirely cured of the phobia.

Walking Meditation

When I walk alone in the beautiful orchard, if my thoughts have been dwelling on extraneous incidents for some part of the time, for some other part I bring them back to the walk, to the orchard, to the sweetness of this solitude, and to me.

—MONTAIGNE

In the Blue Mountains, on the north shore of Sydney, on the south shore, I used to escape to write. And after grappling for hours I'd clear the air, or so I thought, and walk—by the ocean, through the forests. And as I walked the ideas would whirl, what I'd written would shatter and recompose, I'd retrieve forgotten fragments, discover out of the air new felicitous phrases. It was a sort of séance. A continuation of intensity. I remained the nerdy kid who studies too hard and anxiously right up to the moment of the exam. And then in the exam, or back at the writing desk, many of the discoveries would disappear, all the ideas would be sucked back into the genie's bottle, irretrievable except as a ghostly memory. Then I learned some techniques of meditation and how to disengage from the octopus grip of writing. How to break free, let it go, breathe, notice, feel the sensations. I'm pretty good at noticing, but the temptation for me is always to name, to catalog, and for those things I cannot name, I either put them into the "later" box (back home look up that plant) or, if walking in the neighborhood, stop and ask if lucky enough to see a person in their garden, say. Now I see the walk, the break for a cup of tea, the pause to review what I will cook tonight as a real break, all thoughts of what I'm writing are banished. But particularly this is so with walking. And it isn't as though I don't notice the plants and, particularly in a wild place like here at Dorland, how their leaves are structured, say, so I can guess their genus or family. But the cataloging drive is less intense. And the details which spring out and draw me into their sensory orb are often surprising, unrehearsed, unfamiliar. And I return to the Mac Air refreshed.

A Ticket for Tuppence

59

A week before departure for Australia, for the big trip—to the Red Centre and Arnhem Land in the far north and to remote Cape York in Queensland—Dr. K drops a bombshell. He advises me to reconsider. Given your latest test results, he says, and given the dangers of travel, especially of the long flight. I'm aghast, argue with him. Eventually he says, I would never tell you what to do and in fact I don't know what you should do, but think of this: You surely want to finish this book, and I'm sure you have more books to write and more traveling to do, and if I were you I'd weigh that up against the dangers of taking this trip.

I burst into tears and cry like a six-year-old. Weep and wail, as I see all that planning and saving and excitement, that dancing balloon of expectation, punctured. Hope goes out of me in a whoosh.

This is how it began. Or at least let's decide to start this episode here, at a relatively high point, a point of relief and euphoria. I get home at the weekend from the hospital episode that began with gut pain and ended with the discovery of a pulmonary embolism, and pick up where I left off—making kimchi. This brings me back into the sensuous world of ordinary smells and tastes, it levels me back onto an even keel. Then on Monday Sheila from Dr. K's office calls to check in and to make sure I have stopped taking the Revlimid. Actually I haven't because the hospital had told me to continue until I saw Dr. K and discussed it with him. No, no, stop immediately, says Sheila.

A few days later I see Dr. K. We are both despondent. It looks like this is the end of the Revlimid. After the intensive treatment, combined with Rituxin and subsequent good results, I went off it for a while, to be drug-free, and then returned to a much lower maintenance dose. What Dr. K was particularly interested in was not only its ability to tackle the CLL but also its probable ability to actually enhance the immune system. A twofer, as he had said. He is upset and disappointed, I was doing so well. He says that in the early stages of trialing Revlimid for CLL there were some issues with clots, but since it's been combined with a small aspirin daily there have been no incidents. I am the first. I feel bad for upsetting his trial. It takes a long time and a lot of research to get a drug to trial. Many trials fail, sometimes complications and deaths are involved, and I imagine that this must entail a barrage of emotional responses for the doctors and researchers as well as the patients. I feel upset for me too: Whatever next? My heart starts sinking deep down through my legs into the floor. There is no proof that Revlimid has caused this embolism, as the doctor in the hospital pointed out, it might have been there for some time and if it hadn't shown up accidentally it might have eventually dissipated by itself. But Dr. K is adamant that it's not worth the risk of continuing. For the moment let's take a break from CLL treatment, he suggests, until symptoms return and need attention. For the moment we will concentrate on the clot in my lung, get me onto a regime of blood-thinning medicine in the hopes of stopping further clots while we wait for the body to get rid of the lung clot in its own time.

He thinks traveling to New York next week will be OK but is more worried about the big trip to Australia. This is because weekly monitoring of the blood thickness and flow (necessary when on the blood-thinning drugs) will be difficult, it will be hard to maintain a constant diet, and I will frequently be far from any hospital. He has himself recently been in Melbourne and Sydney, but because he gave nine talks, he saw nothing outside conference rooms and lecture halls, though he would have liked to, he says, and he would like me to see more of the continent.

Dr. K wants me to take warfarin rather than Lovenox, but you can't just terminate the Lovenox injections, there has to be a transition period. Sheila books me in to the Coumadin clinic, Coumadin being the brand name for warfarin. This is a nightmare for me. Initially, it means blood tests every two days, and it has to be a vein in the arm, because the flush is incompatible with the port.

We take off for the Berkshires and New York with a bag full of injections. Walking through greenness, the balm of friendship renewed. I have known Kari and a number of her dogs, all of whom we have outlasted, over almost thirty years of friendship. First there was Idaho, when we shared a rental in Orange County where we met, both of us as young visiting professors at UC Irvine, then Gustav in Los Angeles, and now Mathilde. Gustav was my favorite. The general consensus seemed to be that, though large and loving, he was a little dim. Yet he appreciated my reading aloud to him and would rest his large head on my lap while I intoned from Nietzsche or Hannah Arendt. Perhaps it was the cadence of the language he liked rather than the philosophical implications, I do not really know, but an attunement to cadence is a sensitivity many humans lack.

Now it is Mathilde who leads us through greenness, through meadows and woods and away into a pond in pursuit of a stick. I search for the New England Red that Katie writes about and at first do not recognize it, as I am looking for bright red like the blood that spurts out from the injection that morning. But here red is rusty and once I see it is everywhere—on barn doors, rooftops, gates. Michael and Kari take us to the legendary Berkshire Mountain Bakery in the town of Housatonic. Richard Bourdon was a mentor to Chad Robertson, of Tartine Bakery in San Francisco, and an inspiration for the slow ferment. We buy, for our lunch on the bus to New York City, a couple of mini ciabattas spread with cream cheese and dill and tomato. And then just as we are leaving, almost out the door, J and I turn back simultaneously and add two *pain au chocolats*.

Back in San Diego the tests indicate that the transition to Coumadin can proceed. Coumadin comes in the form of tablets so you'd think it would be easier than constant blood drawing and daily injections. Moreover, it's a common drug, many people are on it (some permanently) so you'd think it would be a breeze. Not for me. Generally speaking a balanced diet is indicated, with a moderate consumption of leafy greens (and absolutely no liver or mango). Leafy greens, tending to contain a lot of vitamin K, a natural coagulant, lower the effect of Coumadin (although the vitamin is not immediately available to the body, it is gut microbes that convert leafiness into vitamins available to the body). My problem is immoderation; I love and grow and consume leafy green vegetables like a rabbit. No problem, they say at the clinic, for of course we are in an accommodating age and environment. The thing is, you have to be constant and systematic: Eat the same amount of greens every day, and then through trial and error they can figure out the dosage required. OK, so I try and stick to one cooked green vegetable a day, one salad, and one green drink. But it's hard to regulate, to get a constant reading, and my consumption turns out to be in excess of moderation. Normalization is the goal. And here is the other problem: The INR has to be tested very regularly, daily to begin with. INR stands for international normalized ratio, and the test is administered to check on how fast your blood clots. The aim is to maintain an INR in target range and to adjust your Coumadin dose so that it falls within target. The test is simple—a pinprick on the finger.

But being blood phobic this sends me into a spin. The more trivial it is—just a pinprick—the worse the reaction. Or at least the struggle. You walk into the clinic and panic starts rising as you anticipate your own uncontrollable bodily response. You know it is wildly incommensurate with the simplicity of the test. And this just makes matters worse. You balk at confessing your weakness and asking to lie down for the test. You feel like such a big baby. Personnel at the clinic change daily it seems, there are many trainees, the more senior doctors are nevertheless very young, harassed, and keen to impress upon you the importance of regimes.

My worst reaction was with the best, or anyway, most agreeable doctor. It was the only time I saw Dr. W. He explained things with calmness and clarity rather than with punitive zeal. Feeling at ease I didn't ask to lie down.

But as soon as she extends her finger, like a princess in a fairy story, she starts transforming. First: a vague wooziness, morphing into nausea. The barriers between her body and space start disintegrating, a jagged blackness enters into her. Sweat is pouring off her, her clothes are soaked. He is kindly, this Dr. W, he stays quietly by her side, he is not overly fussy, he lets things take their course and doesn't seem perturbed when she vomits into the wastebasket.

She drives home shivering. So much time lost. She is exhausted and cold, wants to get under the bedclothes. She beseeches Elvis to come to bed with her, makes a hot water bottle to comfort them both, hoping the warmth will absorb and disperse the residue of guilt and shame and humiliation.

. . .

Eventually, after what seems like a long, long time but is actually only weeks, my IRN falls within the target range, the Coumadin dosage is stabilized, and I don't have to visit the clinic so frequently. We breeze along. Then, something slips. I forget to take a dose one night and my unconscious finds this a much happier state of being, and so do the warfarin or Coumadin tabs. For four days they have a vacation, or call it a reprieve, swooning happily, pillowed in their little pillbox which looks exactly like all the other little pillboxes, all jumbled up on the bedside table, perching on and under and round about raggedy rascally piles of books. My IRN plummets. But at the clinic they are fairly confident that it can be brought back into range fairly easily. A week later, when I see Dr. K, which is a week before getting on the plane, it has hardly edged up.

He throws a wobbly. I start crying.

I have been planning this trip for a year. Tickets have been booked, are nontransferable, and almost everything has been paid for—hotels, car rentals, internal flights, tours. J is already in Australia, and I am scheduled to meet up with him in Adelaide in a week. There is no way in the world I can give up this trip. But I also don't want to die just yet.

Then, as the howling turned to hiccoughs, I had an idea. Dr. W! He is a Coumadin specialist, maybe he would have a suggestion about what I could do within a week to get the warfarin into an acceptable range? But there was no way I could get to see him officially within the week. Then I remembered that my neighbors Bob and Barbara, the doctor, had mentioned once in passing that he was a friend. So I knocked on their door and asked for help. Barbara sent him an email. We waited and later that night got a reply: The best thing would be for Lesley to go back on Lovenox for the duration of the trip. Although the transition from Lovenox to Coumadin is slow and subject to testing, the other way around is straightforward. She should start a few days before traveling and will still have to be careful on the plane trip and indeed in long car trips. Barbara advised on restriction stockings and the need to exercise every hour, if possible, while traveling. Sheila fast-tracks a supply of Lovenox injections from the pharmacy and helps me negotiate the insurance, initially trying to charge me thousands of dollars but in the end settling for the correct thirty-six-dollar copay. Jane W and Lynne T and Leslie D offer a gift: to pay for an upgrade to business class to make the travel easier. Qantas will not under any circumstances allow this. At the eleventh hour, while I am scrolling through Air New Zealand, a flash sale pops up, and I get a business-class ticket for tuppence!

The next day I hop on the plane, bound for Yirrkala.

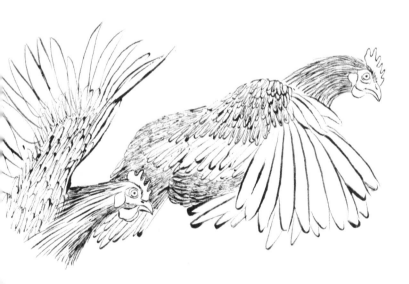

Reaching Yirrkala

60

To Yirrkala July–August 2015

We are here. Here in Arnhem Land, not there, or over there, or thereabouts, but here: in Yirrkala. On the edge of the world and at the center of the world. Oceanic Arafura blueness stretches out beyond the bay, merging with blue sky, reaching toward Indonesia. Behind us: stone country, a dry and stony continent. The dust, though, swirls in the wind, fueling images, imagination.

The obsession began as I wrote those words, the last words of "Blue/Shimmer": "Next time I return to Australia it will be to the Northern Territory, to Arnhem Land, perhaps even to Yolngu country, where the land and the sea are continuous, where boats come and go." Perhaps it began earlier, as I walked out of the New South Wales Art Gallery, stood on the steps, after-images shimmering, etched in the air. More than anything I wanted to get there, to Yirrkala, a center of Yolngu *rom* (law), *manikay* (music), and *bunggul* (dance), to the place where early land claims were so indelibly tied to art, I wanted to see the bark paintings for which Yirrkala is famous.

Do it now. Now now now, said a stentorian inner voice. Now while your blood count is good and your energy up, before the symptoms start creeping back. I started planning: reading, calling, getting quotes, weighing up dates and prices, coordinating friends, charting a journey across the continent, a journey that grew and grew and that would take us much further afield than Yirrkala.

Poor chickens: once the object of a magnificent obsession, now abandoned, bereft, scratching for worms in an impoverished landscape.

To Melbourne

Iron lacework on the buildings in Carlton and Fitzroy sets my heart aflutter.

In the Bella Bar at Trades Hall, a grand Victorian building, tattered now and frayed at the edges, we celebrate a new book (John Cumming), films (John Hughes, the Australian one), friendships.

Big Cities—Melbourne and Adelaide and Brisbane—portholes, ways in and out of a continent, spaces to flit through and perch for a night.

To Adelaide

I arrive in Adelaide just in time to hear J's talk and to share a meal with Denise and Mark at an African restaurant.

To Alice Springs

We board the train midday in Adelaide and alight twenty-four hours later in Alice. The train is called the Ghan, an abbreviated version of its previous nickname, Afghan Express, referring to the Afghan camel drivers who arrived in Australia in the late nineteenth century to help the British colonizers find a way to reach the country's interior. Waking in the dark at 5 AM, the train stops at Marla, we get out and take a walk, the sun comes up over the desert redness. Bacon and egg sliders, good coffee, braziers.

Redness. This is the dominant sensation of the center. But other colors exist.

Olive Pink. Imagine a grevillea or protea, deep-pink flowers and silvery olive leaves, thin and long, their shape and oliveness designed to cope with the heat. Olive Pink, however, is not in fact the name of a plant, but the name of a person and the name, now, of the Botanic Garden in Alice Springs. It is a lovely garden, concentrating and distilling the desert flora of the region. There are a variety of benches and chairs and intimate covered picnic areas where you can pause in your wandering. I sit to meditate and find myself listening to the birds, to the trilling and whistling, the burbling and cooing and raucous bantering chatter.

Olive Pink, a young botanic illustrator and art teacher, in 1926–27 visited the anthropologist Daisy Bates (who had earlier been befriended by the journalist and travel writer Ernestine Hill) at her camp at Ooldea, South Australia. Subsequently, Olive Pink spent much of her life among the eastern Arrernte of Alice Springs and the Warlpiri of the Tanami region, returning in between times to study anthropology in Sydney. Her work with the Arrernte was published between 1933 and 1936, but because her Warlpiri research relied on descriptions of secret rituals, she determined that her research notes be locked away for fifty years. This infuriated both her teacher, A. P. Elkin, and T. G. H. Strehlow and brought her anthropological career to an end, though not her outspoken advocacy for Aboriginal rights. The garden was founded in 1956 after lobbying by Miss Pink, who lived in the garden in a small tin hut and worked to develop it with Warlpiri gardeners, especially Johnny Jampijinpa, until her death in 1975. The garden was opened to the public in 1985.

A daisy chain of intrepid controversial white women, born in the Victorian era, marginalized from recognizable professions: Ernestine Hill, Daisy Bates, and Olive Pink. It is fitting that such a lovely garden should serve as a provocation to curiosity, as a modest memory palace in the desert.

. . .

In the museum at the Strehlow Research Centre I see a startling poster of a gigantic domestic cat gluttonously consuming lots of little feral creatures. It is part of a campaign against the domestic cat, an invasive species. The domestic and the foreign, native and invasive: categories that seem so distinct when you write the words and place them side by side on a pristine page.

To Uluru

In the darkness of the early hours of the morning a long line of red lights snake slowly through the desert. A convoy of buses carrying hundreds of tourists to dune viewing sights, platforms rising above the sandiness, where we will crowd together to witness the sunrise at Uluru.

It is cold and dark when we get out of the bus. From the platform the shapes of both Uluru and Kata Tjuta begin to take shape. Dark immense presences. Redness seeps into the desert, the rocks become luminous. The sky is lit up by the popping of a million cell phone flashlights.

Even so, even though our seeing is organized in an almost military manner, the experience of the Rock, and of Kata Tjuta, is extraordinary and indescribable. My first visit in 1984 was provoked in part by irritation at all the people who declared it indescribable. What a cop-out, I thought, such craven subservience, such genuflecting before the gatekeeping gods of sublimity. Words are tricky. Words sometimes weigh you down, stuffed in your backpack, and so you chuck some out, sometimes you scrabble around but for all your scrupulous and exhaustive packing fail to find those words that would do the trick, that would conjure into being the experience. And so I settle, like others, for indescribable.

In 1984 the resort had just opened, and I watched tourists climbing the Rock and walked in places now forbidden. In 1985 the land was handed back to the Anangu traditional owners. Uluru became the official name for what had, since the colonial era, been called Ayers Rock. The Olgas became Kata Tjuta. Pretty much immediately after the handover there were changes, such as the closing off of certain areas around the rock and Kata Tjuta to tourists, the rerouting of the main roads through the park to avoid sacred sites and also for preservation of the environment.

Later in the day, on the Indigenous Tour, I asked about a light-colored swath down a cleft in the rock. Someone said "lichen." That is the white fella story, Sammy said. His commentary is laconic, wry, edgy. As we walk he tells about the serpent woman and another tale about the venomous snake man. The stories are part of an intricate meshing of many stories that tell of Uluru, how it came into being. We reach the "lichen" just as Sammy's story reaches the point where multiple spears, thrown at the venomous snake man by a group pursuing him for the wrong he had done, created a light-colored swath down a cleft in the rock. Sammy always stressed both particularity (*this* place, *these* people, *this* language, *that* time) and the meshing of stories. The past and the present, the "real" and the mythopoeic. Entangled.

Talking of spears, nowadays, Sammy remarks, although there is still some hunting of animals, mostly we use our spears and make spear holders for something other than wallabies and kangaroos. We hunt, he says, tourists.

. . .

All around the resort the lush native plantings are named with labels as in a botanic garden, and there is even in each room a sumptuous guide for a garden walk. This is in accord with the tourism promotion of the whole of this area as a garden. In Hollywood westerns the garden and the desert are oppositional categories, but here, now—in the center of Australia, and other places in the world too—they are conflated. The official discourse presented by the Uluru–Kata Tjuta National Park in pamphlets and on the coach is unfailingly respectful, constantly acknowledging the Aboriginal ownership and stewardship of the land.

For all of that the Aboriginal presence appears to be pretty minimal. There are some receptionists at the hotel and in restaurants, but seemingly the woman who manages or front-of-houses the gallery in the village complex is white. A group of Aboriginal women bring in some paintings and leave with blank canvases and paints and they all pile into an old dusty car. At the sunset site there are some women selling small tourist paintings. They look poor, like any people selling trinkets to tourists anywhere in the world. But of course it is not so simple to say who counts and who doesn't as Aboriginal and what constitutes presence. Nor is the "village" here, nor the coach commentary, an adequate indication of the struggles and negotiations and bureaucratic maneuverings that undoubtedly shadow the tourism veneer and that have also brought about change.

If harmonious collaboration is foregrounded (there is much talk of joint management of the national park, of consultation between the government and representatives from the Aboriginal community) so too is the environmental discourse, with particular emphasis on fire management, on traditional methods of patchwork burning. Such methods ensured food and shelter for the nomadic Aborigines and wild creatures, rotating new growth and preventing major fires. Today, this traditional knowledge is being deployed as rangers work with traditional people and methods for fire management.

But new methods as well as traditional knowledges are required to fight fire and pest invasions. If tourists are both an economic boon and a pest, so too is the beastly buffel grass (*Cenchrus ciliaris*), a strong, deep-rooted, perennial grass which is believed to have come to Australia with camels and the Afghans in the 1860s. A century later a new strain of buffel, called American, developed at Texas A&M, was introduced to control dust problems. It was indeed successful in mitigating the dust storms that plagued Alice Springs, but it brought its own woes. Prior to the introduction of buffel grass, sandy creek beds acted as firebreaks, but now the opposite is occurring. An aggressive invader, buffel grass is choking out native grasses and sedges along riverbanks, alluvial flats, and moist localities, providing channels for spreading fires rather than stopping them.

. . .

Walking around the base of the great rock Uluru we hear about the sorry rocks. Despite the warnings about sacred land and fines for theft, people take bits of the rock, or sand, or twigs, as souvenirs. Then, often years later, they suffer remorse or sometimes bad luck that they attribute to the theft and they send the rock back with a sorry note. Sorry rocks are returned at the rate of one a day, from all over the world. Can rocks be returned? Can "sorry" compensate for theft? What happens to the returned rocks? Parks Australia has a fact sheet on sorry rocks in which they write, "The care of returned materials is taken seriously by *Anangu* and the Parks Australia staff. Each returned item is catalogued on a database. As it is impossible to identify the correct origin of the rock, these returned souvenirs are used to assist in repairing areas of erosion and flood runoff in the park."

"Maybe the story you remember," writes Zach in response to my email query about a story we recall him telling about rocks as we walked in the Anza Borrego

Desert near San Diego, "concerns the Navajo prayer or wishing stones, I'm not sure exactly what they are called. Some years ago I traveled from Gallup to Chinle on a remote dirt road with a Navajo family who stopped out in nowhere at a pile of small stones, searched around for some suitable stones which they added to the pile, making their private wish for a safe journey. I was told that there are such wishing stones found across the Rez, thought to originate from chance meetings of travelers, mostly long ago. May you go in beauty the Navajo say, hozho."

. . .

Wishing stones . . . sorry rocks . . . rock art . . .

To Mount Borradaile, West Arnhem Land

This part of our trip, the safari tour to Mount Borradaile, is the big-bucks extravaganza component. Scooped up in Darwin into a flashy four-wheel drive, we cruise through Kakadu National Park to the Border Store (that has a good Thai menu), where we cross over into Arnhem Land at the East Alligator River. Here we see our first crocodile, the first of hundreds—estuarine and saltwater—that will, for the rest of our trip, continuously puncture my serenity and continuously delight J. At Injalak Arts center in Gunbalanya (formerly Oenpelli) we see some beautiful bark paintings by Glen Namundja, and when we walk out to the veranda, there he is, an elderly man sitting cross-legged on the floor painting with ocher. It is a deep red earth color, the color that saturates the desert area all around us. His painting has other ocher colors too, including black and mustard yellow. Slowly, meticulously, with a very fine brush, he is *rarrking* or crosshatching. Later I will read that he comes from a distinguished lineage of artists. I buy two small bark paintings, one for Page, who gave me, before we left, a book of color that talks of the ochers of this region, and one for Chandra, who will soon be celebrating a major birthday.

From a small six-seater plane the world is intensely green and blue: mighty rivers and their tributaries, billabongs, wetlands, jungle. We are flying from Gunbalanya to the remote camp at Mount Borradaile. As you swoop closer to the earth, the blue of the water segues into a murky brown, and the surrounding bush lands, washed out by the sun, appear as dull khaki.

Floodplain, escarpments, jungle, various swamps and waterways, sandstone country, savanna woodland: The proximity of different topographies here is amazing.

Our cabin looks out onto dry woodlands where a single kurrajong (*Brachychiton megaphyllus*) blooms. In the Malvaceae (hibiscus) family, it drops all its leaves before blooming—each flower composed of five flame-red petals.

We are woken in the night by shrieking. A long cry, as though it is the last cry, as though a razor is being swiped slowly across a throat drawing out that murderous shriek. But it is not the last cry, it is repeated again and again. It is not a person dying but a bird singing. In the morning Luke, the ranger, tells us that it is the bush stone-curlew. Then as the sun lightens the sky the corellas, small white cockatoos, start their banshee-esque cackling.

The rangers take us out in Jeeps to rock art sites, or we go by boat, and then we walk and sometimes clamber over boulders and through the bush. In overhangs and caves galleries unfold, paintings and petroglyphs executed over the past fifty-five thousand years. Some walls are dense with figures and abstract patternings and much superimposition, though occasionally a drawing will be isolated with a frame drawn about it. There are now-extinct animals, hand prints, stick figures, fully formed humans, ancestral beings, therianthropic creatures combining human features with those of kangaroos, fish, dingoes, snakes, and other animals. There are ships and guns depicted during the contact period. The animals and humans are often naturalistic and sometimes depicted in the X-ray style, where broad fluent outlines are filled in, sometimes with anatomical details and sometimes with elaborate hatching and crosshatching and color variations. The ocher colors range through various shades of red, some slightly purply or brown, deep yellow, and burnt umber. White is obtained from various clays; black pigment from ground charcoal or manganese ore. Some humanlike figures have long elegant arms and legs that form arcs, they seem to be dancing or floating in the air of the rock. There is one overhang that appears to be covered in female forms dominated by breasts and huge vulvae, and in some figures the womb is featured. Variants of the creation story feature a First Mother or Fertility Mother, often articulated as two women; in legend, two sisters. Elsewhere is a creature with two heads, one at each end of the body, and there a man with a dingo head and a massive erection. On the last day we are taken to see the Rainbow Serpent, identified as Aburga, twenty feet long, terminating in a dragon-like head, a great gaping jaw wide open and filled with huge terrifying teeth. There are no superimpositions here, and no other figures.

Some of the scenes are enigmatic and mysterious, sometimes delight and recognition are provoked by the incredible detail in which a crocodile or echidna or sailing ship is rendered, but mostly there is simple wonder: at being in the presence of a profound and complex cosmology.

All of Arnhem Land is Aboriginal country and so requires permits to enter. Mount Borradaile, extending over seven hundred square kilometers, is a registered Aboriginal sacred site, owned and managed by its traditional custodians the Amurdak people. The safari business and eco resort was set up by the owners with Max and Philippa Davidson.

On the way to the galleries of rock art, we pass through and pause at burial sites and places where signs of ancient inhabitation still exist. When you see, or almost tread on, these remains you know what it is to be a trespasser. I feel as though we should declare our presence to the ancestors, say who we are and reassure them that we come in peace. But the ancestors are not mollified. I feel my half-formed declaration returned as a question: Can we, after the history of modern Australia, ever claim peace as our emissary?

. . .

I can't believe that I am here, but at the same there is also something familiar about being in this savanna woodland, about scrambling over rocky outcrops, coming upon cave paintings. I am back in Zimbabwe, *bundu* bashing, looking for caves and rock art—usually we would have a rough idea of where the caves were to be found, or sometimes we would go with more experienced people or with the history society at the university. Once in the Goromonzi area we asked some local kids for directions to a site, they sent us up a hair-raisingly steep, densely wooded, jaggedly stony kopje. After a perilous climb we made it into a clearing surrounded by a gallery of magnificent paintings. What relief, what pleasure. The kids were there waiting for us, laughing. There was, after all, a very easy way in to the hidden area, no need for such an extreme adventure.

A frisson of memory, of deflected déjà vu. But also I experience something unexpected, a painful itching sensation. I have been reading Elena Ferranti's *My Brilliant Friend*, where the emotions of childhood—envy, covetousness, passionate identification, hurt—are summoned into the present in incisively precise language. The memories that return to me now are not like this, they are hazy, half-formed, inchoate. More like the feel on your skin of wood smoke wafting through a savanna forest. Insofar as I have made sense to myself of this compulsion to visit Arnhem Land I've seen it as something to do with Australia, my connection to Australia that was incomplete, knowledge that was gaping. But what I find here is a sparking of somatic memory. Being in the *bundu*, as we called it in Zimbabwe, walking through this savanna bush, encountering galleries where ancient art is etched deep into the cave walls. I wonder if there is something of that old country, of Africa, that drew me here, some spirit of place that set me going on this journey to Arnhem Land.

There is a deep chiseling of grief into the body when you leave your country and yet all that shows, all that you can feel by running your hand over flesh, is a narrow almost invisible scar. A puckering of the skin, the closing over of a wound that could be a scratch or could be a chasm: You cannot tell by reading the skin alone. Something is scratching at that scar here. The grief that never entirely heals, grief and mourning for the country that grew you, for the country you have left, to which, now, you will probably never return.

The trees, though unfamiliar, are reminiscent. Here: stringy barks and wooly-butts, paperbarks, ghost gums, bloodwood, ironwood, grevillea, cocky apple. Back then: stinkwood, msasa, monkey apple, mopane, mufuti, marula, mahobahoba, mukwa. Say the names out loud, let them ripple through your mouth, through the years, into the air.

. . .

Today on the way to Jabiru Rock we stop at what they call the duck pond, see little fawn-colored rock wallabies, elegantly hopping, and once the hop has elevated them into the air they seem to fly. Then to a great stretch of water on the edge of the floodplain shortly before it opens into the Alligator River. Here, thousands of magpie geese are all calling out and the air is vibrating like the sound of swarms of bees circling all around us.

At dinner a woman from Europe who has been on many safaris around the world declares that she and her husband are vegetarians for ethical reasons. She complains about how expensive Aboriginal art is. Especially the big ones, she says, I hear they get paid twenty-seven dollars an hour . . . that's why the bigger ones are so expensive.

At sunset the water shimmers with bird life. Bridget, one of the guides, says that because Borradaile is the only area in this part of the Northern Territory that has all-year water the birds are drawn here as it dries up in Kakadu and else-where. We see purple neck swamp hens, pied herons, ducks, and white-bellied sea eagles—beautiful large birds, perched high in the trees, they take off and soar over our heads in circles, disappear as though heading out to sea, only to reap-pear sitting motionless in another tree. The snake neck darter swims underwater and then its head shoots up like a submarine periscope. The red-crested jacana, a beautiful little black bird with delicate legs and enormous feet, is called the Jesus bird because it can walk on water. I love the white egrets with elastic necks that they can undulate into any elegant shape. Pelicans mate in the desert and then return to the wetlands where they make huge nests high in the trees (sometimes returning to an earlier nest which they use each season for years). The jabiru is a gorgeous, graceful, black-necked stork, though up close the blackness is more like an iridescent green. I'm reminded of Funny Face, my lovely black Australorp who died.

A sudden jab of homesickness for my familiars, those domestic birds, those fat San Diegan chickens.

Birds birds everywhere, but also crocodiles, lazily cruising, opening their jaws. Waiting.

To Darwin

In Darwin there is a musicality in the air. The sound of Aboriginal voices, voicing Aboriginal languages, rhythms, and intonations you seldom hear in east coast cities. Outdoor markets, a sensory reminder that we are closer here to Southeast Asia than to Melbourne or Sydney: Tastes and smells and the heat usher you into a seemingly different country. We meet up with my old friend Helen Casey and her husband Tony (with whom we will travel for the rest of our trip) at Parap Village Apartments. It is tropical, with palm trees and a pool and Parap markets across the street, where we eat laksa and Thai salad and buy mangoes and paw paw to eat later. We find Ruark in the gallery setting up the show "Rrambaŋi/Together as Equals," a joint installation with artists from Yirrkala: Barayuwa Munungurr, his mother Bengitj Ngurruwuthun, who is also the linguist for the show and has written a catalog essay, and Jeffrey Ngurruwuthun, who sings the song lines, the stories.

The show is made up of several elements: a bark shelter, videos, a series of graphite drawings by Ruark (*Star Shelters*), and a drawing/installation by Barayuwa of a whale occupying the entire wall that faces you as you enter the gallery. Most of Barayuwa's art revolves around the whale and is generated out of a key ancestral story embedded in the site, of which he is a custodian—Yarrinya, where the open seas join at and in Blue Mud Bay. The story involves the ritual carving up of the flesh and body of an ancestral whale, Mirinyungu, by Munyuku spirit men (Wurramala or Matjitji) who are brothers of Mirinyungu. The whale's demise, and its kinship with the hunters, is the basis for this important site and clan design: The bones from the skeleton are imbued with cultural and ceremonial significance to Munyuku people and are manifest through myriad features of the Yarrinya coast. The installation sets three of these component parts, covered in the design for that area, against a backdrop of that same design in such a way that they "disappear" into the water, the way that the reefs, which are the manifestation of those bones, are invisible under the sea, made from the same fabric.

Star Shelters, Ruark's graphite drawings, are abstract, geometric designs. They derive from studies made while he was in the Royal Darwin Hospital. Made to chance formulae, they grew out of discussions on Aboriginal astronomy with the late anthropologist Dianne Johnson. "Constellations" of lines in the drawings may resemble maps of the starry sky. However, they also relate to Ruark's idea of building shelters for patients and families awaiting/visiting patients—temporary structures to house possessions. The linear design of Ruark's drawings resonate with the preparatory drawing in light and dark pigment made by Barayuwa, now hidden beneath the surface of his painting, disappearing under the blue water, the blue whale.

On Sunday Ruark fetches us in his rental car, and we head off for Rapid Creek Market. We meet up there with Barayuwa, his wife Whaiora, and their three daughters. Whaiora is a Maori, a warm woman used to mediating between cultures and facilitating exchanges. The Darwin Festival is happening and so is the Darwin Aboriginal Art Fair. We make it to the art fair on the last afternoon: a fabulous immersion in art from all the indigenous art centers in the Northern Territory and even as far away as the Kimberleys.

Seven men in red sarong-type pants move in unison swaying shifting the center of energy. The men only ever look like men, never like fish, but watching these dancers from Indonesia, this performance, *Cry Jailolo*, to do with the degradation of the coral reef, you experience the *sensation* of moving together under water with shoals of fish as you snorkel. You imagine the sea between Australia and Indonesia.

Festival Park is a magical space: lit by fairy lights and magnificent lanterns (some in the shape of fish) strung between large old trees; around the circumference of the park there are food and drink stalls and, scattered throughout the space, lots of long communal tables. We see a show called "Prison Songs" in the Lighthouse—a performance venue set up as a circle with enclosed walls, a stage, and collapsible chairs for the audience. Above, it is open to the air and the stars, the illusion of a big top created with fairy lights. When I try and leave to pee before the show starts I'm stopped and interrogated by a very tall Aboriginal man in a uniform. He is initially slightly threatening but also jokey, and as we talk the bantering exchange turns more and more into a surreal improvisation. Consternation soon ripples into delight as it dawns on me: This is the great actor Ernie Dingo!

"Prison Songs" was comedic at times but also poignant and dismal, much of it based on testimony, on interviews with prison inmates in the notorious old Berrimah prison in Darwin. Aborigines constitute 3 percent of the overall population in Australia, though in the Northern Territory that figure rises to 20 percent. Of the inmates in Darwin prison 86 percent are Aboriginal.

Magic and musicality and fairy lights . . . irretrievable loss . . . the noise of history . . . the losing of frequency, darkness.

One night we bought lots of meat and salad and potatoes for a barbecue and invited Ruark and James, whom we happened to bump into as he was passing through Darwin, and Bengitj and the Yirrkala crew, who it turned out were staying in the next-door apartment. No one came, and no one came, and then suddenly everyone arrived and the place was filled with children. They ate quickly, stacked their plates, and disappeared, though later in the evening, when word got out that there was ice cream, the little people reappeared one by one. Lots of dramas going on behind the scenes: Yolngu business and then more dramas to do with the business of art. And then, someone had gone on a bender and was missing.

We will fly to Nhulunbuy, the nearest town to Yirrkala. Barayuwa and Whaiora will drive with the girls, eight hours without stopping, taking two trucks in case one breaks down. A good precaution as, it turns out, one does indeed give up the ghost an hour from home.

To Yirrkala

We are here. In Yirrkala.

Flying in to Nuhlunbuy you see the promontories and bays, fingers of brilliant blue water. You have a sense of this stone country fringed by the sea.

We check in to the Gove Peninsula Motel and drive to Yirrkala, twenty minutes away, to the Buku-Larrnggay Mulka Centre. The Arafura Sea is as blue as I imagined. The bay is calm but filled for me always now with a whale, the story of the great whale that Barayuwa paints.

Buku-larrnggay means the feeling on your face as it is struck by the first rays of the sun. The phrase conveys the location of the art center in the most easterly part of the Top End of Australia. *Mulka* means a sacred but public ceremony.

Two days of immersion. A beautifully designed space in which there are bark paintings, logs, prints, acrylic and oil paintings, as well as sculptural pieces. We are able to move slowly through the small gallery and museum, to pause, absorb, register echoes of familiarity as well as differences of technique and style. Each section of perhaps three or four works lists clan, group, surname, moiety, language, homeland: such complex networks, ways of being in country. Beginning to notice small differences, experience moments of incipient recognition, echoes, a sense—fleetingly now and then—of shimmer. In the museum we see the famous Yirrkala Church Panels of 1963 (two petitions, representing two moieties, or land-owning clans, attached to sheets of bark with borders painted with designs belonging to the respective moieties) that were sent to the Australian Parliament making a case for Yolngu rights to the land since time immemorial. We buy a print of Barayuwa's, a story of the whale (like all his works): intricate blue and green pixilated patterning shadowed by soft feathery browns. Helen and Tony buy the same print, though because of the print process they are slightly differently realized, the colors not identical. One will hang in Melbourne, one in San Diego, sustaining friendship and memories of Yirrkala. Later, at home, I will gaze at the print, imagine the story, imagine the bones of the painting, the elements of the whale skeleton, the sacred designs, hidden in the work.

How much money, I wonder, does Barayuwa make out of these transactions? He is described as "a rising star" in one of the catalogs, so his paintings are beginning to command a good price. But the center must take its cut, and then, in certain instances, the dealer or gallery also takes a percentage. The centers have overheads and also are often cooperatives, so the money that comes in gets shared. Often very skilled and highly respected artists don't sell much. Clearly Yirrkala is a highly functioning community, and Buku-Larrnggay Mulka is run efficiently (reaching out to and representing separate clans and subclans and homelands spread over a circumference of two hundred kilometers), with live links to the land, to custodianship.

Aboriginal art became an international phenomenon and an industry with the emergence of acrylic dot painting in the 1970s. Like all art it is subject to the market. But unlike much Western art (though like many other indigenous art movements), it rises out of communities that have long histories of culturally embedded noncommercial art making, out of communities that have survived the ravages of invasion. So the circuits of commerce and fame are complicated in particular ways. So, too, the distinctions between tourist art and high art.

Undoubtedly there are abusive modes of tourist art production. There are art centers in Australia where the artists are made to work long hours, not properly fed, and coerced (by hourly rates) to produce paintings according to the logic of factory-line production. The artists and the paintings are tradable things, you might imagine them stacked up against the wall, stuffed into piles, rammed into corners, draped over every surface, bunched up like carpets in a carpet shop, like a pile of dominoes. Then, like dominoes, they fall, are shifted shuffled attached to labels, prices affixed, amended, raised, they are exchanged, disappear, and resurface.

Writing this brings to mind my friend Sylvia Lawson and two paintings that she brought back from a trip to Alice Springs. I remember her showing them to me and talking about Alice, about her experience of the culture and politics, about trying to understand and about the paintings, one of which, unsigned, would be called tourist art and the other an original and beautiful piece by an artist with a name. She turned this musing into an essay, "Budgerigars, or Positions of Ignorance," which appeared in her collection of essays, *How Simone de Beauvoir Died in*

Australia. She writes, of the two paintings, "What's important is that they should be in the same space."

. . .

Standing on the seashore I pick up and pocket a sliver of red rock to take home. Guiltily, already sorry as I walk away, but not repentant enough to return it. Collection, theft, appropriation, representation, and the right to speak: These are tricky and contested arenas. And of course it isn't only rocks that are at issue. Museums all over the world—but especially those situated in cities where once great empires gathered their plunder—are subject now to scrutiny and to demands for repatriation. I ask R about the blockbuster British Museum show *Indigenous Australia: Enduring Civilization.* Much publicity had been given to a strident critique, by a white journalist, leveled at the museum for building the show around stolen objects. R says that, though it was expected, in the end there wasn't so much of a furor. Apparently the museum had traveled to communities and discussed with them the question of return. He and W were on a panel with some Aboriginal elders and senior painters, and the latter said it's been sorted, (effectively) figured out, if the objects are looked after they can remain.

Ruark had urged me to send "Blue/Shimmer" to W for the center's archives, and so I tell him about the piece. At first he is enthusiastic but then launches into a mini tirade: No white person can ever get it right, it's no good thinking you can just get onto a computer and look up a few things and then write an article and you've nailed it. I include myself, he says, and I've written screeds over twenty years. The Yolngu will always have another way. You can never ever understand if you have not grown up in country as part of a clan. I asked him about his journey to here. He came as a white lawyer for the land-rights movement, married a Yolngu woman, and has stayed.

He has persisted. I know that I will never know. Everything there is to know. But I'd like to be able to scrabble together enough scraps of knowledge and insight to face up to the shame engendered by ignorance. And the complicity that ignorance spawns. To be able to negotiate the rocky terrain between the arrogance of entitlement (that you can speak about anything) and a cowed silence.

Yes, it has really happened, this line tenuously traced from San Diego to Yirrkala. But it has also been and still is and always will be a phantasmatic journey, incited by curiosity and ignorance, sustained by a treacherously empirical promise, impishly perverse: that to be here, in person, to feel the ground beneath and to breathe the air, as though all this would be to see. To see differently.

To Cape York, Queensland

Thundering up the coast from Cairns, on a gravelly road, Peter Casey, Helen's brother, at the wheel of his four-wheel-drive ute. We are headed for Quinkan country in Cape York, in the far north of Queensland, where there are hundreds and hundreds of rock art sites. Peter has got to know Steven Trezise, son of Percy Trezise, who explored this remote area and wrote about the extensive galleries of art, most famously in *Quinkan Country: Adventures in Search of Aboriginal Cave Paintings in Cape York* (1969), written with his friend the Aboriginal painter Dick Roughsey (born Goobalathaldin, meaning "the ocean, dancing," a member of the Lardil language group from Mornington Island in the Gulf of Carpentaria).

Up through the rain forest, through the Daintree, up into the Cape York Peninsula. In the Daintree unlikely ecosystems—mangroves and rain forest—edge into one another, and two other quite different ecosystems abut them: savanna forests inland and, not far away in the ocean, the Great Barrier Reef. It is one of the few places where plants representing all stages of the evolution of land plants over the past four hundred million years are found. We pause at Cape Tribulation, an elegantly curved bay, white sands fringed by coastal forest, brilliant blue sky and equally brilliant blue sea, where crocodiles surf and sun themselves. "This is where our troubles began," wrote Captain Cook in 1770. His ship, the *Endeavour*, after scraping on a reef, was done for, though it managed to limp into what was to become Cooktown. We vroom into the town just in time to check into a pretty caravan park where we have cabins, and then we shoot up the mountain in the ute to the lighthouse. The sun has just gone over the tip of the world, and within a few minutes it floods the sky over the sea deep red.

In the night I think it is raining softly, but it is just the sound of wind through the leaves of the palms and the paperbarks. In the early morning the birds screech and whirl.

We drive further north—beyond Cooktown—to Elim Beach. It's a slight detour, says Peter, but he promises something mysterious and magical there. It takes a couple of hours, but when we get there we do indeed experience a surprise. The remote beach is gorgeous, a bay in the Coral Sea. The magic is this: In a few spots near the edge of the shore freshwater bubbles up into the salty ocean. You can cup your hands around the bubbles and drink, drink deeply of crystal clear pure spring water.

Peter wants also to take this detour in order to drive through Hope Vale, the Lutheran Mission where Noel Pearson grew up. Pearson—a spell-binding rhetorician—is an Aboriginal lawyer and activist, author of *Up from the Mission*, a collection of essays ranging from land rights to his controversial views on the detrimental effects of what he calls "passive welfare."

Driving to Trezise country we see a streak in the bush, it's a dingo running—there and gone in a flash.

We reach Jowalbinna, now a deserted camp, but there are huts with bare bunk beds, and a clean kitchen with basic utensils. It is eerie, as though this place, once lively, has been stripped of human presence, now there remain only ghosts. The truth is banal and has to do with changes in tourism trends. Percy Trezise, as a young man in the 1960s, heard about some rock art, came and stayed, eventually buying two large properties in the area with the aim of conserving the art. The country is filled with sandstone escarpments revealing endless galleries of rock art. The way to make a living out of those properties was to establish a safari camp and have a rock art guide service run by his two sons (who had grown up exploring and studying the art with their father), which would include young Aboriginals. But the trend for boutique safari camps, such as the one at Borradaile, had put the venture out of business long before we arrived.

We settle in for the night—with the ghosts of tourists past and with the Quinkan, ancestral spirits that inhabit the landscape here.

Peter heaps huge branches onto the fire, we eat a meal he largely prepared before leaving Cairns—fresh angel hair pasta with a marinara sauce of local Moreton Bay bugs and calamari and mussels and prawns. Good wine. We sit gazing into the fire, listening to the sighing and gentle whooshing of the trees. Potatoes roasting in the embers, tin foil turning black. Peter wants to keep the fire going all night so that in the morning jaffles can be cooked in the embers.

Potato flesh, scraped with ham into jaffle irons between slices of bread, and cooked. Coffee is made in an old stovetop traditional Italian espresso maker. We are well set up for the day's hiking ahead.

Before setting off we hear the sound of black cockatoos, occasionally a group wheels into the sky in the distance, looking like ordinary blackbirds.

Black cockatoos, these birds fly in and out of my dreams, have done so for forty years, sometimes just spinning on the periphery so that their image has almost disappeared by the time I'm awake, though the sound persists, building to a crescendo and then softening, fluttering into silence.

. . .

In the shrine room the sound of the gong fills the air and slowly dies away, rippling into outer space, ushering the body in or out of a meditative state.

. . .

In escarpment country Steven Trezise drives his old ute with the utmost care at five miles an hour through the valley along the edge of a creek. Stony ground sometimes segueing into sand. A steep incline to a crossing and then, on the other side, a hill that appears to reach into the sky. This is a scary hill, he mutters. We all hold tight and lean forward as though on horseback.

We make our way on foot through the bush, into and up and around the escarpment. Gallery after gallery of art unfolds, often in overhangs rather than caves. These paintings are again more reminiscent for me of Zimbabwe rock art, though I can't quite say how or why, perhaps it is the surrounding landscape. Haunted by the skeleton of the whale beneath the surface of the sea yet shaping the contours of the shore, these paintings and pictographs appear to me as the bones of the land. Engravings are frequently superimposed in many layers, suggesting a very long time period. Red ocher dominates, though white, yellow, black, and a rare blue pigment also exist, stained into the rock, sometimes manifesting as just a vague shape or outline and, at other times, clearly delineated. Echidna, emu, crocodile, kangaroo, wallaby, scrub turkey, snake, tortoise, fish are recognizable, sometimes as stick figures and sometimes in dense detail, the interiors intricately patterned with lines and dots and crosshatching. In a trompe l'oeil gesture, a line of fruit bats appear to be hanging from a cave ledge. There are humans too and composite yam figures and spirits. In one cave gigantic penises take us by surprise, as does a depiction of intercourse in which a man and a woman hover in space, feet touching, penis touching the woman's sex. Steven tells us of various interpretations that have been made, but ultimately meanings escape.

Steven is an oddly likable, contradictory, and rather sad figure. Percy Trezise, his father, was the big character who tells a big flamboyant story, a story of discovery and exploration. His extensive writings embed many Aboriginal stories and legends and creation myths; he campaigned for the area to be declared a national park and called for it to be administered by the local Aboriginal community. The national park idea did not eventuate, but the Quinkan and Regional Cultural Centre (QRCC), just outside of Laura, offers guided tours by local Aboriginal people. The Quinkan Reserves, owned by Aboriginal Trustees, are closed to public access.

Steven knows the topography of the area well, he grew up exploring with his father and family, he learned from the last of the "old fellas." He has been dedicated in keeping alive his father's spirit. Although animated when talking of the rock art, he sinks easily into sadness. For six months of the year (the dry months) he lives here in what looks like a brutally basic house, open on four sides to the elements, half of it shared with machinery, satellite dishes on the roof. He's been doing this for thirty-five or -six years, and he is done. He says, I'm sick of living in the stone age, I want to be a city boy and chase girls. A little rueful, he knows he's rather long in the tooth for that. What he would like to do is to sell the station to the traditional owners of the land, but that means that first they have to establish native title, and then the government has to be prepared to pay. This is a fiendishly complex process.

His station, a huge expanse of land, is situated in a part of the country where terrible massacres occurred during the period of colonial settlement and conquest, virtually wiping out the Aboriginal population. Those left were dispossessed of their land, rounded up onto mission stations or local cattle stations where they worked in an unwaged capacity; others moved to camps on the fringes of Laura, Cooktown, and other settlements, where they lived under the surveillance of the local police.

Prospects for reclaiming land, then, are not good here. Loss of continuity, a severing of traditions, the smallness and dispersion of the Aboriginal population—all this is exacerbated by the proliferation of applications in Quinkan country for exploration for coal and other minerals. Some people believe that the best way to protect the region would be to have a World Heritage nomination. But I am not sure how this would address Aboriginal land rights and sovereignty. And given the current government, it seems likely that mining interests would be privileged over all other claims.

There is no counting on the Labour Party either these days. Steven thinks the party is too ideological, a statement that invites us to jump to conclusions about his political affiliations. He is, after all, a Queensland station owner. But he surveys us quizzically, no doubt eyeing us up as small "l" city liberals, clueless, earnestly expanding our horizons, adding nuggets of "otherness" to our store of knowledge and stories. He is, as Helen says, a man who is happy to share his opinions but not set to win an argument.

. . .

The cockatoos track us, and the higher we climb the closer they come until at last they swoop in front of us, a huge flock, cackling and screeching, and then they take off, their tails flashing red, blocking for a moment the piercing blueness of the sky.

To San Diego

Back home: back to routine, to writing every day, to ordinary life. The front garden is dry, spaces opening up between plants, Bermuda grass taking hold, turning brown. It looks brown and dead but nevertheless is growing tenaciously, choking other plants. Peggy shows me her legs, red, inflamed, untouchable. Her neighbor sprayed the lawn with Roundup, her dog rolled in it and then brushed against her legs. But the roses, all the roses, are blooming. What a miracle in this drought.

What tough beauties they are. I pick a bowlful to put in the center of the dining room table, and as I set the bowl down I hear Peter Latz's words, from Alice
Springs, words brought in on a dusty gust of wind: "What we learn [from growing and observing native plants] will enable us to develop and use plants that will
produce new foods and medicines, replace roses and other introduced plants in
our gardens, and provide refuge and a seed source for the desert's rare plants."

The vegetable garden is morose and sad and deadened. But my foraging gathers more than I imagined was there: eggplants, some red peppers, a few tomatoes,
basil, sorrel, dandelion. Kale continues, and there is amaranth, and New Zealand
spinach in the shadier bits. The small bush of habaneros is weighted down by the
vivid orange fruits. I will dry most of them in the dehydrator. I haven't cooked for
six weeks, so it is with great pleasure that I take forever grinding spices and assembling eggplant stuffed with lamb and pine nuts.

Today I at last start dealing with insurance and read that as far as drug pur-
chases go I have entered the "catastrophic zone." To find out what that is I have to
consult a booklet issued by the insurance company.

Propped up in bed with the Mac Air and my pot of tea and Elvis snarling, the
energy of Australia persists. It began a little shakily. Anxious on the long flight, I
got up and walked every hour for sixteen hours. After that, after a day of rest, the
world started brightening up, and as we traveled I got stronger and stronger. The
daily injections proved easy to manage. Now I am totally convinced of something
I knew but had never experienced to the full: New experiences, doing things you
have never done before, going places you have never been, never imagined, being
provoked by curiosity, all this wakes up your brain cells. Ping! Ping! They spark,
glow, become infectious, activate your sluggish bodily cells.

All travels have an imaginary dimension. You project. You bring with you, even
when startled by the unrecognizable or visited by ghostly resonances and associations from elsewhere. And then later as you narrate and describe your experiences—to friends, in a journal, in a book—even as you aim to be faithful you bring
into being a phantasmatic journey braided from skeins of desire and memory.

Of course I know that I will never know. Probably as time goes on I'll know
less and less. Of this other Australia, these other ways of imagining and living in
the world, and of rendering that Yolngu world, this world now, in paintings on
bark and rock and bodies and in the sand and funeral trunks, in murals and installations, in legal/political cases. The journey, tenuous as it is, will become even
more gauze-like and imaginary. Yet I am glad to have been there, my feet on the
ground in Yirrkala.

The ghost of Lévi-Strauss is snorting with derision. I am laughing with glee.

Chookless

61

In the supermarket, rushing between work and dinner, she is juggling in her arms several cans, a bottle of wine, box of spaghetti, and packet of vacuum-sealed, pre-washed baby spinach leaves. Suddenly she is jolted as something hits her from behind. With considerable force she is driven into a stacked display of super-sale-priced miniature bottles of gourmet olive oil, fragility incarnate. Everything flies out of her arms, bottles smash, wine and oil erupt, liquid gold spurts from the supermarket jugular.

Operatic sobbing fills the air. On her butt, in a sticky mess, she looks up and is met by a weeping face looking down, anguished, into her face. It is a woman's face, probably—when not contorted by tears—a genial face. The face says, "Sorry, sorry." She speaks with a foreign accent. "Sorry," the nice face says again. "I am chookless, chookless, all day I am chookless today."

She doesn't know what "chookless" means, but somehow it resonates, seems to mirror exactly how she is feeling. Once she gets home, after she has washed and eventually after she has eaten, hours and hours later, and had a glass of wine, the sense of the word *chookless* begins to percolate, eventually rising to the surface of her mind and settling there, a gem of condensed clarity. Running around like a chook with its head cut off, that's what today has been like. The woman has managed to compress two words, *headless* and *chook*, into a new concept word, thus adding a crystalline shard of perspicacity to the English language.

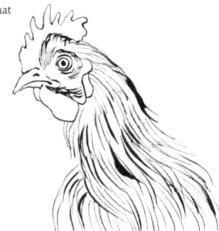

Chicken Shit

62

There is a Shambhala saying, "You do not just want to work with chicken shit; you want to work with the chicken itself." I take these words to mean something like this: Chicken shit may be messy and stinky and time-consuming to deal with, but as a task it can almost invisibly become routinized, easy, predictable, and satisfying. Samuel Beckett nailed it:

> *Habit is the ballast that chains the dog to his vomit.*

The chicken is another matter: Flighty, opinionated, even though her opinions are impenetrable, or rather, the logic of her opinions seems to bear no relation to the material conditions of her existence. She imagines she is a queen and should be treated thus by loyal subjects, or she imagines she is a hawk, a bird destined to prey on all smaller creatures and insects and even invisible beings who plague and torment and also add spice to her life. Or she may be perfectly healthy, apparently happy and cooing one moment, and then just like that, without warning, dead as a dodo. Understanding the chicken, loving her through thick and thin, is not always easy, though you might say that this is all projection—human projection of our own or my own crankiness and unknowingness—onto the chicken. The Shambhala saying (Chögyam Trungpa Rinpoche's riff on the Buddhist maxim "Work with the greatest defilements first") is, after all, a saying, a slogan, a deployment of metaphor. To take it too literally is to stray into minefields of our own making.

Many cultures and storytelling traditions and philosophical orientations utilize animals in this way. Think of Aesop's fables, think of African folktales, think of a philosopher like Jacques Derrida. I remember hearing Derrida talk, over many weeks, about the cow, in the context of "eating the other." And in Sydney, delivering a lecture on friendship, he spoke about cats, taking a very concrete, quotidian experience to play with the notion of friendship. Well, he said, it's irritating and a pain to deal with other cats in the building who come and eat your cat's food. But you can work on your attitude and eventually see this cat as existing in a continuum with your cat. Instead of contiguity breeding contempt and hostility and erecting domestic barricades, you might eventually entertain the notion of a feline continuity and welcome the other cat into your home, not grudgingly, but with generosity of spirit. However, he said, and I remember how Derrida played out this moment dramatically, using the pause, the tilted head, the glinting eye and raised eyebrow: What if one day you hear a scratching at the door and you go to open it and you open it and there sitting on the mat is a cat, but this cat is a lion. This image was so vivid, it has stayed with me as a complex thread unraveling over time.

Was this a metaphor? Or was it an example grounded in the material world? I have come to think it was both. And so it is in many of these traditions or inflections of moral precepts or teasing out of philosophical conundrums. The lion and the chicken are not to be taken literally, but neither are they merely metaphors. They are at once familiar, quotidian (the lion is a kind of cat, the chicken is connected to chicken shit), and their dramatic performance is surprising, unlikely, has the capacity to wake us up, to confront us with the unexpected and alien and difficult.

Chicken shit happens. Chickens, on the other hand, can take us by surprise, provoke unhappenings.

All I wanted when I first went to the Shambhala center at the end of my street was some help with meditation, some hints on how to integrate the body with a calming of the mind, some training in how to foster a practice, a routine. I wanted to subdue the panic, find some way of coping with illness. Trained in the hard knocks school of high theory I felt I did not need any more mind-training.

Today I pull *Training the Mind* off the bookshelf, to check on that chicken shit reference, and two slogans printed on flimsy bits of paper fall out: "Work with the greatest defilements first" and "Don't be so predictable."

On the one hand, there is sitting meditation, a concentration of the mind on the breath. On the other hand, there is contemplative meditation. Theoretically the focus on breath, on the body, grounds one for contemplation. I still haven't quite figured out where the practice of sitting-and-breathing-and-not-thinking intersects with sitting-and-breathing-and-thinking-about-things, about, say, the slogans. I just muddle along, helped by teachers, by the structure of the sangha.

Training the Mind by Chögyam Trungpa Rinpoche explicates the seven points of mind training (lojong) attributed to the Indian Buddhist teacher Atisha in 982 CE.

The list of fifty-nine mind-training slogans is often referred to as the Atisha Slogans. Pithy, practical, a way of training our minds through both formal practice and everyday life as a means of awakening. Waking up entails coming to realize the habitual nature of the self, realizing the "other" as other. The slogans bear repetition because of their capacity to change: They double back, dodge, and creep up on you from unexpected angles.

You should work with whatever is your greatest obstacle first—whether it is aggression, passion, pride, arrogance, jealousy, or what have you. You should not just say "I will sit more first, and I will deal with that later." Working with the greatest defilements means working with the highlights of your experience or your problems. You do not just want to work with chicken shit, you want to work with the chicken itself.

Good habits, repetition, the assurance of a routine, all this is necessary to maintain a meditative practice. It is very hard to learn to breathe without this kind of structure. The structure facilitates: How much easier the day becomes if every day you manage to find even a short time for slowing the mind, for breathing peacefully. But, but, but . . . it is also all too easy to settle, via routine, into the fatness of certitude:

> . . . his certitudes perched like fat chickens.

How do you grapple with the tenacious grip of the ego and yet avoid positioning the other as the predictable obverse or prop to one's glorious egolessness? How do you avoid interpreting the slogans through the lens of a moral universe? How to preempt the snarkiness, the judgment, the relentless drive to control everything, the frustration and irritation and despair with those around, with myself, with Israel's assault on Gaza, with immigration policies in this country, with the global environmental catastrophe engulfing us all? How do you engage with the world? How do you avoid grand generalizations and self-righteous litanies of complaint about the bad other? For this we know: Mindful shifting of the habitual can in itself become a habit, promoting a comforting quietude and detachment from politics both quotidian and public.

> From the farmyard in which his certitudes perched like fat chickens, every night of the siege, one or two were carried off in the jaws of rationalism and despair.

Chicken shit happens. Chickens transmogrify. Between the cushion of contemplation and the world out there is an ocean, an ocean where we surf and are tossed by the stormy waves of birth, old age, global catastrophe, genocide, sickness, and death.

It's all very well to realize and to see the lion or the chicken as merely a projection of self. But to fully recognize the lion or the chicken as something other than a projection of self? Not so easy. Not so easy to do this off the cushion, out there or in here, in the world.

Oh the world, the world.

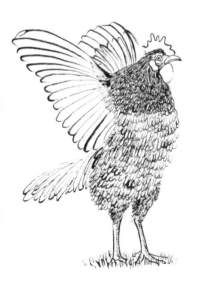

Mimetic Pain

She outlines the options: We can amputate or try radiation.

My heart races toward the precipice. He is trembling, his entire body shuddering, his nose buried in my hand as he tries to hide from the world.

Panic, shame, guilt, terror.

I should have made this appointment months ago, as soon as the tumor on Elvis's right rear leg started growing again, but I couldn't face the thought of him going through another surgery. It is less than two years since it was cut out. We were told it would likely grow back, but so soon? If I had taken him to the surgeon as soon as it started growing perhaps the surgery would have been quick and simple. Instead I chose not to look. His other rear leg is already wonky.

Five years ago he went missing for twenty-four hours and then late one night we heard a weak mewing, he had managed to drag himself into the front garden. His face was mashed and his left rear leg was mangled, dangling. Every tendon around his knee was torn. I carried him in, gave him water that he drank a lot of, and he ate a tiny bit. He lay by me purring, perhaps in relief to be home but, more likely, in pain. He might have been hit by a car or any number of things. But my theory is that he got in a fight with his *enemigo*, the big orange tom cat, a real mean bruiser, and was chased into an impossible corner. The surgical process and long confinement and recovery were torturous. And in the end it turned out that his leg had failed to set correctly. "We can try again," they said cheerfully. "No thank you," we said.

Eventually Elvis the old warrior recovered from the failed attempt to successfully set his left rear leg. He limps and has developed arthritis, though this has not stopped him from jumping with creaky agility on and off the bed. Although the cat door is still open to the backyard and to the bamboo forest, the door to the front garden, the street, and the wide world beyond is closed. We worried that he would not be able to defend himself. He sits sometimes, especially in the evening, looking out mournfully through the screen door but seems reconciled, speculative, musing. He doesn't even go out the back that much anymore, though a while ago I heard a squalling one afternoon in the back garden. Elvis is squaring off against his nemesis, the orange *enemigo*. As soon as I appear the cowardly *enemigo* makes a run for it. Elvis gives chase, moves at the speed of light, as fast as a Sputnik he slices through the air, no sign of his limp. The *enemigo* reaches the back fence and scrambles up and over. Elvis reaches the fence, looks as though he is about to jump, but then stops, growls, and turns, flexes his body, and swaggers back through the yard to the house.

. . .

When the surgeon says to me, Now the tumor has grown too large, I cannot cut it out, the options are radiation or amputation, my body turns hot, waves of shame break over me, over Elvis, over his tumor. Why did I ignore the growth of the growth for so long? Could it be that I was projecting my own fear and loathing of the surgical option onto Elvis? Or, in imagining how much he detests and fears the whole business—being in a cage, traveling in a car, being submitted to pain and humiliation in a hospital room—am I overidentifying with him, my sympathy serving merely to tangle him up in a swaddling sheath of suffocating empathy? Like Jerry Lewis in *The Disorderly Orderly*, who manages to mummify his patient by literally bandaging him from head to foot and rolling him down a hill.

APRIL 7, 2015

We are due tomorrow for the first visit to the pet oncology hospital in Carlsbad. This means that Elvis has to be kept indoors and the cat door blocked, otherwise he will make a run for it. He will also be suspicious as soon as he realizes he's trapped in the house, so I have connived with J to stay up and put the cement block against the cat door after Elvis and I have gone to bed. He can't eat after midnight. So he gets his last snack before we head to bed close to eleven. I get into bed, hoping he will follow me, but Elvis takes his time, sits under the dining room table, looking like he's settled for the night. I know he is just sizing things up, waiting until most of the lights are off and I am drifting into sleep. I'm struggling to stay awake. Then he jumps onto the bed with a little squall that says, I'm here, hello, roll over. He sits at the end of the bed, his back to me, but purring. I get the asthma tablet and slip it down his throat. Then I settle back down, and he sidles up, stares intently into my eyes, willing me to roll over. OK, I say, and roll onto my back. He settles down on my chest, purring, eighteen pounds of him, just like when he was a little kitten. He purrs very loudly, but it isn't the sound so much as the rumbling sensation that moves from his body into mine. When I had the lower lobe of my left lung removed because of the cancer tumor I would lie there in my hospital bed after the surgery and imagine Elvis on my chest, those rolling thunderous vibrations, rippling into and through my body, sending healing waves. After a while I nudge him off, and he curls up in the crook of my leg. I practice breathing normally, but am alert, listen intently for J to deal with putting the slab in place to block the door. It takes forever. I'm nervous that Elvis will cotton on and make a dash for it. But he's sleepy. Eventually I hear J getting to the back porch and can at last relax. This morning, no food for Elvis, so he knows immediately what is going on. Gives one angry snarl and then retreats into the closet. I get up to have a shower and afterward poke my head into the closet. No Elvis! I go to the back porch. The heavy cement block has been pulled away from the cat door and toppled over. I see him sauntering off toward the bamboo thicket, where he will be for the rest of the day despite his terrible hunger. How could he have moved that heavy cement? He must have contemplated it and realized that it was not securely in place, considered his options, tried a few moves, first with one paw and then the other, and then reached out to the weakest point, tapped, and toppled it over.

A terrible fury seeps through me. I blame J. Recriminations and fury rise like vomit, lodge in my throat, escape.

I reschedule. The next morning we sit mournfully around the breakfast table, J and Elvis and I. I am remorseful for my recriminatory disposition, J and Elvis are hungry. Roxy has been fed outside. Elvis cannot have any food. J cannot eat in front of the cats when they have to do without food so he is going out to get a burrito. Stomach churning, I can't face a burrito. I get Elvis into his box, hidden on the bed in the back room. His paw reaching through the grate he snarls, scratches, and tears at the doona cover on the bed, ripping it. I give him some drops of homeopathic fear stuff to lick off my finger and lick some myself. OK, I say, let's go! Check the time: I am an hour early. Anxiety has knotted me into a tight ball and rolled time backward.

There are three alternatives: let him out and then reenact the rigmarole of getting him into his box again; go and wait in the waiting room at the hospital where there are dogs and construction cacophony; or sit at home together, he in his box, I on the bed beside him, reading.

So for the next hour I read aloud to Elvis, trusting that the sound of my voice will be soothing. Now and then we each lick a drop or two of the homeopathic fear treatment.

I have unearthed a diary I kept when I was seven, in 1957, and we went on a trip, driving in our little Mini-Minor to the Gorongoza game reserve in Mozambique. Going there was the most exciting thing that had ever happened to me in all my life, but something even more exciting was about to happen. I read to Elvis, elaborating the childish sentences, embroidering the stories, until I reach the really exciting bit where we are charged by an elephant: "Dad slammed into reverse and the mini shot back like a sputnik in space."

In Sputnik 2, in 1957, the Russians sent a little dog found on the streets of Moscow into the air, knowing she would never survive but hoping to learn for humans something about the conditions in space.

This is not very calming and so I turn to our old friend Montaigne. *The Essays* falls open on a passage about the power of speech and how animals communicate with one another and we with them:

We can see that they have means of complaining, rejoicing, calling on each other for help or inviting each other to love; they do so by meaningful utterances: if that is not talking, what is it? How could they fail to talk among themselves, since they talk to us and we to them? How many ways we have of speaking to our dogs and they of replying to us! We use different languages again, and make different cries, to call birds, pigs, bulls and horses; we change idiom according to species.

That reminds me of a film, *El Circo*, about which I tell Elvis. In this film, the Mexican comic Cantinflas talks to the different animals in a zoo, using exactly the same language for each of the different species; he speaks to them without differentiation or condescension, in exactly the same way he talks to people, rubbishing the language, playing with it in his hilarious and entirely idiosyncratic manner. The animals look at him attentively but with bemusement. Cantinflas has lost his job, and the elephant, not very Sputnik-like, having outworn her usefulness, is about to be done away with. The film ends with Cantinflas and the elephant together, having left the circus and formed a working alliance, on the street, shining shoes.

You Are Mostly Not You

You, like me, probably think of yourself as a human being. You sense and experience your body as a human body, with luck having two legs, two arms, a brain, and what have you, all composed of tissues and organs made up of human cells. Moreover, you conceive of yourself as a distinct individual. Wrong. Your body is teeming with alien life-forms. It turns out that you harbor within your body whole populations of nonhumans that have separate DNA structures to you, and they outnumber you.

The mistaken perception that you are entirely and unmistakably human is understandable because we are not aware of these other life-forms that inhabit our bodies—they are almost entirely invisible to the naked human eye, and we do not generally *feel* them or even sense their presence. Yet they take up space, collectively weigh a lot, and have an enormous effect on us (digestion, immune responses, emotional states, and behavior, to mention just a few areas). The microbes in your gut are said to weigh as much as your brain, around three pounds. Even though our skin, nose, mouth, esophagus, vagina, and gut are populated by something like ten thousand distinct species, the nature of their presence has only recently begun to be understood.

How do we know they are distinct from us, that they are different life-forms and not just generated by us? Because of their genetic material that is quite distinct from us and also much more diverse.

The collection of micro creatures that make their home in and on us is called the human microbiota. And their genes are called the microbiome.

In comparison to the microbiome, the human genome is standardized and limited; the human genome has about twenty-three thousand genes, whereas the microbiome has about two million. In other words, 99 percent of the unique genes in your body are bacterial and only about 1 percent human. If you take a group of people, their genomes will look mostly the same, but their microbes will look very different. And microbe species that are shared across people still differ in terms of specific strains and the genetic makeup of those strains. Microbes are more diverse and have a lot more genetic material than us and other animals and plants. They also evolve much more quickly than us, swapping genetic information with their neighbors (often different species) in a process called horizontal gene transfer. Horizontal gene transfer is one of the most fascinating differences between human evolution, which is predominantly vertical and where change is very slow and gradual, and single-cell evolution, which can be horizontal and extremely fast. This propels us into a very different understanding of evolution than the model we have lived with of vertical inheritance.

"Animals and plants are far more similar to each other than they are to all the other kinds of Earth life!" said Lynn Margulis. We have more in common with chickens than with microbes.

"You are mostly not you"—this phrase is taken from Rob Knight, but you can find variants of it all over the popular science pages of newspapers and internet sites. But what's the big deal? you might ask. If we assume that people are not simply biological beings or at least not entirely biologically determined, then surely this is not a novel proposition.

> You do not of course you do not really believe yourself why should you, you know so well so very well that it is not yourself, it could not be yourself because you cannot remember right and if you do remember right it does not sound right. You are of course never yourself.

Gertrude Stein, empress of the avant-garde, wrote this in 1936. Philosophers and poets throughout the twentieth century and before—stretching way back to the gnostics and throughout Eastern traditions of thought and spirituality—have been reconfiguring the "you" and the "I," positing not a unified and autonomous self, but a "you" made up of bits and pieces, of social and cultural, conscious and unconscious, influences. So is this current biological understanding of ourselves, what we might term the microbial perspective, fundamentally new and different? In some ways, no—twenty-first-century biologists are not the first to unsettle the sovereignty of the human ego—but in other ways, yes. What this biological turn does is introduce a fundamental breach, not just into the way of seeing you, the human body, but into the way the human is situated in a larger environment and in relation to other ecosystems. In a time of devastating global warming it introduces a potential reframing of the world.

The human body isn't just what you see in the mirror. . . . It's an ecosystem, just like a forest, just like the ocean, where microbes of many different species are interacting to support the whole.

Just like a forest, just like the ocean. Linking the human body to a forest or an ocean is not just a poetic metaphor, though it is this as well; it is performing a conceptual acrobatic maneuver. The effect is not just to dethrone "man" from his pedestal, but to insert the human into a web of associations. While it may be the case that, genetically speaking, we have more in common with chickens than with microbes, we do have very intimate and enmeshed relations with microbes, especially the microbes that live in and on our bodies, and these relations mirror the symbiotic relations that sustain ecocultures, such as coral reefs and forests.

It might be a common refrain today to hear that microbes rule the world. But "microbes don't just 'rule' the world: they make every life form possible, and they have been doing so since the beginning of evolutionary time." The scientist Lynn Margulis argued in the sixties and seventies that cells with nuclei, including all the cells in the human body (except mature red blood cells), descended from bacteria that formed symbiotic relationships more than two billion years ago. Although this view is now commonly held, she was ridiculed at the time by other scientists and virtually ignored until recently.

They sentenced me to twenty years of boredom
For trying to change the system from within.
I'm coming now, I'm coming to reward them.
First we take Manhattan, then we take Berlin.

Rather than a neo-Darwinian account of the motor of evolution as driven by random mutations, the alternative she proposed was "a symbiotic, interactive view of the history of life on Earth." The key words here are *evolution* and *symbiosis*. Although in this new schema these two words—*evolution* and *symbiosis*—can't easily be separated, for the moment I'm going to treat science like poetry and parse the verse. First we take symbiosis.

Symbiosis is the scientific term for two different species of organisms living closely together in a way that benefits at least one of the species. Examples of symbiosis are a species of small fish that cleans parasites from much larger fish, or a fungus that grows on a person's skin, or the microbes that digest the grass the cow chews so that the nutrients that she cannot herself digest are made available to her. It isn't that scientists didn't know about symbiosis long before Margulis, nor did she coin the term *symbiogenesis*, but she was the first scholar to draw attention to symbiosis as a major developmental and evolutionary force.

And so to Berlin: Then we take evolution. In contrast to the vertical view of inheritance and descent, symbiogenesis proposes that evolution is a function of organisms that are mutually beneficial growing together to become one and re-producing. Swiveling from the vertical orientation, where the precept that man evolved from apes reigns, to a horizontal orientation, we might say that man and apes evolved from a common ancestor. The precept that all life-forms share a common evolutionary origin induces a swerve, a refocusing of attention toward relations between apparently complex and seemingly lesser organisms.

There are no "higher" beings, no "lower animals," no angels, and no gods.

Although the concept of symbiogenesis was proposed a century ago, the hypothesis could only be tested relatively recently. In the past scientists focused their attention on microbes they could see—in a lab, in a petri dish, under a microscope—so they focused on a single species at a time. In the early 2000s researchers developed genetic batch sequencing techniques, allowing them, say, to catalog all the DNA in a rind of cheese. Suddenly microbes became visible in startlingly new configurations. And what emerged is evidence that symbiosis is much more common than was previously thought and, indeed, that it is "not a marginal or rare phenomenon. It is natural and common. We abide in a symbiotic world." During much thinking of the twentieth century, and particularly in neo-Darwinian ideas of evolution, the imagined autonomy of the individual was tied to the autonomy of the species. Each species was thought to rise and fall through the fitness of the individuals it produced—the "you are you" perspective. Today these ideas of separation and autonomy are being questioned. A major engine of accelerated adaptation and evolution, it turns out, is hybridization. Cross-species interaction has been shown as essential to development, evolution, and ecology. "Genes are jumping around"—the "you are mostly not you" perspective.

. . .

Microbes actually have a propensity for horizontal gene transfer, for exchanging information, grabbing genetic material, jumping around, whereas multicellular organisms have a propensity against horizontal gene transfer. However, new discoveries in the realm of the human genome—instances where human cells migrate—are endorsing the idea that you are not all you. It seems that we all contain a small fraction of cells from someone else. During the birth process the cells of the mother infiltrate horizontally across the placenta into the child, and the cells of the child infiltrate into the mother. Thus we all are more like a "we" than an "I."

The horizontal has upended what we thought we knew about gene transfer, and it has caused a radical rethinking of the Darwinian tree of life, with species branching out and separating. A web of life, or network, seems a more appropriate model with genes moving between close branches as related species interbreed. As Lynn Margulis put it:

In reality the tree of life often grows in on itself. Species come together, fuse, and make new beings, who start again. . . . The tree of life is a twisted, tangled, pulsing entity with roots and branches meeting underground and in midair to form eccentric new fruits and hybrids.

One of the areas opened up when we view existence as a web rather than a tree, and when we bring symbiosis into the foreground, is the coevolution of species, an aspect of life as crucial as the actual exchange of genetic information. We now know that many of the microbes that live within us have coevolved with us, enabling us to live in a variety of ways, for instance, through digesting for us what we ourselves cannot digest. Take human milk: One of the major nutritional ingredients of human milk is a complex of sugars called oligosaccharides or HMOs—that babies cannot digest. Why do they exist? Scientists have discovered that they feed certain microbes that produce nutrients for the baby. "So while mothers nourish this microbe, the microbe in turn nourishes the baby." The human body is a series of nested ecosystems. Many species of coral have microbial symbionts that live within their cells and provide them with oxygen and sugars. Pollutant stress and thermal stress, caused by global warming, can cause the symbionts to die. Without them, the coral cannot survive; it whitens and dies. We know of many damaged natural systems where the return of species, once plentiful, has restored ecological balance to the environment: gray wolves to Yellowstone National Park, for instance, and sea otters to coastal regions. In areas (islands particularly) where otters were killed off it followed that the kelp forests were denuded by sea urchins. Sea otters, by eating sea urchins, enable the growth of lush and productive kelp forests that have the capacity to absorb billions of kilograms of carbon, thus contributing significantly to global environmental health.

. . .

So in the end does it mean much to say you are mostly not you? Does the turn toward the horizontal view signify a major shift in our apprehension of the world? Yes, because it reframes, rejigs our image of the world, the map, if you like. (As Gregory Bateson famously said: The map is not the territory.) In upsetting the established hierarchy of the tree of life it introduces into the picture new and unexpected relations. As Ursula Le Guin puts it:

And now, both poets and scientists are extending the rational aspect of our sense of relationship to creatures without nervous systems and to nonliving beings—our fellowship as creatures with other creatures, things with other things.

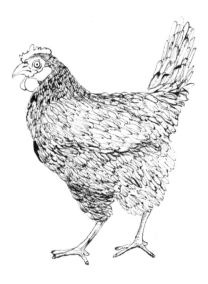

RIP Elvis, the King of the Cats

I know of course that all things pass of course I know and know too that passing takes time and time and time. Yet I do not know how I will face a world in which Elvis is not there. When I wake in the night and he grunts and nudges with his nose, purrs snortingly. How I will miss him.

December 21, 2015. He remained a gentle warrior till the end, we were together on the bed where we have spent so much time together, he was purring as I read aloud to him before the vet came, though I doubt it was the story or even affection that moved him so.

After about ten years (say, four years ago) Elvis decided to stop his campaign of indifferent malevolence toward J, and they became friends. J is digging his grave in the garden. He is wrapped (Elvis, not J) in a beautiful cashmere shawl in jewel colors of green and deep sea blue. This afternoon we will go to the nursery to find a camellia to plant for him.

When he came to Herman Avenue, fourteen years ago, I wrote this:

Feline Transmogrification

[Plutarch] states that it was not the cat or (for example) the bull which the Egyptians worshipped: what they worshipped in these beasts was an image of the divine attributes . . . in the cat, quickness, or . . . its refusal to let itself be shut in: by the cat they represented that freedom which they loved above any other of God's attributes. —Michel de Montaigne

J goes back to Australia in June. I drive home from LAX feeling bereft and lonely. Almost home I pass the large ANIMAL SHELTER sign, which looms over the freeway at Solana Beach. Poor Lulu, I think, she too is lonely and grieving for Barnabas. On impulse, I take the next exit and double back to the shelter. And that is how it came about that I fell in love with a cat called Elvis.

When I fell in love with Elvis, however, he wasn't yet Elvis. Or maybe I only fell for him once he was named, once he *was* Elvis. Prior to that he was not exactly nameless. But he might as well have been. In the shelter he was called Chester, which seemed an indignity. Not that he was dignified. A white and apricot tabby he had inordinately long skinny legs on a tiny body. Passing along the aisle of adorable kittens I did not give him a second look. It must have been that indifference that provoked him. He flew out of his box like a Sputnik, landed on my chest, wrapped his little paws around my neck, and purred so loudly it was hard to imagine how the noise was fueled in such a tiny body. So that was it, he chose me, and without further ado I signed the papers paid the money put him in his cardboard box on the seat beside me, and off we drove. The moment the car started so began an unholy bloodcurdling yowling. I spoke soothingly to the kitten, I sang lullabies, I tried turning the name Chester into a magical incantation. But there is nothing remotely magical in the name Chester, and the caterwauling only got worse and worse. And then it came to me. The sound of rock 'n' roll, a sound that changed the world. Elvis Presley filled my pubescent years with exhilaration, with longing, with the beginnings of desire, with a sense of a world beyond the farm. But to my father's ears the sound of Elvis Presley was the sound of caterwauling. He would rant and rave and fulminate against the evils of rock 'n' roll. But rock 'n' roll has rolled on through the years for me, and nowadays the name Elvis evokes that later incarnation, Elvis Costello, particularly in his album *Blue*: a transmigration of the Elvis soul. You too are a transmogrification, I tell the cat, "You shall be Elvis." And so he is.

Several weeks have passed and all is not so rosy on the domestic front. I expected Lulu to be thrilled by the advent of a new feline companion. But no, it seems that she had become accustomed to and was enjoying being top and solo cat. She turned on this little kitten with a savagery I had no idea she possessed. She watches him with what seems to be a mixture of fear and loathing, and then at some moment when he is most vulnerable, she pounces. J says cats do not have emotions, and I tell him he should see Lulu, I do not know exactly what emotions are gripping her but something grips her: hatred, malice, jealousy, resentment. I have not been able to leave them alone together and the first week put Elvis in the backroom with his litter box. Each morning the room was covered in litter as he dug furiously through the night it seemed, scattering sand to the four corners of the universe, over furniture, in the bed, on the rug, in pairs of shoes. Last week I introduced him to the garden. He was delirious with joy, made a beeline for the camellias, frantically dug several holes, raced into the vegetable patch, and picked his way through every bed, nose in the air, sniffing, comparing all the different smells, mapping out the territory, digging more holes. In the front garden he made a dash down the street and disappeared up a tree. My heart stopped as I envisaged him disappearing into the black hole of suburbia. But after trying out several trees he raced home, made a nest in the dust, and rolled around, purring. While I held my breath watching him race away, Mrs. Tam giggled like crazy, clapping her hands. "Lulu," she says to me. "Lulu," she splutters, shaking her head with glee, putting her nose in the air and sniffing, imitating Elvis. *Lulu* is the generic English term she uses for *cat*. I think that she has recognized in Elvis a kindred spirit, a denizen of the garden.

. . .

We were together a long time, Elvis and I. Since coming to live in this country in 2000 and moving into Herman Avenue in 2001 (J only moved to the U.S. properly in 2004), I have spent more time with him than with any other being. I'm so used to sensing him, at night, on one side of my body, the weight of him, leaning in. And now he is not there, there where he was there is just the feeling of nothing. After some days the pain—a heavy contracted sensation across my chest—mutates into anger. Anger at Elvis. For some years after being diagnosed, and especially in those times when I was less well than now, I imagined that both Elvis and J would be with me for the rest of my life. I never imagined that I would outlive them. I wrote him a poem:

> Fur of my fur where are you?
> somewhere
> without
> me
> catless
> spurned abandoned blubbering
> or
> oftener and oftener,
> as hours and nights and already etiolated days
> stretch and shrink
> feelingless
> why the fuck Elvis
> did you have to go and die
> and leave me thus?
> beloved cat
> furless
> skinned

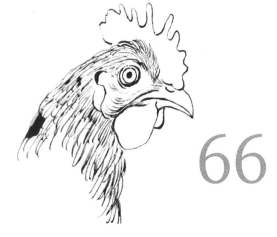

Afterlife

We had two cats when we lived in Newcastle. . . . They departed within a
month of each other, and I remember looking out into the garden from my
study thinking—it's so empty out there. Cats are somehow always on your
peripheral vision—or just out of it. Sitting behind you. Sleeping somewhere,
half hidden. Prowling out there around the fence. Settled under a bush, feet
neatly together, looking upwards at the birds. Missing them becomes part
of their extended life cycle—keeps them just there, out of reach but never
quite out of mind.

Jane G wrote this to me after Elvis died. I am now in Dorland again, grappling
with words, trying to finish this book. Delusional, I had imagined it was almost
done. Just a few touch-ups here and there. But there are great holes, and passages
of garbage, and occasional words that shine but as I reach out they vibrate with too
many associations and memories and then when I'm ready to commit they have
slithered out of view, into the past, or into someone else's book. I complain to Eileen, she writes back, I know that kind of writing delusion. Once you accept it's
not there I think it gets there quicker don't you? Total collapse, total acceleration.

It feels more like a crawling out of collapse. But I keep hoping for acceleration,
and her words are a kick start. No distractions here, no one to talk to (though an
email comes from J: Lula May and Holly continue laying eggs, accompanied by a
photo of Elvis's scarlet camellia bush in full bloom). The hungry ghosts are here,
everywhere, tempting and tormenting. But so too is Elvis, in my peripheral vision
all the time. I was so used to running things by him—phrases and turns of phrase
and sometimes convoluted ideas. They'd run right past him, he'd maybe look, listen, yawn, but the ideas would run and run like rabbits in a field of stubbled corn,

right past him. And I was so used to the weight and warmth of his body against my leg as I sat propped in bed with the Mac Air. Sometimes he would get fed up and nudge it off my lap. And all the years we spent in the garden together, and all the time he spent in the garden alone, in his own world; often he would disappear—especially in the summer—for days and nights, sequestered deep in a lair within the bamboo jungle, impenetrable to humans. Then, when least expected, he would wander into the bedroom, jump onto the bed, and make a squalling sound: I'm back! What's up? What've you got to show?

Here at Dorland I continue the habit of waking early, making a pot of tea, and writing through the morning in bed. I started this habit because I found it a way to preserve energy when I was unwell. I never noticed this when I was well: that sitting up at a desk and working takes energy, just like driving. Now I am better than I have been in the past six years since I was diagnosed. Amazingly better. Apart from the permanently wonky immune system, all my results are stellar, no flags. Dr. K gave me the green light to go off all the remaining drugs a few weeks ago, not long after Elvis died. Now I just take vitamin D each day. How ironic, even perverse, it seems, that I should become so much better as Elvis's health declined. Of course my symptoms will return. But Elvis will not. And how will I manage then? I ask myself. As I am now, I suppose, still talking to Elvis, feeling and hearing him. My feline muse.

I know that habits are best broken rather than clung to. I know how expert we are at weaving cocoons of custom. But from my bedroom here, with the Mac Air and a pot of tea, as always and wherever, I see the sun come up over the hills and in the distance the snow-covered mountains where we were not so long ago.

I have never been here with Elvis, he hated traveling in a car, which is not to say he did not travel, on his own four legs, around the neighborhood, knowing parts mysterious to me. It is curious, however, that his presence is very strong here. In the afternoons a shaft of sunlight comes in through the side door. I can't actually open the door to the sunlight because the bees gorging on the hedge of rosemary come buzzing in. But I stand in the warm golden pool, basking, feeling as though I am becoming Elvis: how especially in his last days when he did not go outside he would wait for the sunlight to come into the living room, and there he would lie, stretched out, sometimes flexing his paws, arching his back, feeling the light enter into him, loosening the pain.

Or so I imagine. Of course I do not really know what he was feeling. I don't know what was going through his mind on those occasions when he looked at me so quizzically. I can only guess at the nature of his fear when coerced into a box and taken in a car to the veterinary hospital, and when we played with that well-chewed toy creature, half airplane and half dog, stuffed with catnip: Was he really in the grip of ecstasy? Remember Montaigne: "When I play with my cat, how do I know that she is not passing time with me rather than I with her?" I'm sure that Elvis was often passing time, indulging me, or simply trying to let me know he was hungry. Nevertheless, there was between us an empathetic energy, an understanding. Charlie Aarons wrote to me, speaking perspicaciously of rhythms: "Ah Les . . . How you enjoy and get used to each other's rhythms, patterns, habits. How even though they 'don't speak,' you learn each other's language and talk to each other every day."

J points out to me when I become angry with Elvis for going and dying on me that he didn't just die, that it was we who made the decision to euthanize. It isn't as though I didn't think about this before the event, it isn't as though I don't think we should be cognizant of the divide as well as the shared terrain between humans and their animal companions. But for the moment, now . . . I can't yet think or write it.

After arriving here at Dorland, all day I heard the soft dull sound of a braying donkey. How strange it sounded, where can it be coming from, how can it carry across the canyons and mountains? I walked around trying to locate it. It was like being back in Mexico in the village of San Agustín Etla near Oaxaca, or walking along by the train in Marathon, Texas. I loved the sound. At night it continued. Eventually it dawned on me that the braying was coming at very measured intervals, a gentle muffled rhythm. I put my ear to the fridge! That was it—a burro in the fridge! What a strange delusion, how I managed to rearticulate sound and space so that the image of the burro was stronger than any logic. Even after I located the source of the sound I had a strong sense of the burro as a presence, not in the room but somehow in the space in which I've been enveloped. The burro and I, wrapped together. A comfort in being brayed. Perhaps Elvis is taking on the form of a burro, braying, the sound of him in my peripheral hearing.

Earlier this month, not long after Elvis died, I saw Laurie Anderson's film *Heart of a Dog*, revolving around the life and the passing of her rat terrier, Lulabelle. "Drizzled with sadness," the film is also enjoyably playful and silly. It is also a meditation on memory, on forgetting (on occasion evoking jagged and painful relationships, as with her mother), and a tribute to those she's loved and lost in addition to Lulabelle. Ghosting the whole film is Lou Reed, with whom Anderson was involved for twenty-odd years (five of them married), who died while the film was being made. He flickers only very occasionally in and out of the frame, but he is heard, his voice and music, in the closing track of the film: "Turning Time Around." Me, I couldn't help conjuring the Lou Reed I saw on stage in Glasgow in 1974, just after the release of "Sally Can't Dance." Prowling around the stage, close-shaved, bottle blond, all in slinky black with aviator shades, he blazoned: a match flaring in the deep dark Glasgow gloom. It is love, he intones in 2015, that turns time around.

Laurie Anderson tells how, after Lulabelle died, she observed the forty-nine days in which her dog was in Bardo. Bardo is the gap, the liminal zone, the afterlife between this and other lives. I didn't do this for Elvis, but I did and still do tonglen for him, to ease his passage into another world. When I do this meditative practice for Elvis it is of course as well and even more so for myself that I do it. To feel that constriction in the chest loosen a little, a dissolving of the brittleness. I have brought *The Tibetan Book of the Dead* and dip in and out of it. It is the little pocket edition that, wedged in behind some larger books, fell out of the bookcase the last time I stayed here. By mistake it got into my suitcase when I left, and so I brought it back with me this time, to return to its proper place. But it is worn and grubby because I read it while eating, so probably I should replace it with a new copy. On the other hand, perhaps there is no proper place for a book of the dead. As Chögyam Trungpa Rinpoche points out in his commentary, it is not really a book about death, it could equally be called "The Tibetan Book of Birth."

When I do tonglen I have a very strong sense of Elvis being present, his spirit being physically here. Sometimes at home at night I hear him scuffling around on the wooden floorboards and then padding toward the bed, I talk to him and in his way he responds. When I say his spirit is here it's not exactly that I apprehend him as a ghostly imitation or replica of his living self. But, rather, that the distinction between the living and the dead is indistinct, blurry, like the soft under feathers of a chicken fluffed in the wind.

And it is not only Elvis. Other spirits return—my mother and father—vividly present as they have not been for many years. They are not quiet ghosts, and for me their presence, as in life, is unsettling. But I am getting used to them being around, am beginning to listen, to discern through the accusations and vituperative exchanges some other tones, more tender. It is as though Elvis is now my guide through the world of the dead, my Virgilian cat, leading me through the liminal zone where life and death blur into one another.

. . .

Missing them becomes part of their extended life cycle—keeps them just there, out of reach but never quite out of mind.

. . .

Even when you have become mindless, or turned your attention totally elsewhere, he turns—or is turned—up. Reading again that remarkable book *Tristes Tropiques* I turn to the last chapter and in the very last words discover Elvis, on the periphery, looking back over his shoulder at me. But before that I am surprised at something that never registered before, perhaps because in the past the allure of structuralism was stronger than the provocation of poetry. These two aspects are condensed in a typically tossed-off bit of bathos: "Florence, which I visited after New York, did not produce any first effect of surprise: in its architecture and plastic arts, I recognized the Wall Street of the fifteenth century." That makes me laugh (not least because of the way a high-flown theoretical point is undercut by a recurring grouch against travel writing), but what surprises me, what had not really registered before, is the hint of Buddhist sentiment in the Lévi-Strauss of *Tristes Tropiques*. You might say, but this is simply an aspect of his structuralist view of history and culture, perfectly rendered in this analogy: "Between the Marxist critique, which frees man from his initial bondage—by teaching him that the apparent meaning of his condition evaporates as soon as he agrees to see things in a wider context—and the Buddhist critique which completes his liberation, there is neither opposition nor contradiction." Perhaps, but there is also something in the jaggedly poetic summoning of images, the descent into a calmer cadence. The end of the book is initiated by the observation, "The world began without man and will end without him." The human species is not the only species, and in fact what matters in the end ("Oh! Fond farewell," doffing his cap with a splash of irony, "to savages and explorations!"), and what every human has in common, is the possibility of *unhitching* for a moment, of being able to grasp, in those brief intervals between frenetic activity, "the essence of what it was and continues to be, below the threshold of thought and over and above society." Of being able to grasp this in the contemplation of a mineral more beautiful than all our creations, the scent of a lily more imbued with learning than all our books, or—and the book then comes to an end with these words:

> In the brief glance, heavy with patience, serenity and mutual forgiveness,
>   that,
> through some involuntary understanding, one can sometimes exchange
>   with a cat.

Art Alive

67

APRIL 2016

"This is like Costco," mumbles the young man in front of me. "Is this Italy?" shouts a young kid, excitedly. Suddenly boring old San Diego becomes mysterious, the museum reveals itself simultaneously as a big box store and an exotic locale, resplendent, teeming with people and art and sublimity.

We are squished together, art devotees and flower lovers, kids and adults, Asians and San Diegans, and Asian San Diegans, and people in wheelchairs, and docents clutching big books full of notes. We try to edge toward the art and toward the flower arrangements and try not to obstruct each other's camera view.

It is the "Art Alive" show, in which flower artists are asked to respond to a work of their choosing on display in the Asian art collection. I'm here to see the flower arrangements, particularly the piece by my ikebana teacher Donna West. I respect her enormously and am in awe of those ikebana masters who can distill all the energy of the universe into an austerely exquisite arrangement, but I'm predisposed to find the whole concept of arranging flowers in response to works of art rather kitschy. The participating artists include florists and event orchestrators as well as ikebana practitioners. I'm here to roll my eyes a bit, to pick up a few tips, to whizz in and out and away.

But it's as though I've entered into an unfamiliar super-charged universe. It's at once quotidian, jam-packed with weekend tourists, full of elbow poking and gossipy exchanges, and otherworldly, resplendent with saturated colors and sensations: celadon pottery glazed in oxblood, mustard yellow, lapis blue. Room after room reveals amazing surprises.

Very few of the arrangements mimic or copy or even try to represent the works of art to which they speak. Imagine a wild snarling cat, crouched, ready to pounce, configured through a composition of calla lilies, iridescent velvety purple; an artichoke, deep burgundy; red spiky proteas; cat's tail willow; dried flattened mushrooms. A structure of chicken wire and kangaroo paw, reeds bent at sharp angles, speaks to an intricately geometric sandstone *jali*, or perforated screen, from seventeenth-century Northern India. In the Buddhist rooms there is a wooden carving of a "Bodhisattva Guanyin of the Southern Seas." The verve of the carving—drapes and scarves flowing around the muscular and still body of the Bodhisattva—is evoked in the gestural echoing of the floral arrangement that includes roses and proteas, lilies and burgundy leaves. Flattened calla leaves reach out swooningly, like the arm of the Bodhisattva.

I'm charmed by the use of local materials, such as small succulents actually planted in the base of an arrangement that speaks to a Korean pickle jar (with lid and facets), gorgeous in green and brown stone, edging into burgundy. The shape of the jar, with a flattened top, is suggested by a green protea, and the colors are elicited by sunflowers with celadon petals and burgundy centers. The floral composition echoes the artwork but within itself is also murmurous with echoes. The succulents at the base are like a mirror image of the sunflowers towering above them: burgundy flesh unfurling from green centers. The best room of all is "Tombs: Art for the Dead in Ancient China." All artifacts here are recovered from tombs dating from 3000 BCE to the eighth century CE. "They pertain to the feeding, protection and entertainment of the dead who are in transition from this life to the next." There is a brightly colored prancing horse from the eighth century and two camels that, except for their size, seem to have wandered in out of the desert. There is a section on entertainment in the afterlife that includes dancers, a polo player, and figures engaged in various athletic games. There is a rich cosmology in many cultures and religions in which the afterlife is not the end of the road, not dedicated to deadness, but is rather an intermediate zone where life goes on and where the living can accommodate to the idea of death, to living without their loved ones. Think of Aeneas in book 6 of *The Iliad*, where passage from this world to the next, on a boat steered by the boatman Charon through the inky Stygian waters, through a place of shadows, of sleep and dreamy night, is terrifying. He is in search of his father, Anchises, but is warned that though the path to hell is easy, the hard task is retracing your footsteps, finding your way back to everyday life. In the process of searching he, and we, encounter a densely populated world where figures from history and mythology come to life. Eventually he finds his father, who, prophetically, teaches Aeneas how to avoid or face each trial awaiting him in the future, in the known world. Other cultures might describe Aeneas's journey as a form of ancestor worship.

The conjunction of living plants and dead things—sculptures, artifacts from vanished civilizations—reminds me that ikebana is a communicative as well as a meditative art, we do the flower arrangements for our community but also for the shrine, to remember, to encounter the ancestors, to find ways to survive the future.

Bodies in Pieces

68

Hung by the neck. Heads hacked off, chests sawn open, hearts wrenched out. Bodies in pieces.

It's 1789 in Paris.

Reading, in France today, in September 2016, about these severed bodies, you'd think would be unnerving. I'm reading this in the countryside, so bucolic, an endlessly streaming sense of space and light. Friendship, reunions, long slow cooking of apples that fall off the tree, and figs squishy and oozing, rabbits and sardines brought home from the market, the bunnies smothered in mustard, the little fish tossed in fruity olive oil and lemon juice sharp as razors. Wine from the village, pale and flinty with an aftertaste of sweetness. Indolently time unwinds, confessions dribble out, memories clash, laughter laced with stress, how foolish we have grown instead of wiser.

But no, it isn't France that is unnerving. It's the U.S. I have escaped the vaudevillian horror of this election year: to spend a few weeks in late summer with old friends. Who would have thought that Les Ruda, my oldest friend from childhood days in Zimbabwe, the sporadically penniless but always-resourceful artist, would land up with a share in a beautiful eighteenth-century house in a village in the Dordogne. A few changes have been made, the kitchen updated, but the old veranda remains. We eat all our meals there and sit and watch the light fade each evening, and it is almost like being back in Zimbabwe. But not quite. The sliver of violence that was always snaking through the air there is not here. Or perhaps it is, but the sense of elsewhere is more pronounced.

The noise of the U.S. elections was deafening, like a schoolyard scrum, with bullies and cheering mobs, never-ending, a bright assaulting sound-and-light show. A sense of horror and disbelief that it can have come to this: a fairground shyster in the limelight, gathering votes like a fisher of men from pools where the fish are plentiful and swim with their mouths open, waiting eagerly for the taste of a hook.

In France there's a lull, the screeching subsides, no radio or television. Your in-box is still crammed to overflowing with emails begging for money money money to keep democracy alive. Social media doesn't go away of course but you only go there once a day, like a visit to church—keep it short and sharp. No more babble.

It's Hilary Mantel's *A Place of Greater Safety* that immerses me. A huge and utterly engrossing novel about the French Revolution. I'm about halfway through and have this dual sensation: of greed, on the one hand—please, good Buddha, good heathen god of words and stories, fairy godmother magicked out of the moment, please let this go on forever, these words that stretch caressingly into sentences and then recoil and whip you across the face, these characters that oh so slowly expand their tentacle dimensions, curling and uncurling and expanding in ways you never anticipated even though you know, roughly speaking, the story. On the other hand, a parsimonious withdrawal: If everyone leaves me alone for the next hour, then I can finish part two and will be satisfied and socialized again and able to put the French Revolution out of my mind and make a start on the dinner. I only need a little hit, a little bit of time, a taste of the story.

Eventually I have to leave the French Revolution to attend to my body. I am feeling far from sick but still need the monthly infusion of immunoglobulin. I have been learning—like an old dog, slow, and on some deep level, stubbornly resistant—to administer this myself "at home." I was lured in by the company that provides the drugs and training by the promise that traveling would be easier. But there are many bottles to travel with, not to mention the needles and swabs and wipes and tubes and scissors and pump. Trying to fill the minuscule transparent pipes with transparent liquid, to gauge the level, is a nightmare, and each week there is the traumatic encounter with needles and stomach flesh and the possibility of blood. More like a big baby than an old dog, if the truth be told, or perhaps some sort of antiquated baby–dog hybrid. Most people seem to learn quickly and manage fine. Eventually I will give up and confess my ineptitude to Dr. K, who is unconditionally sympathetic and writes the letter to return me to my friends at the infusion center. Back home Judy would sit with me during the setup, a calming presence. But here, in this paradisiacal escape, I recruit Virginia and Helen to help. Better, it turns out, than being hung by the neck.

In fact so far the bodies are few and far between. There are long long passages of intimate encounter with names we know so well: Danton and Robespierre, and less well Camille Desmoulins. Common and garden names. And names we do not know: Lucile, Gabrielle, Angelique, Annette, Louise, women brought into the picture by Mantel. In the process the names are denatured, reconfigured. How it all begins in a populist uprising, the women storming Versailles—dramatic, bloody, horrifying; and then the politics, the refining of strategies, distinguishing strategies from tactics, the taming of impulse, the romance, the friendships and alliances and betrayals and ambition.

Leslie Dick gave me her copy of *A Place of Greater Safety* when I mentioned needing a novel for the plane. I thought it kind of her but far too weighty to carry on board and probably also not thrilling enough even though she claimed she couldn't put it down and carried it with her to the supermarket and to class. Then Tershia saw it sitting on the table at home and said, It's the best book I've ever read. And so I ordered it on Kindle. And while I'm here in France, Tershia's book, *The Man Who Thought He Owned Water*, is being released, such a different book, about water rights and farming and the city and her father, but I think I can see why she loves the Mantel, and Leslie too, perhaps it has something to do with the story of politics, the telling of stories that intertwine and complicate, something that emerges in the details—gestures, obsessions, the toss of a head, languishing looks, cutting remarks, everyday survival (how the books are balanced, say), what is read, the jokes that are flipped back and forth.

. . .

Now it is the early hours of Monday morning, back in San Diego. I have made my tea and been to stand at the front of the house and the back where everything is glistening, wet, smelling of earth.

. . .

It is almost as though the night, filled with horror, never happened. We were woken at 3:30 AM by a huge shaking thunderous din. Or was it the night sweats that woke me? Boiling, tearing off clothing, swamped by sweat. On and on it went, the earth tumbling, a rumbling in the desert, my body feverish. Earthquake! I grabbed for J. It's the end of the world! We lay there wrapped around each other, shaking, until we realized it was a storm, whipped up out of nowhere, great claps of thunder and lightning, car alarms going off up and down the street. It poured, it poured rain, for about half an hour. And my body poured sweat, drenching the sheets. Then suddenly, in a matter of moments, the feverish heat turns into an arctic freeze. Layering on clothing—socks, sweaters, vests, articles of clothing worn in the day and discarded at bedtime. But it's impossible to warm up.

Although there is no warning, I knew of course that the CLL symptoms would return. But somehow I am unprepared, psychically, for another bout of the beast. I know that there are far worse things going on in the larger world than in my body, yet somehow at 3:30 in the morning it all seems conflated into one big miserable mess, leaking into the room, invading the bed, creeping up over my pillow into my mouth and ears and eyes and anus and vagina and through the pores of my skin. J rolled over and went back to sleep. I was wide awake and returned to reading *A Place of Greater Safety*. I almost wonder if I didn't dream all this, if I didn't conjure up, out of the French Revolution, a local apocalypse. Once I stopped shaking and the flashing and bellowing ceased and the sweating and freezing subsided, I lay there listening to the rain, happy for a moment, imagining a brighter future.

Of course many utopias are conceived of and brought into being through coercive means. The revolutionary impulse so often aims too high and, as a result, falls short or even lands up betraying the very principles that inspired the uprising. Revolutions and wars signal historically dramatic high points, but the quotidian existence of many, even under peaceful and often democratic regimes, can entail intolerable poverty, habitual struggle to survive, and disenfranchisement.

I have to gloss many of the pages told from the perspective of the guy who wields the guillotine, practical stuff like how his salary doesn't cover costs, how he has to order more carts to drag the bodies away, how much blood there is to deal with, how he can't pay the wages that would attract people to the job. The French Revolution degenerated into a bloodbath "and yet," as Rebecca Solnit observes, "when that revolution was over, France would never be dominated by an absolutist monarchy again; ordinary French people had more rights, and people around the world had an enlarged sense of the possible."

The nightmare that rocked me in the night now seems phantasmatic, a haunting rather than a real occurrence. Planetary despair finding an ally in my body. Collusion, consolidation. As it turns out, the storm is an aberration, not the longed for breaking of the drought. And the night sweats persist for only a few nights and then mysteriously disappear.

False alarms or intimations of things to come?

A Prospect of Consolation

Fran, Les's mother, is dying. Les and Diane are flying home from France. In the meantime, since I returned earlier to the States, I have come to San Francisco to sit by her side. I have known her most of my life, but I don't know if she knows who I am. I don't know if she is in pain. She says not, but sometimes she shudders and screws up her face, and mutters I don't know I don't know I don't know. Is this a deep existential realization in the face of death? Maybe. More likely, I think, it is disapproval and confusion: I don't know what the fuck is going on (though she would use another word, any word, rather than *fuck*); I don't know how they can be such idiots; I don't know who this fuckwit is sitting here all day long. Sometimes she smiles and there seems to be recognition. But mostly the expression on her face is crumpled disgruntled confusion. So hard to form words, let alone sentences, though sometimes a coherent burst. Like when she stares fixedly at something on the end of her bed. I think it's the brightly colored crocheted blanket. She mutters, disdainfully, It's overdone. Yes, I say, it is pretty bright. She looks at me as though I'm a complete idiot. What? What do you mean? I could move the blanket, I say. Why? And she shakes her head. Slow-motion exasperation. I realize there is no possibility of conversation, of an exchange, though I keep falling for what seems like a trap once I've fallen. She has no memory of the words she's just spoken, they evaporate like the smell of hospital alcohol. But these bursts seem so cogent and hopeful that I blunder on trying to draw out a thread. She can speak clearly the phrase "I want." But all she wants now is ginger ale. I spoon it into her mouth and she savors it. She's not eating. In the morning she was better, sparks of recognition. We looked at her photos and she smiled now and then. I said, "Look at Richard, doesn't he look handsome?" Richard her son, young in the photo, now on his way home from Europe. "Not anymore," she mutters. I feel relieved, can almost discern a sardonic grin. It's the old Fran Ruda back in form. But after this any mention of Richard produces pained incomprehension, as though she has no idea of what I'm talking about but is somewhat grasping for comprehension. Richard calls from the airport in Italy and I put him on speaker phone so he can talk to Fran and she can hear his voice. She looks at me as though I'm out of my mind, trying to torture her: Where is this voice coming from? Who is it? What does it mean? Take it away. She has a toy dog, which she clutches and sometimes strokes; he has silky ears. Where is he? she sometimes asks, and she means the dog. He's constant, but he doesn't always behave, it seems. All I can discern is "behave himself." The old language of a white Rhodesian madam.

On the day that I leave Fran seems more in the world, she asks where J is. I say he's home looking after the chickens. We have three chickens, I explain. "I know," she says, indignant, "I know, I've met your chickens." I remember she has indeed. I've been situating her back in my childhood, back in Zimbabwe, forgetting her long and difficult journey, leaving the country she'd lived in for more than eighty years, learning to live in and accommodate to the U.S. of A. She has a photo of Obama on her picture board along with images of family and family dogs.

She is in hospice, but what this means in the nursing home is simply that she is on hospice care. Everyone is extremely busy, mostly filling in forms, doing paperwork on the computer. It's very hard to get any attention, to talk to anyone. Some of the nurses are gentle and observant. Others might as well be trash collectors, those people in official orange waist jackets who carry a trident and inch along the street spearing bits of rubbish and chucking it into a bin. Fran is simply a scrap of rubbish, an inert dummy. They put her bed up or down and rearrange her without asking her if this is what she wants. The tubes fall out of her nose, and they are shoved back in as though they are cigarettes being stuffed back into a pack. It isn't properly hung over her ear, it falls out again in five minutes. I cringe mimetically, involuntarily. What? barks the nurse. You could be more gentle, I say, she glares at me and flounces out. When I call in the evening to check up on how Fran is, the nurse says, Oh she's all right, sleeping now. Has she had any food or water? No food, but she drank her milk. You wouldn't know that this was a woman dying. Just a good girl because she drank her milk. I had a mistaken idea of hospice as a serene place. God save me from such an exit. I don't want to be ninety-three and not in control of many faculties. And at the mercy of nurses like this. I'd rather go quickly. But I look at Fran and am reminded that choice—that thing we cling to in the so-called greatest democracy in the world—is a thing that becomes so easily fragile and ragged, hard to grasp in your hands.

. . .

I gloss the gory pages of the novel and move on to how Robespierre is furious at the ranting of the atheists, taking away the last shreds of hope from the poor and dispossessed. How he writes to Danton, who has gone home to the country. He wants help from his friend, but he does not want to be patronized, he wants an ally, but he does not want to be dominated. He thinks, I should get Camille to write it, remembering himself and Camille as boys. Camille could put his case so simply, had put it so simply earlier that day: "We don't need processions and rosaries and relics, but we do need, when things are very bad, the prospect of consolation—we do need, when things are even worse, the idea that in the long run there is someone who could manage to forgive us."

Perhaps Fran, by letting me sit with her, giving me this space to perform as a surrogate daughter, is extending consolation, healing the regret, the shame, of being not-there when both my own parents died.

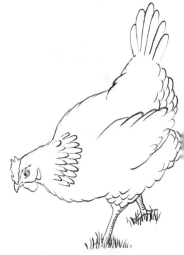

Fig Future

On November 8, 2016, the results of the U.S. presidential election are announced. Donald Trump will be the next president.

We started watching on television with Elana and Brian and his parents and a supply of fried chicken and beer. Parastout and Bahram are in other cities, they call in throughout the evening, increasingly agitated, as are we all. We pack it in early, in shock, seeing the writing on the wall. There is still a margin of chance when we go to bed, but J gets up after a couple of hours to check on his iPad and returns to bed ashen. This is not any ordinary flipping of the electorate; this is an unimaginable and catastrophic paradigm shift, though of course only those lacking in imagination can invoke the unimaginable. That'd be us: those of us taken by surprise, not alert to all the signs.

The next morning I rise early, get a shovel from the garage in the dark, and plant a fig tree as the light comes up, before the heat and the Santa Ana winds get going. It will turn out to be ninety-six degrees. When I first came here that would be unusually hot, even for summer. It is a Black Greek that Steve got as a cutting on eBay and nurtured in a gallon pot. I replanted it into a larger container, and now, replanted again, it is firmly in the earth, ready to be espaliered against the fence where the bamboo once grew so rampantly. Virginia M, who helped her parents plant hundreds of trees on their farm near Sydney, writes from Australia to say her daughters are frightened by the election results, what this means for the world. She tells me that many of those trees are now mature and beautiful, though her dad is not faring so well. I, on the other hand, am doing better but without trees. When I imagined that I might not have many years to live I wanted to plant things that would grow quickly and afford quick gratification. But now that it seems I am surviving, and now that the planet is heating up I feel compelled to start an urban forest filled with edibles.

In the last weeks J has been muttering about how, if Trump wins, we will go back to Australia. After the Brexit vote a Zimbabwean friend, living in London, wrote, with typical drollness: Fuck Democracy, let's all go back to Zimbabwe. But J surprises me this morning by saying, "This is where we live now, so let's stay and do what we can."

The fig tree will join the other fruit trees planted in the last year as gray water and rainwater tanks have been installed at Herman Avenue: a nectaplum with gorgeous deep burgundy foliage and pink flowers and tasty fruit called Spice Zee, a Parfianka pomegranate, an Australian finger lime, an improved Meyer lemon, a fuyu persimmon, a Wax Jambu that I buy on impulse from the Vietnamese nursery because of its beautiful spidery white flowers and rose-tinged green fruit, two pineapple guavas (feijoas), and two gifts—a Surinam cherry from Brian, grown from seeds that fell under his tree, and a mandarinquat from Nan. In addition to the trees, six blueberries have been planted in pots and six blackberries against the fence behind Elvis's grave. These all join the minimal orchard planted over the years we have been here: a Eureka lemon, the grapes that grow over the arbor at the back, the three espaliered apples, and the Gold Nugget mandarin. There are plans to round things out within the year with a Cara Cara orange, a Kishu mandarin, and a strawberry fig.

It is something to do, planting a fig tree, something physical to assuage the sense of paralysis and nausea that is creeping through my body. But it is also a tiny act of resistance, a statement, if only to ourselves, that we are here to stay.

Although, Samuel Beckett warns me against even a whiff of righteously hangdog triumphalism. It surprised me to learn that he was a digger, always digging and filling holes or planting trees in them in his plot of land outside Paris. He wrote to his American publisher that he had not been able to look for some weeks at the new play, *Endgame*, "But I have dug fifty-six large holes in my 'garden' for reception of various plantations, including 39 arbores vitae and a blue cypress." But this is not the last word. He adds: "They'll probably all die long before the Spring to judge by the look of the holes."

Between Fresh and Rotten

Between repetition and compulsion, between obsession and curiosity, between habit and ritual there is a thin line. I walk that line, into the valley of fermentation. First it is bread and then yogurt and then cheese and then all those really-almost-rotten ferments like kimchi and sauerkraut. Nose twitching, taste buds quivering, I walk the line.

Between fresh and rotten there is a creative space in which some of the most compelling of flavors arise.

My interest in learning how to conjure the solidity of cheese out of the liquidity of milk grew in tandem with a curiosity about microbes and fermentation and an urgent desire to strengthen a weak immune system and to promote and nurture a healthy gut. But as any fool knows, cheese—especially in excess—is not unmitigatedly healthy. It wasn't just an earnest devotion to self-help that plunged me into cheese making. It was a love and taste for cheese that was nurtured early.

My childhood was not festooned with an array of delectable and exotic cheeses. But what I do recall vividly, what pierces the smoky shroud of memory with sharp pungency, is a particularly strong cheddar. When the farm was in strife, losing money fast after a couple of seasons of failing tobacco crops, my parents replaced the habitual Sunday lunch—a huge roast and vegetables followed by a rich chocolate pudding—with what they presented as a very special, indeed extraordinarily exotic, meal called a ploughman's lunch. They in fact had never been to a British pub and had never eaten such a run-of-the-mill meal, but my father, in particular, was intrigued by food from all over the world, was always trying out recipes he came across in the *Sunday Mail* and even adapting and concocting dishes. When I turned twenty-one my parents did not have the resources to throw an elaborate party, but Dad did cook six dishes from different countries for ten of my friends, which we ate in the garden at Hillmorton Road in Harare (where my parents then lived), under the large old jacaranda tree through which was threaded a bougainvillea vine. In bloom together: a cascade of purple and flame red. Four years later his ashes would be scattered under that tree. During those bad seasons on the farm when Duncan and I were little kids, the exotic feast Dad prepared for us was in actual fact an extremely thrifty meal. There were jars of small brown onions that he had pickled, fermented watermelon rinds, bread, and a fabulous strong cheddar cheese, and to round it all out he had brewed some beer, and us kids were allowed the tiniest taste, each in our own glass.

He had not made the cheddar but did explain to us how it came from cows just like ours. In those days and on that farm there seemed no need to draw attention to the primarily grass diet of the cows. It was par for the course. The cows grazed on pasture, occasionally their grass diet augmented by lucerne hay (called alfalfa in the U.S.) and by silage (maize and sorghum and hay compacted into huge piles or pits in the ground and fermented). We had a herd of seventy-two Friesian cows (known in the U.S. as Holsteins) and a bull called Hero. Every cow had a name, and at three in the afternoon, in response to the ringing of the *simbi*, they all lined up in the grassy paddock, they lined up voluntarily in order and started trotting toward the dairy where they would wait impatiently, snorting and crapping and grunting and farting, each waiting for her name to be called so her heavy udder could experience relief. The *simbi* was a plough disk hung from a tree and hit with a piece of metal. Its reverberations, gong-like, would ring out all around the farm.

Microbes work in the gut—human or animal, caterpillar or aphid—and among other things, they digest fibers and things that the host cannot digest, and subsequently they make nutrients and vitamins available to the host. Look at cows lazily chewing the cud, munching endlessly and mindlessly on grass. It's a long slow process because, despite all the munching, the cows themselves cannot actually digest the grass. But the microbes in their stomachs can; it is they that digest cellulose from plants and produce nutritious acids for their hosts to absorb. Happy cows, happy people who eat those cows and their milk, as opposed to cows forcefed in feedlots, stuffed with grains they cannot digest properly, fed antibiotics that make them fat and that we absorb in drinking their milk.

Until that ploughman's lunch I had never made a connection between the cows delivering up their milk in the dairy and our daily visit to the row of calves in the barn at feeding time. They would stick their heads out of the small pen in which each was caged and open their mouths, nuzzling, reaching for our hands. We would slip a small hand into a calf's mouth—and experience a frisson of pleasure, the sensation of the ridged corrugated roof of the mouth and the rough sandpapery tongue and the soft slobbery slurping as the calves sucked. Then would come the pails of formula milk and they would duck their small heads in and drink greedily, lifting their frothy faces when finished: gorged, replete. We found it curiously satisfying. We knew where calves came from, had seen cows birthing, we saw human babies all the time on the farm suckling at their mothers' breasts. Yet it never occurred to us to ask why the calves were not with their mothers. Or maybe it did but I don't remember. As we ate that sharp cheddar and Dad explained where it came from, how it came to be on our table, the satisfaction of our harmonious union with the calves was shot through with sharpness. As is goat cheese sometimes today when I think of those kids yanked from their mothers so we can have milk and of all those boy kids disappeared. The violent edge of dairying and cheese making.

It was that strong cheddar that got me going on a path that before many years would lead me into the realm of squishy stinky cheeses redolent of the smells of childhood on a farm.

When I went to live in Glasgow as a graduate student with my then husband NS, we were cold and poor and hated the stodge that was dished up as food at the university. Eventually we lived with ten others in an old large Victorian house. NS had a number of skills, not the least of which was his talent as a shoplifter, a selectively ethical shoplifter. He never stole books, even though we spent a lot of time lusting after books. He only pocketed luxury food items. When misery and hunger were beginning to escalate he would return to the house, a bit aromatic, his corduroy pockets bulging and squishy. Then he would unload his foraging finds: smoked Scottish salmon, Italian salamis, plump succulent olives, and cheeses—smelly, soft, moldy, blue, and redolent of spoilt straw. Then we would feast.

Those were good days. Eventually, as is sometimes the way with marriage, those days deteriorated. We split up and I went to Australia. About six months later NS appeared. We tried to reconcile, but my heart wasn't in it, and maybe if the truth be told, neither was his. He got caught leaving the gigantic mid-city branch of the largest hardware chain in the city, trying to conceal a small chainsaw under his corduroy jacket. This was the man who could carry off plundering peregrinations with aplomb. He had never been caught in his life.

Although that was the end of the road for us, I was grateful for the symbolic rather than literal dimension of his acting out. And I will be forever grateful for his conjuring of food out of the bleak midwinter and for our sharing of early adventures in the illicit tasting of cheeses.

The years passed, and then I was diagnosed with CLL. I became interested in fermentation as a possible way of stimulating an immune system under siege. Some foods—sourdough bread and fermented pickles, for instance—were relatively safe to make, but cheese making seemed much more dicey. So I began with something easy and known to feed the immune system.

Yogurt—milk that has been cured into a tart, semisolid mass as bacteria ferment lactose (milk sugar) to produce lactic acid—is how it all began for me, the start of the slippery slope. It is very easy to make, and I was brought up to believe in its goodness as an almost biblical fact. Early in the twentieth century the Russian microbiologist and Nobel winner Ilya Mechnikov (who, incidentally or perhaps not so incidentally, discovered that white blood cells fight bacterial infection) gave a scientific rationale to the ancient belief that yogurt and other cultured milks (buttermilk, crème fraîche, sour cream, kefir . . .) can actively promote good health. He proposed that the lactic acid bacteria in fermented milks eliminate toxic microbes in our digestive system that otherwise shorten our lives. He was, as Harold McGee says, "prescient." McGee also writes, "Particular strains of these bacteria variously adhere to and shield the intestinal wall, secrete antibacterial compounds, boost the body's immune response to particular disease microbes, dismantle cholesterol and cholesterol-consuming bile acids, and reduce the production of carcinogens."

The basic cultures or probiotics in yogurt can also be taken in the form of pills that many believe to be more comprehensive and potent than yogurt. For a number of years I took an expensive probiotic recommended by my naturopath, but after disability retirement, with less income and more time, and working on the assumption that you might get an even more diverse microbial flora by making your own yogurt, I decided to ditch the pills and started making yogurt on a regular basis. Soon it became a habit. I felt rather pleased with myself for this self-help initiative, particularly as a defense against frequent exposure to antibiotics that notoriously deplete the population of beneficial gut microbes as well as harmful ones. And, as added benefit, J would swoon before a bowl of fresh creamy yogurt into which scarlet berries had been crushed, Roxy would greedily lick the bowl clean, and the chickens would go crazy for a dish of bread and yogurt, scarcely lifting their beaks to breathe, but when they did they'd look like gloopy ghosts dripping ecstasy.

Then, all of a sudden, my self-satisfaction was punctured. Ed Yong, in a series of articles, later condensed in *I Contain Multitudes: The Microbes within Us and a Grander View of Life*, reported that the microbes that Mechnikov idolized don't do much good in the gut. And other doubting voices were raised—about the efficacy of both yogurt and over-the-counter probiotic pills. Skepticism about the efficacy of the microbes in yogurt and probiotics is due to several issues. The first is that they are being added to the human gut, where they do not reside naturally; you cannot just add good microbes, they need to be in a community of microbes that work well together. Second, the few hundred billion of bacteria per pill is a drop in the ocean, the gut already holds a hundred-fold more. The debates continue, and though I'm prepared to share a degree of skepticism about probiotic pills, about yogurt, J and Roxy and the chickens and I preserve a frisson of faith.

After yogurt I turn, inexperienced and rather cautious, to the easy "fresh" cheeses. They, however, are also the cheeses most vulnerable to contamination. Most fresh cheeses, unlike aged cheeses held for weeks or months, are aged for only days. This, it is generally believed (though the claim is controversial), is not enough time to change the pH of the cheese to kill any harmful bacteria that may either have been in the (unpasteurized) milk at the beginning of the process or gotten in (to either the unpasteurized or pasteurized milk) during the making.

So, with all the precautions in place in my kitchen, my bleak theater of sterility, I set out to make cheese. It's the unwanted bacteria you have to watch out for, as they can zip into the milk and spoil it. I buy the milk in bottles, making sure it is pasteurized but not *ultra*-pasteurized nor homogenized. I have my beautiful kitchen range, where I can get the heat just right to bring the milk slowly up to the required temperature. In my fridge I have the rennet and additive or culture that comes in frozen form. The kitchen bench and all the implements, such as the whisk and ladle and thermometer and the old blue Dutch oven and the jars and molds, have all been sterilized. Actually, a stainless steel saucepan would probably be safer than the Dutch oven, but I like the blueness of the latter and its solidity for keeping the goat milk warm.

Yet, despite all these fetishistic precautions, magic happens. Somehow the milk turns into cheese. It is this element of magic that lures me, turns me into an obsessive. Funny thing about magic, like special effects in the movies, you become curious about how it happens, you too want to become a magician, and getting to peek behind the scenes does not spoil the show at all, on the contrary, you find that there are always more tricks to learn, a whole bag of tricks, in fact, endlessly unfolding.

I begin with goat cheese, ricotta, paneer, mozzarella, cottage cheese, various Mexican cheeses, such as *queso fresco*. You can make ricotta with your hands tied behind your back and an eye patch over one eye if you have some milk and lemon or white vinegar and even a few spoonfuls of cream, though this is not necessary. Invite friends over and present it in a colored bowl, and they will go gaga because the difference between store-bought ricotta and the warm creamy version that has just been made is incomparable. Plain is perfect, but you can also add all sorts of things: The combination of chopped mint and lemon zest pops or try lemon thyme and chopped walnuts. Best to eat straight away, however, because once plant materials are added, and if the ricotta sits out in the heat, you are creating conditions for an inauspicious visit by bacteria. Paneer is fun to make because you need to weight it down, and not having a professional press, you use books and can play a game imagining which fictions or essays will best enliven the saag paneer for which this cheese is destined. Because J cooks much Mexican food I attempt *queso fresco*, but though I enjoy the cutting of the curd with an adapted coat hanger, it never tastes better than bland. Certainly it tastes nothing like the cheese we bought in the markets of Oaxaca. I am proud of my homemade goat cheese, even though it mysteriously lacks the piquancy of the cheese we buy from the Little Italy farmers' market.

So there I am, tooling along fairly contentedly, when I see a film that sets sparks flying:

We are in the bleak Sardinian mountains. The sound of wind and fire, the feel of snow on bare skin. The cold is sonorous. Here the shepherds herd their goats, huddle together, bodies of men and animals merging. In a small stone hut they milk the goats, milk and snow and flames: large vats over an open wood fire. As the milk separates, solidifies, as the screen fills with fire and steam, hands shape the cheese and turn it into wooden molds. Perishable milk is magically transformed into a preserved product that can be transported back down the mountains.

The film is *Pastori di Orgosolo* (1958) made by Vittorio De Seta, part of a series of short documentaries he made in the 1950s, mostly in Sardinia and Sicily, to record aspects of peasant culture before it passed away entirely.

I don't yearn to be in the snow nor actually to be milking goats, though I would love to rest my head on the stomach of one of those small fat silky creatures. But warm milk, the splashing sound as it hits the tin pail, the frothing of the milk, the noise of the goats—all that is enticing. So much more enticing than the sterility of pasteurized milk. I realize my yearning is utterly romantic. Nevertheless . . . I turn again to a book that on the first time around, before I took up making cheese, struck me as cloyingly romantic and precious: *Goat Song: A Seasonal Life, a Short History of Herding, and the Art of Making Cheese*. This time I can't put it down. In the book Brad Kessler documents his life as a shepherd and cheese maker in rural Vermont (having moved from New York City). It is a self-conscious pastoral and, as such, is fully aware of the romantic longing for paradise (always already lost) that is intrinsic to the genre. There is a passage that resonates this time. Every pastoral since *Gilgamesh*, he writes,

has been part elegy, a yearning for a time when humans weren't separated from the animal Other, but understood implicitly what each one "said." Every pastoral is the dream of a common language; and I've been searching for such a language all along. I've caught fleeting glimpses here and there on walks in the woods with my goats when we share a footprint, a rhythm, a key. When I sing to them and they sing back I think I know what they say—but the only way to tell is in psalms.

I want to find some way to bridge the disconnect experienced in my palace of purity, between the realm of human intervention or creativity and those other realms involved in cheese production: on the macro level, animals and plants; on the micro level, bacteria and fungi.

Even though I am not herding and milking and mucking out the dairy, knowing that the milk I'm working with comes from real goats rather than from unreal cardboard containers makes a difference, not only to my state of mind but to the quality of the cheese. Of course the milk in the cardboard containers is not entirely *unreal*, but stripped of its cultures, it is edging toward *dead*.

I start thinking about how, even though pasteurization might improve food safety, it also removes much of the indigenous microbiota of milk that imparts distinctive flavors. In killing off the live culture and enzymes it diminishes the health benefits of the cheese. In shopping for recognizable cheeses in the supermarket, you can be sure, because of standardization, of what you're getting, but you close your door, as you do in using pasteurized milk, to the rich diversity of microbes that might give a particular inflection to the flavor. You miss out on all the subtle variations in local artisanal cheeses, you deny yourself the pleasures of experimentation and surprise. Many critics argue that pasteurization is not the only way to guard against food-borne illnesses; much of the research indicates that our best protection against the undesirable microbes is not to sterilize the milk or the aging spaces in the hopes of killing them off, but rather to ensure that the desired microbes are able to thrive and form a steady bulwark. This means healthy animals and a scrupulously clean dairy and aging facilities—be it a professional cave or a plastic box in a fridge. A developing cheese that has a thriving population of desirable microbes already resident is a much harder target for invaders.

Of course things can go awry in the cheese-making process if you use unpasteurized milk. The wrong bacteria might find their way into the cheese, producing certain molds or smells that might be virtually indistinguishable from the effects you want to achieve. You could land up giving your friends and family one of those dreaded diseases that nevertheless have marvelously luscious mouthfeel names: listeriosis, brucellosis, and salmonella. You might even land up killing yourself.

Luckily I do not have to contemplate such disaster since I do not know anyone with goats. Until . . .

One day I am wandering around City Farmers, my local nursery, run for forty-five years by Bill Tall, who started the business when he was sixteen. In addition to the wealth of plants there are ducks and chickens and horses and a miniature cow. And free advice from Bill. When I first came to San Diego and moved into the house at Herman Avenue and began developing a garden in this strange land, Bill was my go-to advisor on everything. Mortgaged to the hilt, I could scarcely afford plants let alone tools; Bill lent me pruning shears and ladders and saws. On this occasion, as we wander through the camellias, I see there is a new animal house with new animals: goats! glorious goats! Bill tells me that there is a small group of cheese makers, a club called Queso Diego, that meets once a month in his house. Come along he says, you might learn something new. And so I do, come along, and so I do learn something new.

In Queso Diego I discover a world of true fanatics. My obsessive instincts pale into insignificance in the light of people who have entire basements stacked with cheese caves (actually dismantled fridges ingeniously tweaked and rejigged), who are making ten or more different cheeses at once, who have the patience to wait months or even years for a cheese to mature, who can express irrepressible glee at a mistake that yields new and unexpected flavor combinations.

In the club I meet people with goats. I visit and peruse the funny furry beasts and the meticulous cleanliness of their environments. I think about my damaged immune system and for a short while pirouette on the horns of a dilemma. I want to bolster my immune system and believe that raw milk is healthier, not least because it contains a much greater microbial diversity than dead milk, in which all indigenous cultures have been killed in order to then add back in some of those cultures in frozen or dried form (the destroy-and-replace method). On the other hand, I have a weak immune system and working with raw milk is potentially more dangerous. True, there are less brutal ways of rendering the milk safer than harsh boiling, and I try these out, but in the end, confident in the sources of my milk, I throw caution to the wind and start making cheese with fresh unpasteurized milk. In the U.S. you can't sell unpasteurized cheese that is less than sixty days old, after which the bacteria will have died. But you can make and eat it. J is the valiant taster. If he survives I dive in, and then we share with close friends. It's an intimate undertaking.

On different occasions I try adding different cultures, and I also try adding nothing but rennet, letting the indigenous microbes ferment at will. The results are delicious and surprising. Rennet causes the milk to form curds that are less fragile than acid curd. Traditional animal rennet is an enzyme derived from the stomachs of calves, lambs, or goats before they consume anything but milk. But plant-derived rennets have also been used in traditional cheese making for thousands of years, and you can buy vegetable rennets that work perfectly well. Enzymes extracted from the flowers of two plants that grow in my garden—*Cynara cardunculus* and *Cynara humilus*, commonly known as the cardoon and the globe artichoke—are still used in the Mediterranean region for cheese making, especially in Spain and Portugal. I would love to know if it is possible to somehow distill or extract the rennet from the brilliant globular purple inflorescences. I have never been able to find quite the right word to describe the color of those flowers, but Pantone's Ultra Violet seems perfect. The company characterizes it as a "dramatically provocative and thoughtful purple shade" that evokes the "experimentation and non-conformity" of Prince, David Bowie, and Jimi Hendrix.

When you drain the cheese it separates into curds and whey. The curds go into the making of the cheese, and the whey—considerably in excess of the curds—is usually treated as waste. Sometimes I use it as a base for soup. Try cooking white beans in whey. Then, keeping some of the beans aside to add in at the end as crunch, whizz most of the whey and beans in a blender for a tangy soup, finished with a swirl of olive oil and scattering of parsley or rosemary. You can also add in toward the end a handful of kale or collards or mustard greens. Improvising with what is in the garden or the fridge yields surprises; one of the best for us was a tossing together of the slightly acidic beans with tuna and the first broccolini of the season.

If I don't use the whey in the kitchen I sometimes feed it to the tomato plants. A much more ingenious method of recycling whey was developed by Frère Nathanaël of the Trappist Abbaye Notre-Dame de Tamié. This abbey, founded in 1132 in Haute-Savoie, high in the Alps, is where the monks, since 1863, have made the cheese we now know as Tamié. Cheese production at the abbey produces one thousand cubic meters of whey annually, and Frère Nathanaël developed and installed a methane-generating system that transforms the whey into enough energy to heat water for the domestic needs of the abbey and its dairy for a year. A number of creameries in this country have followed suit.

You can eat the goat cheese within four hours of draining, but you might want to dry out small logs for longer in the fridge so you can roll them in lavender and fennel seeds or pollen, or you could set taste buds popping by rolling the loggettes in a Middle Eastern spice-and-herb like za'atar or dukkah. In the fall there are pomegranates, which love goat cheese. For nibbling with pomegranate mimosas, and providing you are not a cheese purist, you can try this concoction: Combine fresh goat cheese with some cream cheese and a small quantity of strong blue, fold in lots of chopped-up sage, roll it into a log, and then, after it has cooled and can be handled easily, roll the log in pomegranate arils. The outside will be ruby jeweled and crunchy, the inside, shamrock green. Fall is also the time of quince, that yellow, knobby-hard fruit that looks like a misshapen pear. But cook quince very slowly in nothing other than sugar and water for a day and a night and you release into the house the most alluring aroma and can watch as the quince turn slowly rosy and then deep dark vermilion. Eventually you will transform this mush into a paste that will dry over the next several days. And there you have it: *membrillo*, the most marvelous accompaniment to cheese.

After a while I start aspiring to more provocative adventures than those provided by the soft goat cheeses, delicious though they are. Night after night my dreams are invaded by more challenging and mysteriously delicious smells and textures, I wake with a tingling at the back of the throat, tortured by names dancing and twirling, just out of reach: Epoisses, Harbison, Winnimere, Limburger, Taleggio, Red Hawk, Tomme de Chèvre, Stinking Bishop. These are the smelly, washed rind cheeses I love above all others. They are also the cheeses that inspire a veritable cascade of vilification. Not everyone loves these cheeses, but almost everyone takes delight in rolling around in the descriptive excesses they inspire: putrid, fetid, funky, dirty laundry, smelly underarms, sweaty socks, urine, stables, barnyards, rotting flesh. Not altogether surprising, since the same microbes— *Brevibacterium linens*—are found in these cheese rinds as in human armpits and between toes. Stinking Bishop featured in an episode of *Wallace and Gromit* where it brought someone back from the dead. Actually, the cheeses themselves do not usually taste of what they smell. The interior that often oozes out, so runny that a spoon is needed to scoop it, can be delicate and sweet. But to me it is impossible to separate the smell and the taste; it's not that the cheese tastes of gym shoes, say, but rather that there is something very bodily and sensuous about these cheeses, you feel as though you are in the stable or the field, there is a disincentive to gobble, they encourage you to take time sniffing and breathing and feeling the shape of the taste. Michael Pollan would say I am captivated by "the erotics of disgust."

Memory provocations, too. Whenever I visited Milane, even toward the end, when she could barely talk and could not eat herself, even when cash was tight, she would always serve Epoisses on a lovely plate. Now whenever I taste it I am again with Milane, her wicked sparkle, our sharing of an out-of-the-ordinary pleasure.

These cheeses take at least a couple of months to cure, and they ripen from the rind (washed in liquid ranging from brine to brandy to pear cider) inward. The microbes in the rind secrete enzymes and flavor compounds that alter the texture and flavor of the paste. Different microbes and different aging methods produce different kinds of cheeses with different textures and tastes and smells. For most cheeses, the first day of cheese making is centered on the bacterial fermentation of lactose to lactic acid. Thereafter, along the way of aging, from a day to weeks or much longer, a lot can change, including cell death and lysis.

Cell death and *lysis*—these are terms I have become familiar with via CLL. In CLL white cells don't die when they should, won't fall into step with the normal processes of death and regeneration that keep a body going. They conglomerate. During treatment what sometimes happens is that the accumulated cells (clus-

tering in hospitable niches, lymph nodes in particular), under attack from a medicinal onslaught, suddenly die off en masse, instigating a reaction from the body
that goes into a kind of shock (affecting especially the liver and kidney) or what is
called *tumor lysis*. Of course this isn't quite what is happening to the cheese, but
neither is it so radically different. Cheese doesn't just happen by mixing together a
few ingredients and popping the resultant mix on the stove or in the fridge, crossing fingers and blowing kisses. It involves a process of consumption and death and
the generation of new ingredients and flavors. During the aging process of cheese
there is *cell death* or *lysis*: Bacteria die, amino acids in their bodies explode or seep
out. It is this process of *affinage* (finishing), the French term for controlled rotting,
that adds distinctive flavors to the cheese.

Cheese making is inextricably linked to microbiology. And, for me, to CLL.
Just as CLL cells form communities, make alliances, and recruit normal cells in
the surrounding microenvironment, so cheese making crucially involves not just
the additions of particular bacteria, but also the interactions of those microbes as
a community. It is the environment they form that is crucial.

In terms of a larger environment, dry semiarid San Diego does not quite carry
the cachet of Haute-Savoie or Vermont or even Northern California. Much has
been made by food historians and gourmands of *terroir*, the idea that the tastes (in
fermented foods particularly, like cheese and wine, but also fruits and vegetables)
are specific to a region. But San Diego is a Mediterranean climate, welcoming of
goats, of fermenters, of brewers, of Queso Diego, and also, as it turns out, home to
a fast-growing community of immunotechnology drug developers and a concentration of microbiologists (including, at UCSD, Rob Knight, cofounder of the Human Gut Project, and Rachel Dutton, who has attracted considerable attention for
her research on cheese). These individuals and groups don't necessarily overlap or,
anyway, not simultaneously or intentionally. But the links strike me as auspicious.

So when I start obsessing about rinds I make a beeline for the Dutton lab.

Cheese is the object of Rachel Dutton's research, it's what she collects and
tastes and sniffs, but it is not, strictly speaking, the focus of her inquiry. "The reason I'm so interested in food microbes," she says, "is not because they are essential
for the production of fermented foods, but because as they are growing in food,
they work together, they fight, and they communicate." Microbes never work in
isolation; they form multispecies communities, but traditionally it has not been
easy to understand *how* complex communities form and adapt and evolve simply
because of the difficulty of re-creating microbial environments (soil, the human
gut) in the lab. Cheese, or specifically cheese rinds, as this is where the microbes
work, is an ideal model system for studying the general rules that govern complex
microbial communities. A rind represents a relatively simple ecosystem. Instead

of thousands of microscopic species living together and adapting to their environment, a stinky washed rind cheese might contain only a dozen or so. Not too simple and not too complex or diverse. Advances in genome sequencing mean that it is relatively easy now to sequence microbial DNA from cheese, to collect and identify different types of species and then dissect the interactions of a community. Also, it is much easier to observe how ecosystems are formed in a cheese cave than in a forest or coral reef, how these interactions change and evolve over time.

Rachel Dutton is a rock star in the firmament of gastronomy; she's been courted by the likes of Harold McGee, Sandor Katz, David Chang, Michael Pollan, and Jim Lahey. Articles about her have appeared in the *New York Times*, and she and her colleague, Benjamin Wolfe, have written for *Lucky Peach*. It is a propitious moment for the convergence of microbiology and gastronomy. But clearly the reason Rachel has attracted such attention is not only because microbiology is hip at the moment; it is also because she loves food and cheese in particular.

I enter the lab with some trepidation, prepared to be befuddled and overwhelmed. The only other lab I have ventured into in recent years is a research lab at UCSD Moores Cancer Center, where blood samples, including my own, are stacked from floor to ceiling as research samples so that (among other things) the progression of CLL and other blood diseases can be measured. But this is a welcoming environment. Rachel, disarmingly lucid and friendly for a rock star, has made the time for my visit even though she is extremely pregnant. She and her grad students, fired by curiosity, are also adept at explaining and illustrating complex procedures in language I can grasp.

Before coming to UCSD Rachel, with Benjamin Wolfe, set out to map the diversity of organisms across more than one hundred and thirty cheeses from cheese caves in ten different countries, a project that, one might surmise, involved a lot of exposure to turophiles (cheese lovers) and a lot of cheese tasting. She also put in time learning about cheese by spending three months with the cheese maker Mateo Kehler at Jasper Hill Creamery in Vermont. She has never worked so hard in her life, she told me, cleaning and lifting and turning great heavy wheels of cheese. The exchange was two-way. Kehler and his brother, influenced by Rachel's research, have since developed their own lab, with attendant scientists on the premises, and are developing and adapting their cheese-making practices according to their findings.

Dutton and Wolfe had shown that the environment (cows, cheese caves, pastures) and methods (washing, salting, managing acidity) were as important as the ingredients to the development of cheese rinds, if not more so. Pretty much the same microbes, it turns out, occur in the same kinds of cheeses across the world. But the strains vary, and it is these variations that produce the distinctive flavors cultivated by the farmers and cheese makers as they prepare the environment on the rind. These strains can be identified through DNA sequencing and then preserved. As a post-pastoralist, Kehler has been developing his own starters by collecting and sequencing the indigenous microbes in his caves.

Thus, new cheeses may be developed, but current artisanal cheese making is also a means of preserving the diversity that is under threat from standardization and corporatization. And it is not only in the U.S. that this is happening (where artisanal producers have a much tougher time than in Europe and where the only three domestic suppliers of starter cultures are multinational corporations better known for chemicals). Even in a creamery as ancient as the Abbaye Notre-Dame de Tamié, Abbey Frère Nathanaël, he who has been recycling whey into energy, has isolated bacteria from hay and milk of the region and, in collaboration with a commercial culture company, has developed a collection of starter cultures that could be alternated in Tamié production in case the starters became infected by bacteriophage. "Tamie thus is a cheese that stands at the cross roads of scientific and traditional methods of fabrication," writes Sister Noella Marcellino.

As you walk into the Dutton lab you encounter a furiously jiggling machine, sitting atop a workbench. This is a cell disruptor that is shaking glass beads around to break the tough cell walls of the microbes to release the DNA for sequencing. Opposite is a freezer, and when Rachel opens the door, it is as though we have entered Antarctica: Gusts of something like dry ice billow up. Containers of microbial spores from cheese rinds are encrusted, as though they were buried in an ice storm millennia ago. It is as though we are discovering a mysterious hidden cache of treasure. It is in fact a frozen library like a catalog of cheese species, akin to the great seed banks of Kew Gardens and its offshoots around the world, such as the San Diego Zoo. Here cheeses can be preserved for the future, resuscitated, brought back to life.

Rachel shows me a petri dish in which two species are growing adjacent to one another. The scientists are monitoring the dish to see what kinds of interactions might take place, what possible horizontal transfers. Using the cheese rind microbiome as a model system, it becomes possible to explore how horizontal gene transfer works in more detail than before. A better understanding of this process can then be applied to other microbiomes and has important implications in the field of medicine. For example, the problem of antibiotic resistance occurs in part because genes are often transferred between different microorganisms, creating increasingly drug-resistant microbes.

I leave the Dutton lab with a tingling at the back of the throat, my aspiration to more provocative adventures than those provided by the soft goat cheeses, ratcheted up. I have to make a rind-ripened cheese. Somehow. Even though I do not have a proper cave. Fortuitously, Larry Stein, of Queso Diego, offers a class on Brie. We spend an afternoon preparing the milk in its first stage of becoming cheese: heating carefully, watching the temperature, adding the culture and the rennet that will promote the curds and the *Penicillium candidum* that will promote the development of the rind. We cut the curds, we ladle them into our homemade molds, and transport them home very carefully. My cave consists of a plastic lunch box with a base cut from a large white plastic ventilation grid purchased at Home Depot and a mat of plastic canvas (used for needlework) purchased at the 99 Cents store so that the whey can drain. I wet a paper towel and place it in the bottom of the box to provide humidity. Into the fridge it goes. I tend it like a special plant, taking it out and flipping it regularly, moving it after a while to a cooler part of the fridge. And after a few days the miracle starts occurring, it starts growing a white fuzz all over. I take it out and stroke it, patting down the fuzz. This is the wondrous part: touching the cheese, feeling the becoming of the rind. After eight weeks it looks amazingly like Brie and even more miraculous: It tastes good and the texture is squishily satisfying.

On the lookout for a used wine fridge that my friend Curt, a much more experienced cheese maker and tinkerer, will hopefully help me convert into a cheese cave, I watch videos about cheese. I see Sister Noella, dubbed the Cheese Nun, caressing a large wheel of the Bethlehem cheese she makes. She tells how she got into cheese making by falling in love with a cow called Sheba and beginning to milk her. She then went on to get a PhD in microbiology. Her Bethlehem cheese was made from a recipe given to her by a cheese maker from the Auvergne, who advised her to use wooden vats, a reservoir of microbial biodiversity, and to keep the milk—raw, no cultures added—in the first stages, at the same temperature as the cow's body. Sister Noella says,

> It's this sense that we're eating decomposition, breakdown products. You could call it death. To me it's a taste of that but a promise of something delicious. So I think it's almost a subconscious way of being prepared for death and facing our own mortality. And for me the analogy of really a death, a decomposition, creating a wonderful flavor, it's a promise of something better. I experience this over and over again when I look at cheese, when I smell cheese and when I look at the micro-
> bial ecology of cheese.

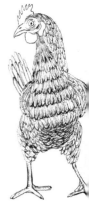

Blood Poetry

72

Haematopoiesis: blood poetry. Actually, the word comes from two Greek words, αἷμα (blood) and ποιεῖν (to make), it refers to the body's capacity to make blood cells. In adults this predominantly occurs in the bone marrow, and when the system malfunctions you get such diseases as leukemia. But to me the word sounds like blood poetry.

The family in *Breaking Bad* is celebrating Walt's remission. He's been pronounced cancer-free. Hank, Walt's DEA brother-in-law, tells of an incident that occurred early in the series. He tells it as a story, with a bottle of tequila, the family gathered around the swimming pool. A giant tortoise ambles slowly across the desert, a decapitated bloody human head strapped to its body. When it reaches a group of DEA agents it explodes. Hank explains that this was the Mexican drug cartel's way of sending a message: The head belonged to a snitch named Tortuga (tortoise). Hank tries to explain the how of the scenario. "It's not a metaphor, not an analogy, it's a, Walt, what's the word I'm looking for?" he asks. Walt refuses to participate, stares stonily into the distance. Hank finally finds the word: "poetic," he says. Softly he repeats the word to himself: "poetic."

Shimmer and Glimmer

73

Remember how she would shimmer and shake, fluff and preen, turn and take up a pose in the sunlight. Flashes of blue and iridescent green, a glimmer of purple, and then she'd turn away from the sun and be simply Funny Face, a beautiful pure black chicken, my lovely Australorp. Donna sees teal where I see green and purple. The color is chimerical because what we see is not solid but has to do with the refraction of light. The other chickens shimmer less, but their coloring is complex, layered, silky, especially Sabrina, the Welsummer, who reminds me of a game bird: elegant velvety browns, interlaced with gold, translucent ochers, the red tinge of deep dark earth, autumnal tones. Her coloring is a key to her eggs: chocolate brown, but never a simple matte, each surprising egg freckled and speckled individually. My friend Page, who has an eye for stylish clothes and a feel for texture, oohs and coos over her, and I imagine that she is imagining wearing Sabrina. The sensation of being swathed in feathers, of swooshing down the aisle in her stunning coat, ruffling into a thousand shades as she swings, then settling into satiny splendor as she pauses, seized mid-step by a thought, probably about birds in antiquity. Holly, the barred Plymouth Rock, is sculpted severely in black and white, she comes from another era, as fashionable as a Mary Quant model. She has, however, grown into a very fat hen who loves to be held and stroked, so although you can look closely at the ingenious sculpting, the delicate deep black scalloping that shivers as she settles into an embrace, she is more like a fluffy zebra than a svelte model. Holly goes through phases when she refuses to go into the henhouse at night unless picked up, cradled, and carried in to be gently deposited by hand on the wood shavings. You have to search for her, but she is usually hiding close by. If it is dusk or turning dark you can spot her easily because her whiteness glitters, bright striations in the blackness of night. Lula Mae is the least striking of the four, but she is the funniest and lays the best eggs: pale blue. I first encountered these eggs in the market in Tepoztlán in Mexico, where the little old women would sit cross-legged under the trees, outside the covered market, and sell you one egg or two, or however many you wanted, in various shades of blue or green or pale turquoise. As they wrapped the eggs individually in newspaper I asked about the birds, what color were they, were they blue and green? They laughed: Oh no, no particular color, they said, all sorts of colors. I felt dispirited, sure that I would never find these chickens in the U.S. But I did. The Tepoztlán eggs were probably from what are here called Easter Eggers, descendants of the Araucana, a Chilean pre-Hispanic chicken. The eggs come in a fairly wide range of colors (though each chicken will lay just one color), and so I opted for a more certain blue by choosing the related Ameraucana. The birds themselves, as the old women indicated, do indeed encompass a variety of colors, so although we knew she would one day lay blue eggs, we had no idea what the little black-and-yellow chick would eventually look like. What she looks like, it turns out, is simply funny. She has a feathery muff and a tufty beard, which you are tempted to tug, but her colors are inviting: Come, her colors say, bury your head in my soft wheaten fluffiness, my buff brown—streaked with cream and ivory—downiness. Moreover, she has magnificent prehensile blue legs and feet.

The blueness of these legs is produced by pigmentation; much of the feathered coloring is brought into the world of sensation through refraction, the play of light on and through the materiality of feathers.

In the market in Tepoztlán you can also buy a plucked chicken to take home and cook. A yellow chicken. Most of the raw chickens I have encountered in the U.S. have white skin, and all the raw chickens I have seen in Mexico have yellow skin. Many people believe this is because of diet, that Mexican chickens are fed marigold seeds and flowers and yellow corn, or sometimes people say it is because yellow is the more natural color, that has been bred out of U.S. chickens because gringos prefer skin color to be white. Both these arguments are persuasive, and the marigold variant is poetically appealing, but it turns out that there is a different, very intriguing, answer to be found to this question of chicken skin color. But that is another story.

I Need an Advocate

74

The plane is delayed in Manchester, New Hampshire. Bad weather. I have a short connection in Charlotte and would really like to get home tonight, as I'm carrying a cache of smelly squidgy Vermont cheeses. Nervousness begins in my toes, wends a wormy way through my body, squiggles under my tongue, and lodges in the tip of my nose.

Eventually the plane takes off and after a bumpy ride reaches Charlotte. The people in uniform say it's very tight but if you run you might just make the connection. I start running but have no idea how long the course is. The plane for San Diego is in a far terminal, a terminal too far as it turns out, and not a terminal at all, just the beginning of an endlessly nightmarish detour, though I do not know this as I run and huff and puff and pause, doubled over with a stitch, and get back on track again, running, bumping into people, reading the electronic signs and arrows that never seem to reach a target, simply direct one down another elusive rabbit hole. I arrive at the gate just as they are closing it. Literally just closing up, but they will not let me through. I imagine that this is what it's like when, after a life of sinning, you arrive at the pearly gates, repentant, reformed, having made a real effort and Saint Peter says, with a malicious glint in his eye: Almost but not quite.

I'm directed to the customer help desk. There are six uniformed helpers behind the counter, some of whom are laughing with their disconsolate customers and clucking with empathetic concern, but I get the one who is tasked with being the bad cop, the one who does not indulge in small talk and who delivers recrimination raw, on a platter. She looks at me as though she's being forced against her will to witness a bedraggled but potentially vicious mouse emerging from a sewer. I understand that I do look like and smell like said mouse. My hair is matted with sweat, skin pukishly pallid, nose unbecomingly roseate. The hard cheeses are in my checked bag, now probably orbiting Earth wondering which remote outpost of civilization to choose as a final resting place. The soft cheeses, however, once tenderly wrapped and carefully arranged in my backpack, have been jostled and squashed on the mad run across Charlotte airport and are now oozing stinkily, their odors infiltrating the clinically clean, antiseptic customer help arena.

Impatiently her fingers fly across the keyboard, now and then punching numbers, and each time she punches she sighs as though this is an impossible demand, an importunate request. Portunis was the God who protected harbors, and perhaps she sees herself as the protector of the airport against all those unreasonable travelers seeking to take advantage of the system. Probably she had her sights set on a post where she could really be effective and mete out punishment to serious offenders. But here she is standing behind a long counter where stand also other people in uniform, in a public space with swarming masses of travelers, untethered, milling around, and here am I in front of the counter, no chair to sit on, exhausted, fraught, not thinking straight. A murky memory sludges to the surface of consciousness, a friend telling me: When you are in a sticky spot, help yourself, don't hesitate to play the cancer card. I need to sit, I tell the bad cop/customer helper, and then I mumble, shamefully, "cancer." This is a bad move, indicating psychic weakness. She shrugs and indicates the floor. Here you are, she says, eventually, in a tone of bored triumphalism, handing me a whole swath of new boarding passes and reeling off places, times. Is this the best route? I ask, meekly now, as befits a humiliated sewer rat. If you can do better be my guest, she snaps back. I get the message: She is telling me I am not the expert here. Water? I squeak pathetically. She flings her arm out in a broad sweep, as though a tourist guide in a city full of opportunities. The airport is full of water fountains, she declares.

I sit on the floor, my head in my hands, dehydrated and despairing. I weep. No one notices, not surprisingly since the area is full of weeping amateurs. Eventually I recover enough to find water and an empty lounge with many hard resilient empty chairs glued together and bolted to the floor. It is a liminal zone through which you pass in preparation for the flight; it is the anesthetic room, preparing you for surgery.

I feel I've failed myself, not represented myself in the best light. I need help but have been rebuked because others need it more. You can't argue with that. On the other hand, the world has turned into a morass of unknowable things. I don't, for instance, know how the geography of the U.S. corresponds to flight paths, hubs, how you make the best connections to get yourself home, I don't know how to avoid sleeping on hard intractable airport chairs in the middle of the night, simply to be flown to another holding pen, there to be suspended again, waiting again. I don't know what questions to ask in order to receive the best attention. This is partly because my brain has turned to fudge after all that running through interminable terminals. And it's partly because I am merely an amateur traveler. Caught in a clogged system, I need an advocate.

. . .

The nurse calls me from the GI department. You've tested positive! she chirrups, as though delivering good news, as though she's announcing a white Christmas. Your antibiotics are ordered, and you can pick them up from your pharmacy. Since they've been running a multitude of tests I have no idea about what has shown up positive. I ask her and she tells me, but I do not understand the long and complicated name, though I do recognize the words *bacteria* and *infection*. And why this combination of antibiotics? I ask. She does not know but says she will look them up online. Thank you, I say, but I'd like to speak to the doctor about the diagnosis and treatment plan. I'll ask the doctor she says and call you back. The next day she calls me back and says you have to make an appointment to talk to the doctor. She tells me to call the scheduler. I do this, though I have to hold for twenty minutes, and he laughs and says, Oh Dr. L is booked up until January—three months away. Oh, that's a problem, I say, squeakily, because I'm suffering from cramps and diarrhea, and I don't think I can wait three months. But I understand antibiotics have been prescribed, he says. I say: But I want to discuss the diagnosis and treatment. I want to know what antibiotics I'm taking. Oh well, he says, his voice audibly shrugging. Hysteria mounting I inquire querulously about spots reserved for emergencies? No, nothing like that. What about cancellations? Ah yes, I could look and see if there are any cancellations. You're in luck, he says, dolefully, she has a spot in two weeks. Thank you, I say, pitifully. I put the phone down and dissolve in a puddle of pain and tears. Later Elana says to me, Why didn't you call MM? She's been an advocate for you before. I feel silly confessing I did not think of it. The system has worn me down so thoroughly by now that my brain is porridge. I can't even help myself to call a helper.

. . .

Eventually I semirecover from the temporary disability brought on by the marathon and from the onslaught of the customer helper. I carefully read the proposed course of treatment. It is now 10 PM. Her rerouting has me running to catch a plane to Dallas that's leaving in an hour (how many light years away, how many terminals to sprint through?), arriving in Dallas at 1 AM, hanging around cheerfully in airport bars until the next connection, a 6 AM flight to somewhere else,

Phoenix perhaps, that gets me to somewhere else and another period of hanging around and eventually home at 5 PM the next day.

All I want at this stage is a fridge for the cheeses and a bed for me. I would even settle for an air-conditioned room, minus fridge, and share the bed with the cheese. So I gather together my diffused particles of personality and worldly goods and stagger back to the counter.

This time I make sure I get a different helper. I tell her, as succinctly as possible, since I know that this part of the hard luck story is not one she wishes to hear in any detail, about my missed connection. I show her the routing I have been given and explain that I would rather stay here in this city in a hotel bed, get some sleep (settle my cheese in a fridge for the night, though I don't say this out loud), and then head home in the hope of reaching a destination sometime before the end of tomorrow. Will the airline offer any compensation, say some accommodation relief? She rolls her eyes. Bad weather, she says. There's nothing we can do about bad weather. I get it, bad weather is my problem, like having a blood phobia and a thing about needles. I slink back to my hard chair, tail between my legs.

I dig out bits of scrappy paper detailing the trip, stuffed into the bottom of my rucksack, stained now by oozing fat from the cheeses. And what do I find but confirmation of insurance! Bought in some lucid moment in another life, done as a routine matter because all the patient advocates in the cancer world remind you to always buy travel insurance. If I'd had a travel advocate she would have reminded me immediately of this nugget of gold, this open sesame, this bit of insurance. Calmer now, perking up, my self-esteem suddenly soaring as a glimmer of hope permeates the gloom. Maybe I can help myself. I call the insurance number and someone in India responds quite quickly, looks up my details, says, Yes you are eligible to have a hotel stay recompensed and meals too. Up to three hundred dollars. Keep your receipts and fill in the form or even just write a letter explaining what happened. Enjoy the rest of your trip, Ma'am, she says.

And I do. Calmer now and relatively clearheaded I ask myself: What would an advocate ask? And it occurs to me that "options" has to be high on the list. Get your options first and then decide on a course of treatment. Of course if it's truly an emergency or if you are unfortunate enough in these times to be an unwelcome visitor, a Muslim person, say, then you do not have the luxury of this stage, the question-asking stage. But in this situation I am relatively lucky. So I screw my courage to the whatever and pretend to be my own advocate. I return to the customer help desk, realizing that whom you get at the counter and how you get routed is basically a crapshoot. I show her the routing I have been given, explain that I would prefer to spend the night in a hotel in this city and travel home to San Diego tomorrow. She clucks when she looks at the itinerary I've been given, impatient at having to correct the stupidities of a colleague but also perking up a smidgen, becoming more cheerful as she realizes she has also been given an opportunity: to come up with a better treatment plan. I'd really appreciate a few alternatives, I implore. She rattles off some alternatives, all convoluted. Please, I say, please say that again, slowly, I do not speak your language. She might as well be a nurse in GI reeling off a list of drugs with unpronounceable names to treat diagnoses that are arcane and incomprehensible and seem to have nothing to do with you. She slows down. Goes over a couple of options. Together we settle on one that seems almost perfect under the circumstances and will get me home before the end of the day tomorrow. Then she hands me some extra bits of paper and says, And here's a coupon for the hotel and a list of hotels where you can use it. Enjoy the rest of your trip, Ma'am.

I get a car to a hotel downtown. The driver tells me that although he has lived here for seventeen years (just as long as I have lived in San Diego) he still misses Senegal. What do you miss? I ask him. You can't really put your finger on it, he says, but it has to do with the way time and work are connected. Time passes in a different way in Africa. You must know that, he says to me. I feel at last as though I'm on the way home.

Nameless

75

Downtown Los Angeles: ER at the Good Samaritan Hospital. J is on a gurney, hooked up to various machines, tubes running in and out of his body, electrodes stuck all over his chest. It is a fairly small and crowded open-plan room.

An old man sits on a chair, maybe an old man, maybe just worn out and chiseled into an indefinable embattled oldness. The social worker talks to him, trying to ascertain his history. Where are your things? she keeps asking. I don't have anything, he says. Your wallet, she prompts, your ID. Let's look in your pockets. All he has is a cigarette lighter. OK, so you were in a psychiatric hospital, and they transferred you to a care home and you walked out. Can't you remember the name of the hospital? No no a blank. And the care home? No no a blank. My problem, she tells him, is that I can trace you up until a few months ago, and then you disappear. You've disappeared, she tells him. There he is in front of her. The he that has disappeared is the he of a paper trail, of institutional records, the he that exists and is sitting here has no past, history, story. Can you remember anything, she asks, about where you were when you walked out of the care home? A street name, a building, anything? Pico, he offers, near Pico. And there was a laundromat. The name, she says, can you remember the name? No, just a laundromat. Mmm, problem is, she says, tired and despairing but patient, Pico is full of laundromats. A name, she needs a name. There are no names in his world. Or none that rise to the surface, none to share. He is given a blanket and wraps himself head to toe, you can barely see that there is a human figure in there. Lunch comes, and he eats slowly but with savage determination, every morsel.

. . .

This is serious, he has to be monitored very closely, says the doctor attending J. It is his seventieth birthday. One moment we are standing in the gorgeous art deco public library, listening to the docent on the conservancy tour, and the next moment there is a resounding crash. I turn to see J on his back on the floor, head bleeding. Suddenly the place seems to fill with cops and security guards and ambulance attendants. His blood pressure is super low and his heart rate super high.

There is another man in the ER, younger and voluble. Though tall and well built, he emanates exhaustion, a billowing tent that has had the air sucked out of it, capsizing. Good-looking, he has some intricate and gracefully etched tattoos. He has been walking walking walking but now his swollen feet are in hospital socks. He's talking to someone I can't see, I guess a social worker, who says very little, just asks the occasional question. No, he says, the man with tattoos, I can't stay in those places, in shelters. I'm not so-she-able, he says, stumbling over the word. I can't be with other people, so I walk around. But I can have sex with a woman after I've had my meds. No problem. Can't work cuz I have to walk, though I have thought I could clean hubcaps. But you have to buy cloths and a bucket. I thought two dollars would be a good price to ask, what do you think? No problem with sex, he says, but I have to have my meds. He asks the hidden person what he earns an hour. There is muffled muttering. Probably I'd guess twelve dollars, says the tattooed man, that's a lot of money to me.

. . .

They won't let me into the ambulance as it sits outside the library. An eternity of torture, imagining . . . The kind man from the conservancy stands with me chatting, offering distractions. A young security guard, she doesn't seem much more than seventeen, is very excited by the event, keeps telling people in the small crowd that has gathered that she actually witnessed him falling. As soon as she has an opportunity she tells me too. I actually saw him falling, she says, and you know what? I was worried that he would never open his eyes again!

In the ambulance they stop J's heart and reset it.

They let me sit in the front of the ambulance as it whizzes the few blocks to the Good Samaritan's ER. Eventually, J's cavorting heart is calmed sufficiently that admission is recommended. J himself seems back to normal, droll, playing down the event. I know I should feel relief, he's alive. But it's as though we have both suddenly been propelled from normalcy into a state of permanent irrelief. At any moment, I feel, things could change. This time it is J hovering on the edge of that other world, not me. And it is much more frightening. One foot is in the old world, it seems, and one in the new, and it's hard to tell the difference. Slipping and sliding.

Later as I sit in the cafeteria eating a lunch of dried-out turkey in a greasy burger bun, I overhear snippets of a conversation between two doctors. On the TV overhead George Stephanopoulos is talking with his guests about Trump's sacking of the FBI chief Comey. The doctors are both young, but the one who has been in the hospital for longer is telling the novitiate stories. They all involve guns and buckets of blood. She leads up to the final story: This guy has been shot in the head, blood is pouring out, and he's holding a gun, waving it around and threatening to shoot anyone who comes near him. No one does anything—because we are not allowed to touch guns, she says. Only the police. So the police arrive and disarm the man, and he's admitted to the ER. That's about as bad as it gets, she says.

. . .

I recall this story now, far away in Marfa, Texas (here this time to finish the book), feel intense relief, relief for gun laws in that hospital, relief that I did not feel at the time, so choked with anxiety. Last week I joined the small march of children and their supporters from city hall to the elementary school two blocks away. Two of the kids made moving speeches, as kids were doing all over the country. They are fearful, shocked by the killing at the Marjory Stoneman Douglas High School in Parkland, Florida, on February 14 that left seventeen students and staff dead—and replaced the 1999 Columbine High School massacre as the deadliest high school shooting in the U.S. Fearful and shocked, but not paralyzed. And they are telling adults that sympathy is not enough, they have the power to vote, they must change the gun laws and stop this violence.

On the news I hear more about the latest unarmed black man to be fatally shot by police officers. Stephon Clark, clutching only his cell phone, was struck eight times, mostly in his back, according to an independent autopsy just released in Sacramento.

. . .

We return home to San Diego from LA on the train a few days later. J will see his cardiologist, and eventually his condition settles down, controlled by an alarming array of medicines. It takes some time to get the balance right. But life for both of us gets back on track.

Almost. While we were having our crisis in LA our neighbor and friend, fourteen-year-old Amelia, went to check on the chickens and found that our Little Lula Mae, the sweetest and shyest of the hens, had died. Her little body was turning stiff by the time we reached home, but her tufty ears were still tufty, her feathers soft and caressible. We do not know why she died, chickens do this, usually without warning. Her life was fast-moving, filled with adventure and discovery;

she always looked so surprised, as though to come upon a worm was a wondrous thing, unprecedented in the annals of chicken life. We hope death outwitted her quickly, before she had time to be taken aback.

No more blue eggs. Now there are just the two big girls remaining: the bully girl Sabrina, the most beautiful of the four originals, who hasn't laid an egg in living memory, and fat and waddling Holly, who still valiantly lays a few eggs a week. She creates a ruckus for about an hour before she is about to lay; it sounds as though roosters have been let loose on the rooftops of North Park. And usually she is joined in chorus by Sabrina, a swashbuckling and arrogant pirate princess, performing as though she is on the helm of a ship leading an armada of boats into battle. She is all front. In the meantime they still give us manure and wander the yard, wreaking destruction where they can, mostly by tearing off the pretty small blue flowers on the large borage plants.

I experience a niggling superstitious sensation: What does it mean that the chickens who came once to save my life are now dying? Reina believes that El Dios let J live by taking Lula Mae. I understand the connection between chickens and divination but take it, rather, as a sign that we are all getting older and that neither chickens nor people live forever.

I miss Lula Mae. I'm glad, and the chickens are glad, we still have J.

Fermentation Dreams

76

Sitting around Diane and Jerry Rothenberg's dining room table, where so many marvelous meals have been shared and friendships ignited, Hiromi and I discovered a shared passion for fermentation. Before you could say "Bob's your uncle" a plan had been hatched, a fermentation party proposed. It would be a reconvening of all present with fermentation offerings.

For starters, as we sat around in the living room, I put out some goat cheese made from Annie's goats' milk, cute little Nubians, and Pragers' walnut sourdough. On my old Japanese shiny black platter:

- a new experimental concoction of jicama, Asian pear, and radish with fresh ginger from the farmers' market and a few grape leaves thrown in to keep things crunchy. All the vegetables were washed in pale champagne pink by the radish.
- from a huge jar that has been sitting in the fridge for eons: green string beans with garlic, red chilies, feathery dill, and some dill seed.
- pumpkin kimchi adapted from a recipe found on the Fermenters Club website. Deep orange streaked with red and wisps of green, the greenness provided by garlic chives which grow abundantly in the garden. They are more pungent than ordinary chives, clamoring always for spicy affinities.
- the remains of another jar found in the fridge, a basic but delicious mix of onion, carrot, and cauliflower.

Hiromi added natto, fermented soybeans. When I lived in Japan this often appeared as a breakfast item along with rice and fish. The sensation of repulsion I experienced then returns to me as the smell rises from the small beautiful bowl

Hiromi deposits on the table, a smell that spreads and engulfs the whole room. It is stinky in the extreme, though not unlike pungent cheese, which I have come to love, even to crave. So I try the natto and find that now that I have fallen for fermentation my tongue dances to the flavor, though the gooey, sticky, slimy okra-like texture still feels funny in the mouth. While driving yesterday "A Way with Words" was on the radio and included a discussion of the word *fungible*. One of the presenters said, Fungible, it's a great mouth-tasting word. Maybe one day natto will be like that too.

Daisuke and Yoko brought Ninkasi beers, Ninkasi being the Sumerian goddess of fermentation. And Masako visiting from Torrance brought a local boutique beer from there: Smog City's Kumquat Saison.

After nibbling and tippling we moved to the dining room table, where Diane put out paper plates and bowls so we could just eat and chuck all the different tidbits without endless juggling and washing of china.

Many containers, filled with mysterious odorous, intriguing-looking foods appeared on the table, and somehow a sequence of sorts eventuated. We kicked off with my cider, made from apple juice purchased from the orchard in Julian, which is bringing back ancient apple varieties. Very dry but pretty tasteless. I don't have the brewing knack. First course: a soup from Hiromi, Polish in derivation: fermented rye bread in chicken soup with a half egg in each bowl. Then my kimchi meatballs and noodles (tossed in sauce and extra kimchi, sprinkled with fresh green scallions and sesame seeds).

A bit of a pause.

Then Hiromi brought out a delectable dish of chicken, which had been marinated in sauerkraut juice, then grilled and sprinkled with green onions and served with young potatoes (boiled not fermented), lightly fermented, small very green Persian cucumbers, and a bowl of similarly lightly fermented red radishes.

A longer pause.

Then Diane brought out a big pot of her famous charcuterie: smoky meats nestled into juicy cabbage.

Still longer pause.

Then Daisuke and Yoko brought out a rich baroque chocolate cake, and Yoko told us about the fermenting of chocolate. A different goddess beer appeared, well attuned to the flavors of chocolate.

Everyone was full. We stopped eating and continued talking.

Then Diane remembered the ice cream and sauce. Oh we'd better just taste it, was the consensus. Out it came: vanilla ice cream (not fermented) with the final fermented dish—Christina Tosi's shiro miso butterscotch sauce (the recipe from *Lucky Peach*).

All the cardboard plates and bowls and cups went into the recycling. Everything was packed up, and we wended homeward, back to our various fermenting stations to dream more fermentation dreams.

And to taste, along with all the fermentation mouth feelings, a sadness that had permeated the evening, leaving an aftertaste that will not pass so quickly. A sense of someone there at the table, someone who is no longer here. On the night of the party which they so generously hosted, Jerry and Diane had just returned from Glasgow, from a conference/celebratory festival in honor of Jerry's work. While they were in Glasgow, David Antin died. They met, David and Jerry, in 1950, the year I was born. So they have known each other and been close, literally living close by, first in New York and then in Encinitas, for sixty-six years. At his memorial service Jerry would read a poem in which he asked, "Can you write a love poem to a friend?" His poem to David was an affirmative response.

. . .

I woke the day after the party feeling charged with health, as though the microbes in my gut were celebrating. Not so Diane; she visited the doctor with outrageously high blood pressure induced by all the saltiness of the food. A case of one woman's ferment being another woman's poison.

The Structure That a Life Has

77

Another friend, David Antin, hits the dust. Someone else diagnosed after I; gone before.

On March 4, 2017, we drive to LA with Becky and wander around the New Getty Museum garden that she photographed in its early stages and where I spent a year in residence in the late nineties, wandering daily through its newness. The structure is definite, always the same and recognizable, but the details and the appearance of the garden change all the time. Today I'm drawn to intermittent patches of deep purply maroon oxalis, punctuated by shocking pink flowers and a smattering of small yellow daisies. Oxalis is an invasive weed in my vegetable garden, almost impossible to eradicate. But this variety of purple oxalis does not spread. I imagine it growing at home in a large celadon pot.

Before the memorial we visit an exhibition on alchemy, the process of taking apart and putting back together again. There is a chart that aligns the alchemical processes with the signs of the zodiac, and I'm tickled to read that my sign, Capricorn, is aligned with fermentation.

And then there is the memorial; many speak before me, and then I say:

. . .

David as we all know was a talker. He could take on all the great drinkers and thinkers of the twentieth century and talk them under the table. What I didn't notice, so busy listening to him talk, was how he listened, his capacity to attend, his capacity to notice, to be alert to the tension between quirky quotidian eventualities and the formality of structure and performance. And what this had to do with friendship.

A few years ago David turned up unexpectedly at a reading I was doing with a few other people. Unexpected because it was a small event and because at this stage David was not going out much, it was hard for him to walk and, indeed, to talk. Elly was out of town, but he found someone to drive him. He arrived late but before it was my turn to talk. He stood in the open doorway, fixed his gaze on a seat in the middle of the front row, and very slowly started making his way across the auditorium. His progress was painstaking. I held my breath, hoping against hope that he would make it. Of course he did. It took a long time, but eventually he reached his seat, sat motionless, like a cat watching a bird, and waited for me to begin. The intensity of his focus was palpable. He marshaled and riveted the attention of the entire audience, channeled their energy, raising the performative stakes. He listened, and they listened with him. I felt like an operatic diva. And then I finished reading, he struggled to his feet, walked slowly across the front of the auditorium, and exited. The end, closure; or, an opening.

The funny thing is it had never occurred to me that David had ever heard or read anything of mine. I was very moved by this act of friendship. And also provoked to go back and look at his thoughts on the tension between endings and closure, the relation between performance and writing and life. In particular I turned to a piece he wrote in 1989, "Some More Thoughts about Structure." This is an almost eerily prescient piece in a number of ways. For instance, he wrote, then:

> it
> seems to me that the state of this country is extremely fragile
> extraordinarily fragile in spite of its banality and blandness
> blandness and banality seem to be the tone in which america
> is presently living   on the other hand we have been surrounded
> at the peripheries of this blandness and banality with poverty
> and the threat of disasters and catastrophes of all kinds   any
> one of which could disrupt our smooth flowing system of
> exchanges and throw it into a panic that could invoke vast
> translations of our situations into something else.

But prescient too because in this piece David reflects on lives in decline, on endings, on the structure that a life has. And he wrote something then that seemed to me to prefigure the way he encountered his own end:

> how do I build something that takes an articulate shape yet
> resists closure while everything else in me wishes to close it on a
> formal note   so I wont do it

Like a Cat in a Hat, Sleek and Brave

RIP RYOKO

Memorial Service, Sunday, September 3, 2017

Imagine this: You have come from another country and you land at UCSD, a typical Southern California university campus. You are appalled by the predominance of desert colors and self-effacing or nonexistent fashion. Everyone seems to be hugging everyone else, which is very awkward for you, having come from a more uptight culture. Then one day there appears an apparition, a spectacle of exotic splendor, a human butterfly who flits around campus dressed flamboyantly in bright adventurous colors, sporting the sort of glamorous hats you might once have seen at the races or English garden tea parties. She is gregarious, spontaneous, and yet she does not squander hugs, she retains a certain very distinctive formality and dignity.

I got to know Ryoko a little, mainly through attending her concerts with Scott Paulson, watching and listening to her play and sing and entrance audiences. Imagine then my surprise when I first started attending Sunday sittings at the Shambhala Center and who was there but Ryoko San? She was dressed exactly as if for a concert or an extravagant public performance. This was not the image I had of Buddhists. But as I stuck around, observing Ryoko and sensing her interactions with the sangha, I realized that she embodied in sometimes eccentric ways a combination that I take to be intrinsic to Shambhala: being awake and cultivating the capacity to listen (without answering back or inserting one's own story). At the end of the first training I attended with Ryoko and others, when it is customary to enjoy a feast and offer, if so moved, a story or poem or song or thoughts, Ryoko burst into the most riveting song, her voice cascading through several registers and reverberating through the room, through all the bodies in that room, creating one body.

. . .

There are many people in Shambhala who have known Ryoko longer or more intimately than I. I cannot pretend to summon or honor all her relationships. But hopefully I can engender a sense of her being, her being in a community. In some ways it is hard to describe Ryoko's friendships precisely because they were all so particular, so different, and often subject to ups and downs. Sometimes you were in her inner circle and sometimes on the outer. Why? Well this you might never know, but if you could stick around, perhaps visit a thrift store with her, give her a ride, do the flowers at the sangha or prepare Sunday tea, or sit with her and meditate, then you would find that she had found a way to invite you back. Ryoko had an intuitive sense, was able to find ways to connect with the most amazing array of people, of personalities, some delightful, some of us difficult—both within the sangha and within a broader community, particularly the music community of UCSD.

Ryoko was at once a very private person and a public extrovert. This private aspect of her person could on occasion be experienced as extremely exasperating, as those who tried to help her know. Take her resistance to learning to drive. When I asked Marin, who was very close to Ryoko, how they became friends she said it was probably through driving, their talking as Marin drove her to and from the center. I thought back on all the conversations I had had with Ryoko driving, and I'm sure that others—who've clocked up a lot more miles than I—can say the same. I realized then that there was a method to her exasperating madness. Not driving meant making friends.

Nevertheless, it cannot be denied that as an aspect of her privacy Ryoko loved secrets. How often did she share with me some snippet of information and then wave her finger in the air, saying, But this is secret, Lesley, no one else knows this. Well as time passed you'd discover that many people were party to this particular secret, or to that one. It could be about the hidden supply of chocolate in the Shambhala kitchen or about her decisions regarding her cancer. In some sense Ryoko was a skilled orchestrater, both of music and people. Take the way she gradually, without pushing or demanding or asking, inserted herself as queen of the kitchen. Not only did she know where everything went, what needed to be ordered, but her sense of style and decorum meant that we all lifted our game. I might put a cake out on a plate that seemed OK, perfectly suitable, only to notice later that Ryoko had discretely swapped it for a much more elegant plate that allowed the cake to shine. She imbued the simple morning tea with shimmering gratitude.

This combination of reticence and flamboyance could also be discerned in her flower arrangements. I remember one of her flower partners saying once in amused exasperation, Ryoko doesn't follow any ikebana principles, she just does what she wants. And yet over the years Ryoko's flower arrangements grew at once more austere and more brilliantly magnetic, drawing the gaze, inviting contemplation. How can that paradox exist? I do not know, I know only that Ryoko embodied it. For those of us who hung with her in the kitchen and with flowers: We will miss you and your spirit, Ryoko.

For Ryoko's spirit was huge, her generosity, though never flamboyant, was immense. As well as incredible service to the sangha, she had a flair for finding for each person she loved small gifts that would touch the heart. And her discretion meant that she never blew her own trumpet (well perhaps she did as regards music, and what a trumpet it was). Amanda was a friend of hers who was with Ryoko, as was Gill Giraud, when she passed into the transitional zone. Afterward Amanda told us how her friendship had developed with Ryoko. Amanda once found herself in hospital in a serious condition after being shot. Her family sat with her each day and night, and one other person sat by her side as well—Ryoko.

Although most of us in the sangha did not know about this incident, I think it was Ryoko's generosity that elicited from others the love and generous attentiveness that she enjoyed, particularly at the end. It was a tough journey, the last week, though peaceful at the end and faced with typical Ryoko determination.

Some of Ryoko's ashes are being sent back to her mother in Japan to join the family shrine. The rest, I believe, will be scattered at Shambhala Mountain Center in Colorado, where she herself scattered some of the ashes of her beloved husband, Joseph.

On her nightstand in the hospital was the gorgeous large-brimmed hat that Ryoko had insisted on wearing when Daniel brought her, in a very frail state, to the hospital. She looked so beautiful, soon after she had passed: a smile on her lips and her rich black hair spread out on the white pillow. I imagine her traveling through the stormy waves of birth, old age, sickness, and death with flair, like a cat in a hat, sleek and brave.

We will miss you, Ryoko, intensely, but we will not forget what we have learned from you and what you have given us—as much in your dying as your living—and for sending us the rain today.

Your spirit will remain with us. Travel well, dear Ryoko.

The Malvolio Gene 79

Fields of gold and orange, marigolds gleaming in the sun in the Oaxaca Valley, just before they are plucked for the Day of the Dead, when they will overflow in the churches and villages and cemeteries. These marigolds swim into consciousness when I buy at the market a plucked chicken, ready to cook for dinner, a chicken that—like all the other plucked chickens in the market—is yellow. These chickens, in their alive state, can also be seen to exhibit yellow shanks. Is it the marigold diet, as many claim, that renders the skin so yellow and the chickens so Malvolio-esque?

Malvolio: Shakespeare's incarnation of myopic pomposity, cavorting around the stage in yellow stockings. An aspiring nobleman, he has been tricked into this attire by a false letter written by those who wish to see him publicly humiliated. The letter appears to have been written by his employer, the Lady Olivia; it implies that she is partial to yellow stockings and likely to bestow her affections on one who exhibits such fashionable taste. So, gullible and self-opinionated, yellow-shanked, he parades and prances.

It pleases me to think I am eating golden marigolds rather than a dead bird so I am predisposed toward the flowery explanation of why these chickens are yellow, whereas the ones I am more familiar with in the U.S. are lily-skinned and, possibly like me, lily-livered. But when I face facts and look seriously into the issue I discover that although marigolds, because they contain carotenoids, may indeed intensify the yellow color, they do not produce it. It has, in fact, long been understood that the difference between white-skinned and yellow-skinned birds has to do with pigmentation and is actually genetic and not to do with diet. Domestic chickens with yellow skin and those with white skin share most genes, but when it comes to skin determination they have different alleles (different versions of the same gene). To grasp the difference between a gene and an allele think of the pea, which is a seed of course. The gene for seed shape in pea plants exists in two forms, one form or allele for round seed shape and the other for wrinkled seed shape. Chicken skin has one of two alleles, and that's what makes for white or yellow skin.

You might think then that color is simple: There is yellow and there is white. But hang on. Red and gray are about to enter the picture, and so are larger questions about origins and domestication. Where do the chickens we know today come from? It has long been presumed that the domestic chicken is descended from one sole ancestor, the red jungle fowl (*Gallus gallus*). However, when tested for alleles, the red jungle fowl were shown to have alleles closely related to the white alleles of our own domestic chickens but lacked the yellow allele. This, however, did show up (in a closely related form) in another wild bird: the gray jungle fowl (*Gallus sonneratii*). The deduction is that, at some point, congress (hybridization) occurred between a gray jungle fowl and an already domesticated chicken descended from the red jungle fowl. Their offspring mated with those chickens descended from the red line, and the introgression of yellow skin occurred. In the report of their findings scientists argue that the fact that yellow skin is present among local breeds of domestic chicken across the world suggests that this introgression to domestic chickens happened thousands of years ago rather than hundreds of years ago.

This is the first conclusive evidence for a hybrid origin of the domestic chicken, and it has important implications for our views of the domestication process, the complexities of both domestication and fertilization. New scientific discoveries about the origins of human companions like chickens contribute to our knowledge of how humans traveled across the planet, about colonization, about different kinds of domestication, and thus, historically and regionally, about different relations between animals and humans. Probably the earliest domestications of chickens were not for meat or eggs, but for feathers and bones and entrails, for sewing, for divination, for religious ritual, for gambling, and, above all, for decoration. As new discoveries, primarily through the analysis of DNA in fossil remains, continue, so too does debate about whether there is a single or multiple origin of the domestic chicken, thus extending and complicating the debate that began with Darwin and Dixon and that circles around the more general question of species and origins.

Since Darwin we know that species change, adapt, diversify. But the idea of *species* as a fairly invincible category, linked to the idea of origins, remains. Yet so does the question: How far back do we go, and how far afield do we forage, for clues of ancestry? Is there a single origin, or might there be multiple origins? Does the *creation* of a species (as well as its domestication) occur in one event or in several over time? In trying to understand where chickens come from, should we look to the jungle fowl or to the dinosaur? "*Tyrannosaurus rex* Basically a Big Chicken," declared Fox News in 2007, following the discovery of a protein in a dinosaur from sixty-eight million years ago to be identical to one that exists in the chicken.

The term *species* designates a class of individuals with the same characteristics. But to what extent is the term really written in blood, and to what extent is it a taxonomic convenience, part and parcel of the Linnaean inheritance, a somewhat arbitrary formula for naming, and distinguishing? Varieties complicate the certainty of species as they diversify and perhaps form new species. Some creatures, bacteria for instance, with their lateral gene exchanges, might seem to represent aberration, unsettling the fixity of species and obscuring or multiplying origins. But perhaps they are also an indication of the less than certain division between all species. After all, we are loaded down with microbes. Rather than thinking in terms of categorical distinctions it might be useful to think in terms of assemblages, collaborations, and interactions between creatures.

It turns out, anyway, that we human beings may not be as straightforwardly defined as a species as we have been accustomed to thinking since Darwin. The assumption for a long time has been that we evolved from a single origin, from ancestral hominids in a particular spot in Africa. New evidence, based on the analysis of remains from different parts of the African continent, suggests that, yes, we evolved from ancestral hominids in Africa, but we did it in a complicated fashion—one that involves the entire continent, since the ancestral hominid was itself widespread throughout the continent and had already separated into lots of isolated populations. We evolved within these groups, which occasionally mated with each other and, perhaps, with other contemporaneous hominids like *Homo naledi*.

Some scientists argue that the fossil findings represent different subspecies of *Homo sapiens* or different species altogether. Others argue that perhaps they really were all *Homo sapiens* and that our species simply used to be far more diverse than we currently are.

Either way, African multiregionalism, as this new theory of origins is called, is a fundamentally different view of how we came to be. "It's saying that no single place or population gave rise to us. It's saying that the cradle of humankind was the entirety of Africa," writes Ed Yong. This can be a difficult concept to grasp because when we think about ancestry we're so used to thinking in terms of trees, whether a family tree or an evolutionary tree, that charts the relationships between species. Ancestral trees have single trunks that divide neatly into branches. "They shift our thoughts toward single origins." But these new approaches to the question of lineage evoke not the metaphor of a tree so much, Yong suggests, as that of a braided river—a group of streams that are all part of the same system but that weave into and out of each other. "These streams eventually merge into the same big channel, but it takes time—hundreds of thousands of years."

I watch the chickens in my backyard as they cavort and parade their splendid and widely varied colors, as they weave into and out of a communal feather ruffling and delirious bathing in dirt, during which all you can discern through clouds of dust is a murky mass of feathers. Then the burbling subsides, the dust settles, they arise individually from the mass and delicately pick themselves up, begin again to prance and show off their fine legs and feathers: once again dancerly dinosaurs.

What Do You Expect? 8o

NOVEMBER 2017

Vale Sylvia Lawson, the Australian film critic and historian, public intellectual, and friend. It was a shock to realize that she was eighty-five, I always imagined that she was just a little older than me. Of course if you'd put two and two together you'd know, but it wasn't Sylvia's way to add things up in a conventional manner, and moreover her energy and intellectual curiosity and political commitment outstripped all of us. Her friends and interlocutors spanned so many different spheres and communities.

I wished, today, hearing the news of Sylvia's death, first from Tom O'Regan and then from Anne Freadman, that I was not so far away. Death is exacerbated by distance. It shouldn't be the case, what difference does it make? You are here one moment and then gone, gone from the world, and whether you took your last breath in Melbourne or San Diego or Harare is immaterial. But when friends and loved ones and even difficult family members depart from this world in some distant place, a place where you once were, with them, the loss seems somehow more thorny, ungraspable. Perhaps this is because of a loneliness, a grieving, that is unleashed: not just for the dead one, but also for another life in which you were connected through that dead one to a particular community, to a social fabric.

So I am grateful to Tom and to Anne for being in touch, during Sylvia's illness and decline, and after she died. And I am grateful to Ian Hunter for writing to J and me in such vivid and moving detail about Jack Counihan's funeral in Melbourne in May 2014. Afterward Ian said, "It wasn't easy—to find something like the words—but I was glad to do it. We are all so far-flung now that it's good to shrink the distances where we can."

I always rather envied Sylvia her ability to write regularly, to be at once cogent and provocative, but above all I envied her capacity for distillation. Her thoughts were capacious, her brainstorming intense and digressive, but the lucidity of her writing suggested a certain facility and ease. I could never figure out how she did it while maintaining an insatiably gregarious lifestyle. There were times when the intensity was too much and I would hide from Sylvia; she could talk the hind leg off a donkey and sometimes that donkey was me. But more often I was woken from lethargy in her company, like the last time we walked together, through the Botanic Garden to the Sydney Opera House, about which she had written, sometimes polemically, sometimes in the guise of fiction, so persuasively.

But that was not the last time I saw Sylvia, that day in the Botanic Garden. When I was back in Melbourne early this year I was able to visit her in Rathdowne Nursing Home. Even though I had been warned about her post-stroke condition, it was a shock. After a slightly frustrating question-and-answer session (Where are you living now, Lesley? In San Diego. Do you have enough to live on? Yes) repeated about twenty times in pretty quick succession, the conversation abruptly shifted into a different gear when she asked me, How is your writing going? Slow, I said, dismally slow. Well, of course it is, she chuckled. Writing, if it's worth anything, is always slow, and mostly difficult, why would you expect it to be otherwise?

I realized then what I always really knew: That every new writing project, be it a film review or a book, was for Sylvia always a complicated adventure precisely *because* of her gregarious and curious engagement in and with a world beyond the word processor. Often as I sit staring at a blank page I hear you chuckling, Sylvia, posing a rhetorical question: "What do you expect?"

Chimera

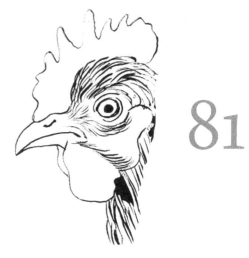

81

The invincible
Chimaira, a beast of divine, not earthly lineage,
a lion in front, a serpent behind, a goat in the mid-part,
fearsomely breathing forth the fury of blazing fire.
—HOMER'S DESCRIPTION OF THE CHIMERA

"Let's make America the country that cures cancer, once and for all." Thus spoke President Barack Obama in his State of the Union address in January 2016. He also announced that he was putting Vice President Biden in charge of carrying out the "moonshot" to cure cancer.

This American aspiration, likened to President John Kennedy's 1961 challenge to put men on the moon by the end of the decade, is not new. In July of 1969 men did reach the moon. In December of that year a full-page advertisement ran in the *Washington Post* and the *New York Times* in the form of a letter. It began, "Mr. Nixon: You can cure cancer." Ann Landers's column of April 20, 1971, asked, "If this great country of ours can put a man on the moon why can't we find a cure for cancer?" That December the Conquest of Cancer Act, to create a national cancer authority, was signed into being by Nixon.

. . .

So grandiose, this persistent optimism, and at the same time poignant. Poignant because, against all the odds, it expresses and inspires hope; grandiose because the analogy, crafted in the rhetoric of greatness and conquest, is misleading. The idea of a definitive cure, once and for all, implies total eradication, posits a country immune to the threat of that enemy, cancer. A clean country.

So let me put my cards on the table, here for what it's worth, is my two bob: The aspiration for a cure for cancer once and for all is a chimera.

. . .

Chimera means more than one thing. In common usage it implies fantasy, delusion, dream, and especially, as Webster's dictionary notes: an unrealizable dream. It is derived from the Greek word *chimaera*, used to describe Homer's legendary hybrid animal. Extrapolating from this specificity it has come to mean any mythical animal with parts taken from various animals.

The concept has also been appropriated by biomedicine, where chimera describes recombinant DNA. In genetics, *chimera* is used for several different cases, but the term alone is most often applied to an organism or tissue with cells derived from different organisms (thus, different sets of DNA).

People can be chimeras too.

. . .

To characterize the rhetoric of the cure as chimerical is not to imply that the words are empty. Various campaigns in this country, often spearheaded by presidential endorsement, have achieved amazing progress in policy and research and funding (for instance, the Precision Medicine Initiative, announced by President Obama in his 2015 State of the Union address, that, without delay, began capitalizing on its promise to revolutionize how we improve health and treat disease). I personally have a great deal to be grateful for, and though there is still no cure for my cancer, treatments and the range of options for bringing about partial remissions have improved dramatically. While it is true that the optimism expressed in the cure rhetoric strikes me as also a refusal, a very American or perhaps Puritan avoidance of pain and death, of recognizing and talking about and living with pain and death, it is also true that, having a chronic rather than an acute condition, I have had more time than many, time to imbibe a modicum of resignation and that alien virtue, patience. Those with a fast-growing tumor or an acute or metastasizing cancer are not offered patience on a platter.

This I know. So it seems mean-spirited to raise a skeptical eyebrow. Nevertheless, the gestural tic is kicked into motion by my own obverse to optimism: Not pessimism exactly, more like an endemic skepticism.

While it seems true to say that many cancer treatments are becoming less brutal and tending toward less toxicity, while it seems eminently possible that medicine will become more personalized and therefore more likely to succeed, that many cancers previously fatal will become manageable, that people will often be able to live almost normally with cancer, it also seems unlikely that cancer as a condition will go away once and for all or that America will be the victorious conqueror.

Optimism looks to the future, but looking to the past reveals cancer (many cancers actually, lumped for convenience under a singular nomination) to be as old as the human race, to be not a foreign invader, but to arise *within* the body, to be produced *by* the body. Cancer cells are mutations of ordinary normal cells, and it is unlikely that the extremely difficult task of distinguishing between normal and aberrant (and determining when one becomes the other) will become very much easier. This is partly because the game keeps changing. Cancers have always been able to develop ingenious adaptive devices and possess a large gamut of survival traits. There are other reasons too. Neither the individual body, nor the country we call America, lives in isolation. Our bodies inhabit environments that are changeable; new environmental hazards, many carcinogenic, are developing daily. And so, too, the U.S. exists within a complex, and far from fixed, network of international relations. All of which implies that any solution—and I believe that there will be solutions if not definitive endings—will only be partially medical.

. . .

Cancer, in one form or another, has been part of the human landscape since the earliest times. We know this from literature, art, science, paleontology, and genetics. Some, like Paul Davies, have even proposed that cancer is "embedded in the basic machinery of life, a type of default state that can be triggered by some kind of insult." He and Charles Lineweaver propose an understanding of cancer that situates it within an evolutionary framework, positing cancer as coevolving with humans as they or us evolved from single-celled creatures to what we are today. Theirs is not a position of resignation; on the contrary: "Conceptualizing cancer in an evolutionary context promises to transform our understanding of the condition and offers new therapeutic possibilities." They argue that

> cancer cells are not newly evolved types of cells, but heirs to an ancient toolkit and a basic mode of survival that is deeply embedded in multicellular life. Cancer, like a lazy poet, when called upon to produce new poems, reaches into its trunk of old poems and pulls one out at random, often finding a good poem, popular a billion years ago. These poems are not shoddy, inefficient, preliminary doggerel, but elaborate compositions with pathways that took millions of years to evolve. Some of these pathways are still in active use in healthy organisms today, for example, during embryogenesis and

wound-healing. Others have fallen into disuse, but remain, latent in the genome, awaiting reactivation.

It tickles me this analogy of the lazy poet. But, I wonder, is that poetic cancer really lazy? Davies and Lineweaver seem, in fact, to be somewhat awed by the inventive capacity of the poet, her mimicry, her facility for juggling old formulae and messing with established generic rules. We might not know what cancer of the future will look like, how it will rhyme, but by looking to the past (as well as to new research) we will discover ways of reading cancer as it continues to adapt, develop resistance to new drugs, cultivate new niches. Reading in this way (as oncologists of course do) becomes a practice—of dealing with cancer as something we live with.

As it turns out, one of the most exciting new developments in cancer therapy today has arisen from a return to looking at an aspect of the body—the immune system—that, in relation to cancer, was in eclipse for a century. It involves viruses and chimeras.

CAR-T is the magic word. CAR is an acronym for chimeric antigen receptor, short for CAR-T cell therapy.

In the early 1890s a bone sarcoma surgeon at Memorial Hospital in New York (now Memorial Sloan Kettering Cancer Center), William B. Coley, noticed something curious happening in some cancer patients: In cases where the patients happened to contract acute bacterial infections they experienced spontaneous remission of their tumors. He postulated that the extent of the fever produced by the infection (registering the stimulation of the immune system) correlated with the reduction of the cancer. Testing his hypothesis, he injected live bacteria into a patient with an inoperable malignant tumor in order to bring about a virulent infection. The patient made a complete recovery, living another twenty-six years until succumbing to a fatal heart attack. Over the next forty years, Coley injected more than a thousand cancer patients (with varying degrees of success) with bacteria or bacterial products (eventually he switched from using living bacteria—which could be quite dangerous—to using heat-killed bacteria, a concoction that became known as Coley's toxins). No one, not even Dr. Coley, had a good explanation of how the toxins worked. *But* the modern science of immunology has shown that his principles were correct and that some cancers are sensitive to an enhanced immune system. Immunotherapy, which has its origins in Coley's insights, is based on the idea that a patient's immune system can be stimulated or enhanced to attack the malignancy.

Unfortunately, at about the time that Coley was making discoveries about the relation between cancer and the immune system, X-ray and radium treatment was entering the cancer stage as a radical new approach, to be followed after the Second World War by chemotherapy. Together they totally overshadowed any interest in the field of immunology.

But eventually researcher-poets, mirroring their antagonists the lazy cancer poets, started reaching back into the ancient toolkit, started envisioning new poems growing out of earlier insights and formulae. Understanding the centrality of the immune system to diseases like CLL has been revolutionary. It might not have brought about immediate cures, but it has provoked further knowledge of how complex that system is, how dynamic, and how, given its strength, potentially dangerous. Since the 1950s the only cure for CLL has been a bone marrow transplant—replacing the patient's immune system with a healthy one from another person—but it is a drastic measure only resorted to when all other options have failed. Some who survive a transplant are cured of CLL (no traces of the disease left in the bone marrow), but debilitating side effects may persist. And some do not survive the treatment. Most often you trade one disease for a slew of other complaints. If you survive you become a chimera. Bone marrow contains stem cells that develop into red blood cells, which means that, for the rest of their life, a person with a bone marrow transplant will have blood cells that are genetically identical to those of the donor and are not genetically the same as the other cells in the recipient's own body.

. . .

People can be chimeras too.

. . .

Rather than attacking the cancer directly, as chemotherapy does, immunotherapy acts on the cells of the immune system, stimulating them to attack the cancer. To understand and situate CAR-T I'm going to backtrack for a moment to earlier developments in immunotherapy that paved the way for CAR-T and indeed are still developing in parallel.

Immunotherapy works in many ways, most predominantly, so far, through checkpoint inhibitors and monoclonal antibodies. It is the latter that CAR-T is a part of.

One way the immune system attacks foreign substances in the body is by making large numbers of antibodies. An antibody is a kind of protein that sticks to another protein called an antigen. Antibodies circulate throughout the body until they find and attach to the antigen. Once attached, they can recruit other parts of the immune system to destroy the cells containing the antigen. Cancer cells, however, are good at fooling the antibodies (by hiding and by disrupting signaling pathways). But with the advent of genomic sequencing, combined with more detailed knowledge of how the immune system works, researchers can design antibodies that target a specific antigen, such as one found on cancer cells. They can then make many copies of that antibody in the lab. These are known as monoclonal antibodies (mAbs).

Monoclonal antibodies are used to treat many diseases, including some types of cancer. To make a monoclonal antibody, researchers first have to identify the right antigen to attack. For cancer, this is not always easy, and so far, mAbs have proven to be more useful against some cancers, especially blood cancers, than others.

Lucky me as a potential beneficiary of this new treatment, to all appearances less damaging than chemo. I was offered the mAb Rituximab as part of my first treatment, to be taken in the form of intravenous infusion. But there was a catch. Rituximab was the first chimeric monoclonal antibody approved by the FDA for the treatment of a cancer (though not initially for CLL, I was on a trial). It was a less exotic chimera than Homer's combination of lion, snake, and goat, but as a combination of part-human and part-mouse DNA it filled me with horror. I imagined my nose turning pointy and pink, my skin sprouting soft white fur, and, worst of all, a long furless skinny tail growing out of my behind. This was in calmer moments; mostly my response was a shuddering repulsion that could not be put into words.

Slowly—over many hours researching Rituximab and confronting my attitude to mice—my revulsion was overcome by a more compelling desire for health. Part of my revulsion was no doubt a surfacing of the horror I'd managed to fairly successfully repress at the knowledge of how many lab mice had been subjected to brutal experiments in the name of conquering cancer. Given that situation, to grumble about absorbing a smidgen of mouse matter seemed hypocritical to say the least. Moreover, my wimpish queasiness reeked rather of the last sailor hanging to the mast of a sinking ship called Human Purity rather than trying to swim to safety. As though we are not, anyway, already containing and merged with all sorts of other beings, from microbes to machines to pollutants, that waft through the air and enter via our skin and nose and throat and other orifices.

Why mouse matter? Or why did it matter that it was mouse? These were the questions I had to ask and to understand. Rituximab is an antibody that is very effective against the protein CD20, which is primarily found on the surface of immune system B cells. When it binds to this protein (think of two bits of Velcro attached to magnets) it triggers cell death. Researchers identified a mouse antibody that had high anti-CD20 activity. The construction of a chimeric antibody was crucial, as the mouse antibody alone was unsuitable for direct use in humans.

While the mouse antibody was able to bind to human CD20, it would not be able to then recruit the immune cells that are needed to destroy the targeted B cells. It would also quickly be recognized as foreign in the human body and destroyed by the immune system. Therefore, by using a chimeric antibody with enough human characteristics, the antibody would not only recognize the human CD20 and mobilize the immune system; it would also remain in the body long enough to destroy the B cells.

I have had Rituximab in combination with other drugs twice (more recently the Rituxin antibody has been engineered with entirely human DNA and is available by injection). The side effects were minimal, and it worked fast in destroying a good proportion of the cancer cells, though they did return, and during one treatment I had a code blue reaction (when you stop breathing).

Rituximab and other immunotherapies, for all they represent as great advances, also, as time passes, have revealed their limitations. Rituximab can't get at cells with low antigen expression and hasn't been able to increase the life expectancy of CLL patients. But it and other immunotherapies have been vital in paving the way for CAR-T.

CAR-T represents a radically new step in that it is customized therapy using the patient's own live T cells, and it deploys a different and much more effective mechanism to eliminate target cells. Blood is taken from the patient and sent to a lab, where the cells are genetically modified by insertion of a disabled virus. These chimeric cells (a mix of DNA from the natural T cell antigen receptor and the introduced virus DNA, also carrying information to disrupt the cancer's signaling pathways) are then infused back into the patient's body, where the modified killer cells are let loose to do what they have been retrained to do: recognize and kill certain cancer cells. The attributes of the virally introduced DNA mean that the killer cells proliferate and reproduce like crazy in vivo and persist long term. As a one-off treatment this is clearly preferable to multiple infusions and doubly preferable in that the CARs (chimeric antigen receptors) are much more effective in seeking out those tumor cells with low antigen expression that elude mAbs.

As I write, CAR-T is being described as a breakthrough, as a frontier treatment, as the "darling" of current research, as heralding an epochal moment in cancer treatment. So why is it not being more widely used? Because "turning the wrath of the immune system against cancer can be a risky endeavor: Sometimes the patient's own body gets caught in the crossfire." At this stage the process takes time and carries many dangers. Producing the engineered cells (from two to four weeks) is lengthy and complex. Then, before the infusions begin, patients get a heavy round of chemotherapy to wipe out their natural T cells and make space for the newly engineered ones. Once those are infused the body can react violently, producing a range of effects, including—most worryingly—neurological problems.

Perhaps CAR-T will not live up to its promise, but then again perhaps it will (quite possibly in a modified form), and even if it doesn't, it certainly does seem to indicate that chimeras are likely to change the face of cancer treatments. I have skin in the game you might say, since the successes so far have been with blood cancers, not solid tumors (though research findings will pretty certainly, in the future, pertain to other cancers). So far, most successful cases have been related to ALL (acute lymphoblastic leukemia, more common in children than adults) but also to dramatic relapses after spectacular remissions. The therapy is not yet authorized for CLL, though a number of trials are in progress and planned.

One of those trials is taking place at this very moment in Seattle. I have been following, with a mixture of trepidation and hope, the progress of Brian Koffman, who has been blogging on the website he runs for the CLL Society, a patient support group that is an amazing resource. At this stage CAR-T is only something you opt for when you have run out of other options. Brian's CLL journey has been extremely arduous, and this is a brave move not least because, being part of a trial, he is contributing to research and helping future patients.

On the day of the infusion of his living cells back into his body he writes: "No bells rang, at least none in the range that we humans can hear. Maybe at a different frequency there was heard a clarion cry to rest up and get ready for the battle of your life." A few days later Brian is less well, and his daughter Heather takes up the blog: "We've been in touch with the University of Washington Chabad, and they're going to bring by a haggadah and Seder plate (vegan shank bone?) so we can celebrate Passover in the room tomorrow. The hospital room has a great view over Portage Lake and Montlake Cut, so we've been looking out at boats and trees and hoping to spot a heron." Two days later (the eighth day after the infusion) she ends her blog with these words: "Next year in Jerusalem." These words, repeated as an incantatory phrase during the Passover service, represent the expelled Jews' hope for an eventual return to a homeland. Given the current configuration of Jerusalem and the Israeli theft of Arab homeland, I'm reluctant these days to utter the phrase at Passover dinner and tend to mutter or fall silent. But reading these words now, written by Heather for her father, hearing the ritualistic resonances— may he live, may he return home—I find that tears are falling onto my computer screen, and soon I'm weeping buckets. Thank you for all you have done for us, Brian. Good luck, may you come home.

Brian is taking big risks, but he has made this choice (and outlined very clearly why). Yet many patients who also have run out of options will never have the opportunity to even make a choice. And herein lie a series of problems of which CAR-T is only a symptom, a series of problems that go beyond the strictly medical or scientific, that indicate that no cure will be achieved solely through medical or scientific means.

The cost of CAR-T is prohibitive. Brian was lucky enough to know about trials and to get into one, thus minimizing the cost (but also incurring risk since the treatment is in the trial stage). He is also lucky to have a family who are concerned to help him make the hospital experience as humane as possible. Trials are becoming smaller, meaning that fewer patients anyway will have access to treatment via this route. If and when CAR-T is approved for CLL, who will pay? It is unlikely that there will be a great deal of insurance coverage (even for those fortunate enough to have good insurance). The question will arise of whether CAR-T offers sufficient advantages to justify the need for personalized medicine, since CAR-T cells need to be manufactured for each single patient while mAbs are off-the-shelf reagents. There is much excitement in the air about the advent of personalized medicine, linked often to the falling price of genome sequencing (from about ten million initially to about one thousand dollars today), but it is not only the preparation of the cells that is costly; the necessary length of the hospital stay incurs an unbelievably huge expense. Personalized treatments may become available only to the wealthy elite. However, there is also a likelihood that combination treatments will be figured out (for example, the delivery form of the CAR-T treatment, the disabled virus, could be standardized, and other aspects individualized).

Whichever way you cut it, the future looks at once promising and scary, particularly given threatened and real rollbacks of the Affordable Care Act under the present administration. The internet of course enables a potentially much more democratic dissemination of knowledge, as does the existence of patient support and information groups like the CLL Society and Patient Power (and other cancer groups have equivalent societies). Yet even now there are many who do not know about or are unable to get to a CLL specialist or to a university research hospital. Given all the drawbacks, it is unlikely that CAR-T will any time soon become the great cure.

. . .

So what does it mean if, however sophisticated new treatments are, many won't come within spitting distance of adequate treatment, let alone a cure? Some patients might be cured, but America will not be able to lay claim to the promise of the country that will cure cancer once and for all.

If treatments are not manageable here, it is very likely that patients will go elsewhere. Even now the hospital tourism to Mexico, Tijuana in particular, is quite extensive. Although it is predominantly the excellent and cheap dentistry that attracts U.S. visitors, people also visit for medical reasons. This is understandable, but there are repercussions. I have witnessed medical waste, including a large amount from hospital tourism, dumped and sometimes burnt illegally in poor areas of Tijuana, especially on the top of one particular canyon, Las Laureles. This canyon is very steep and the patched-together housing precarious, particularly when it floods. When this happens all the toxic waste rushes into the canyon, poisoning the earth and water. It also rushes across the border into the estuary, an area where migrating birds and native fauna are protected. U.S. environmentalists blame Mexico for the pollution. Certainly the city of Tijuana is responsible for not enforcing laws regulating waste disposal, but U.S. hospital tourists, in flight from a precarious medical system, also are responsible. If there is to be a cure, it is unlikely that it will be the U.S. alone that will achieve it. Borders, in the body as well as between countries, are more porous than it seems when we look at maps, at blueprints for Trump's wall, at diagrams of the body organs.

. . .

Living Downstream is the title of a disturbing book by Sandra Steingraber. Subtitled *An Ecologist's Personal Investigation of Cancer and the Environment*, it is a meticulously researched and calmly argued book; what makes it so disturbing, and also compelling to read, is that it shines a glaringly bright light on the carcinogenic aspects of our quotidian environment. Although certain communities (most often poor or ethnically marginalized) are most frequently concentrated in the downstream, Steingraber argues that we are all daily exposed to hazardous carcinogenic chemicals.

You might ask: Hasn't it always been the case that the environment contains or emits some harmful chemicals? The answer is yes; people have probably always gotten sick and gotten cancer both from industrially produced chemicals and from other environmental mutations. The difference today is this: We know that after the Second World War the manufacture and production of petroleum-based goods and a whole variety of newly synthesized chemicals increased dramatically. Soon so many new chemicals were being produced that the government could not keep up with overseeing regulation of their production and disposal.

By 1976, Steingraber says, sixty-two thousand synthetic chemicals were in commercial use. The EWG (Environmental Working Group) has recently reported that since the 1970s, about eighty-five thousand chemicals have been approved for commercial use. Usually we take or absorb them in tandem, in cocktails. New research projects (such as the Halifax project) suggest it's the combination that might render a chemical carcinogenic.

We are surrounded—through cosmetics, packaging, the food we buy from the supermarket, the soaps we use for hygiene, the cleaners we use in our homes—by biologically active chemicals: "Some tinker with our hormones. Some attach themselves to our chromosomes and trigger mutations. . . . Some light up our genes and so enhance the production of certain enzymes." Some, like dioxins, are released into the air through combustion (commercial incinerators, fires, volcanoes, backyard burning of trash), and as a by-product of many industrial processes, such as chemical and pesticide manufacturing and pulp and paper bleaching. Hospital waste presents as a particularly critical issue because during burning a great deal of polyvinyl chloride and aromatic compounds that can serve as dioxin precursors are released into the atmosphere. Once dioxins are sent into the atmosphere they become attached to particles and fall back to earth. Then they bind to or are taken up by fish and other animals, where they get concentrated and stored in fat before they are consumed by us. They suppress human immunity and that immune suppression is associated with several kinds of cancers, most notably leukemias and lymphomas.

We now know how dioxins are produced, and so, since the 1980s, emission controls have limited the amount of dioxins released into the environment. But identifying the cause has come too late for many; they are extremely persistent compounds and break down very slowly. In fact, a large part of the current exposure to dioxins in the U.S. is due to releases that occurred decades ago. Moreover, we do not seem as a country to have learned from these instances to adequately test new chemical products (and products containing new chemicals), to invest as much time and research funds in the prevention of cancer as in chasing a cure. Without adequate prevention the cure will remain forever elusive, and in fact instances of chemically induced cancer are likely to escalate.

When I first started reading about dioxins I experienced a curious sense of relief: as though I had found the cause of my cancer and was ready to dive in and be biomonitored (biomonitoring is a measuring of the levels of pollutants in people, usually in blood or urine). But I soon abandoned this idea as futile on at least two levels. First, biomonitoring, even if a high level of dioxins were to be found, would not tell me where they came from or when. Second, biomonitoring only yields really useful results if entire populations (rather than isolated individuals) can be monitored and tested over time. Only the results from such epidemiological studies can help us understand the causes of cancer and thus enable us to craft prevention. In this sense people are like microbes: If we can only effectively study microbes as communities, in their interrelationships, interactions, and communications, so too with people and cancer and the environment.

. . .

While there is currently intense scrutiny of cancer in the body, there is less investigation of the body in a cancerous environment and more emphasis placed on the cure than on prevention. Medical and scientific "solutions" and "advances" will not alone cure cancer if we do not attend to the proliferating causes that surround us every day. Of course we can put our faith in the Environmental Protection Agency (EPA) to both protect the environment and ourselves, from the environment, when it becomes toxic. But putting our faith in the EPA at the moment (as I write this in April 2018) is a bit like crossing fingers and looking the other way. The person appointed by President Trump to head up the EPA, Scott Pruitt, has reversed or indefinitely postponed chemical bans, rubber-stamped new chemicals, cooked the books when assessing older chemicals, postponed chemical safety rules to protect farm and factory workers, and appointed chemical safety officials who have spent decades defending chemicals for polluters.

It is hard to imagine how knowledge of environmental causes of cancer, or a cure arising out of such knowledge, could eventuate in the current climate. I can't help feeling that there is something superstitious underlying the invocation of a once-and-for-all cure, a national psychic wish fulfillment if you like, akin to closing your eyes, making a wish, and expecting to wake up in a technicolored country free of cancer. Not that I actually have anything against wishing to be with Toto, no longer in Kansas. We need an element of faith, or superstition, of belief in the possibility that things can change. And the question of how to calibrate faith and superstition and optimism and skepticism—that is a difficult question.

. . .

And we are not the first or only country to grapple with this conundrum, though our allegiance to optimism is perhaps more pronounced, and our superstitious inclinations better concealed in rituals of scientific and institutional rigor, than in some other cultures. Paul Stoller is a North American anthropologist who studied the Songhay community in West Africa and in the process became a shaman, practicing sorcery there for many years. After he returned to the U.S. he was diagnosed with lymphoma and underwent treatment here while also drawing upon the shamanistic rituals with which he was familiar. He wrote a fascinating book, *Stranger in the Village of the Sick*, in which he reflects upon both the individualism of American culture and the pervasive optimism, in contrast to Songhay culture. Here, he argues, there is a belief that if you are optimistic then you will conquer cancer; if not, you might bring it on yourself. For the Songhay and many other cultures, however, misfortune and illness, pain and suffering, are a part of life, continuous and ever-present rather than posing a dramatic interruption. "Most Americans," he writes, "don't like to think too much about death. . . . In the world of sorcery, however, illness is a gateway to learning more about life. As for death, it is your constant companion." The cover of the book declares: "Sorcery is a body of knowledge and practice that enables one to see things clearly and to walk with confidence on the path of fear."

Not that I would want to be a cheerleader for the moral superiority of shamanistic practices (though sorcery, I know, takes many forms and does not always involve shamans). During the 1990s I spent quite a bit of time visiting and working with a theater group located in the town of Bulawayo, in Zimbabwe. AIDS was a devastating and constant presence: Men, women, and children were falling victim. Every evening the road leading to the cemetery was blocked by a long line of hearses. Amakhosi was a radical and vibrant group, outspoken on many fronts. One of the taboo subjects they broached—through drama, dance, and music—was AIDS, how to guard against the HIV virus, how to recognize the symptoms and what to do if diagnosed. One by one my friends in Amakhosi fell ill (though some remain alive and vibrant), and not one of them, once ill, would then utter the word AIDS. Was it superstition, as though uttering the word would bring it into being when so far it was just a wraith? Or was it denial? Or was it that they put their fate into the hands of their ancestors and shaman? Undoubtedly they knew they were dying—the shock, when death comes for you, is surely the same whenever or wherever and includes an element of disbelief; and when they consulted the shaman, and often the priest as well, I do not think it was exactly that they imagined a cure would materialize out of the sky. Of course I do not know and cannot tell what people, looking into the jaws of death, were feeling let alone thinking, but I imagine that, by making contact with the world of their ancestors, they were finding ways to anticipate and accommodate, ritualistically, death and suffering.

Perhaps there is a resonance in the rituals and modes of daily observance that some patients in the West adopt and adhere to, a range of practices that are often bundled together and called non-Western beliefs. I know that, in addition to the medical solutions, there are practices that have also kept me alive and opened onto the possibility (albeit in an amateur way) of living with the existence in life of death and pain.

Many in the medical establishment are arrogantly dismissive or patronizingly judgmental about such therapies as meditation, acupuncture, naturopathic supplements, tai chi, and qigong. "If it gives patients a feeling of having control over their lives and bodies, then fine; however, it is nothing but illusion to believe that it will cure cancer." This is almost a mantra (though I myself hear it mostly online, not from my own doctors). As I see it, it isn't an either/or choice. If there are less invasive, albeit complementary, methods of treatment—be it in the garden or my own body—I will always be inclined to explore. I don't think it very likely that the dietary and physical practices that I participate in will *cure* my cancer or be able to intervene in the genetic mutations, but I do believe that they reduce stress considerably, and stress is a killer. Moreover, they keep the body and mind nimble and very likely stimulate aspects of the immune system that traditional Western medicine does not contemplate or indeed fully understand. I am reluctant to offer my body up wholesale either to the overwhelming medicalization of cancer in our culture or to a mono approach.

"It is nothing but illusion to believe that it will cure cancer." What jumps out to me, in such an assertion, is "the cure" as the agenda-setting term. What if we are concerned not to achieve a cure at all cost, but to live as calm and fraught-free a life as is possible with cancer and while undergoing medical treatment? What if we want to find ways to adapt to pain and anxiety that are not merely illusory but that are under our own control, may be beneficial, that don't have to come out of a bottle or be fed into our veins through tubes?

Modern Western medicine has many tools that are sophisticated, but every trial, every new and experimental drug, requires faith as much as certainty. Is a belief in so-called non-Western treatments so much more delusory than the single-minded medical pursuit of a definitive cure? If our bodies are stochastic, neither fixed nor singular, so we might be predisposed to respond to a heterogeneity of treatments.

. . .

In talking of the inflated rhetoric around the cure as chimerical, I was using the term in the more common sense: to indicate an illusion or delusion or unrealizable dream. But my feelings are not as straightforward as they might seem. The biomedical resonances infiltrate everyday common parlance and simultaneously invest apparent scientificity with the poetry of myth, the cadences of magic.

The chimera is not simply an illusion, but a hybrid construction, a multispecies creature. This is what we are. And this is the clue to survival. It is much easier for cancer cells to develop in a body than it is to restore the body to a pristine or cancer-free state. The body is stochastic, and so is cancer. It is a model of evolutionary diversification, mutation, adaptation.

The chimera is a term that comes to us from mythology, and it is easy to think of CAR-T as an almost mythological procedure, as though we were entering into the realms of science fiction, as though the future were walking backward to meet us as we stumble forward in the dark. In the future, more and more of us might find our bodies to be chimeric, made up of recombinant DNA. But in fact it turns out that many people may (now and in the past, if we'd had the technology to see) exhibit so-called microchimerism—when a small fraction of their cells are from someone else. And it turns out too that the way such genetic information is passed along, exchanged, is through a process that was considered to be typical of microbial behavior but not of multicellular organisms like humans: horizontal gene transfer.

People can be chimeras too.

Biologists have long suspected that something is transferred between mothers and babies during the birth process, but they surmised that it was molecules that moved. Very recently, however, biologists have learned that *cells* migrate. The cells of the mother infiltrate across the placenta into the child, and the cells of the child infiltrate into the mother. Thus, each one of us is a chimera of sorts, our bodies containing cell lines of others. If you are a first-born child, you will have a set of cells that come from your mother, including cells that she acquired from her own mother in the same way. If you are a youngest child, not only will you receive your mother's cells, but you will also receive all of your siblings' cells. We are thus not what we thought: Every "I" is also a "we."

The poetry of myth and the cadences of magic pertain to science as well as to other systems of belief. In Shambhala, dralas refer to magical entities. During the 1970s and 1980s, Chögyam Trungpa Rinpoche recovered the drala principle, the roots of which precede the introduction of Buddhism into Tibet and are found in the indigenous traditions of that country—as they are in all countries. Drala is the elemental presence of the world that is available to us through sense perceptions. Trungpa Rinpoche was once asked if the dralas exist. He thought for a moment and then replied: "They *almost* exist."

. . .

Does the big cure exist? *Almost.* Which means not that it's on its way, ambling along, or even rushing breathlessly to a triumphant climax; no, it means sometimes yes, sometimes no. We can retain hope and belief in the possibility of something magical happening; this matters. We know that science is a dance: two steps forward, one step back, and then a twirling. The lazy poet is sometimes cancer and sometimes the ingenious researcher who is investigating cancer. Perhaps it is not just a war zone with this country fighting to be at the forefront, but also a magical realm in which every so often those lazy poets, to our delight or dismay, pull a rabbit out of the hat.

The Last Chicken Standing

82

Sabrina died last night. The third chicken to hit the dust. We always imagined that she, the imperious one, would be the last to go. But in the past weeks she started ailing, eating less, losing interest in dried worms, not responding when her name was called. In the past, when any name was called, be it the name of a cat or chicken or human, she would be the first to come flying, careening into view, laying claim to sovereignty. She was the worst of the egg layers and had given up the habit of pleasing humans years ago, though when she did lay, her eggs were a rich dark chestnut brown, always freckled erratically. She was the most regal and the most richly and intricately patterned of the birds. So sad, then, when age caught up with her and she wilted before our eyes. Up until the end, though, she managed to perk up when offered a squished cherry tomato, cracked open, oozing scarlet juice.

J dug a grave for her on the side of the house, the only place not densely colonized by plants. She will return to the earth in her own time.

Now there is only Holly. And she is bereft. She stalked the corner of the yard today, emitting a strange tormented squawking sound, more like a shriek than a cackle. A haunting sound. I woke at three in the morning thinking of her by herself in the darkness of night, all alone for the first time in her life. So I took the flashlight and went out to speak to her. I chatted, approaching her house, as I always do at night, letting the girls know it's me, and usually they respond with a soft chirruping. But the night was silent this night. All alone on the perch where she would usually cuddle up with Sabrina, Holly sat adamantly with her back to me. My heart is sore and I can hardly contemplate her aloneness, how bare her body must feel without the ruffling feathers of Sabrina. I feel, too, remorse that we did not anticipate this and get more chickens before the end arrived for the old girls. We knew, after Lula Mae died, that the others would follow and felt that when one went, the other would surely follow soon after. But some callous indifference or failure of imagination blocked us from thinking about what it must be like to be left, the last chicken standing.

SIX WEEKS LATER

I found companions for Holly. At a chicken farm in Vista, nearly an hour away, I chose two young birds. Another Americauna (so that we could continue to have blue eggs), though she looked very different from Lula Mae, her feathers more burnished and coppery, her demeanor more saucy. The other is a Buff Orpington, petite and perky, though supposedly she will turn into a large and docile hen. Eliza and Gigi, being different breeds, came from different parts of the farm. They had never met, but in the cardboard box on the way home they bonded for life. Taken out of the box at home they moved together as though a single chicken, they curled up together and rolled around in the dust, and as dusk fell they would sit upon one another. They formed an exclusionary unit, and Holly hated them. War broke out. Holly would not allow them into the roosting house at night. During the day she disdained their company, followed us humans around everywhere in the yard, looking up beseechingly until we picked her up and cradled her and murmured sweet nothings until her neck drooped, her eyes slowly closed, and she began to snooze. She would hang out at the back door and try to slip into the house. She started eating human food. When we ate out in the yard in the evenings she would pick from our plates and try to share our chairs.

Now it seems that peace might be dribbling back into the yard. Sometimes the young ones rush together toward some invisible object and fly into the air, squawking and flapping exuberantly. Holly just ambles. She no longer yearns to be picked up and stroked. I guess she tried the human life, and it didn't, in the end, rate highly. So she returned to her chicken existence.

My estimation of chicken desire was way off beam. My solution skewed. Of course I wanted to ease Holly's pain, but some small part of me, hovering near the surface of consciousness, was convinced that Holly would follow Sabrina into the next world very soon, and this would be an omen that I would die next. So getting more chickens was a way of keeping the chicken lineage alive. And me too.

Sabrina died two weeks short of turning seven. Seven years since I started writing this book. Seven years since the nadir of health. I felt then that the chickens would save my life, and, though a hyperbolic fantasy, there was and is some truth in that conceit. About to embark on my first chemo, the chickens distracted me from dwelling on the six-year prognosis I was given by the first hematologist I saw. Six years to live. In fact, I now suspect he said something like: You will probably live for twenty years, but it might only be six. Yet it was the figure six that assumed a mystically menacing dimension. Even after I migrated to Dr. K, who was much more optimistic and who cautioned against dealing in hypotheticals, even then some part of me remained tenaciously and superstitiously attached to the number six.

The chickens have seen me through those years with casual insouciance. Now they are dying and I am better than ever, treatments have improved, prospects for a longer life seem almost certain.

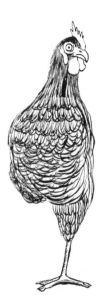

Arrivederci 83

Arrivederci, come le volpi in pellicceria
(Until we meet again, like the foxes at the furriers)

Approaching the end of 2018, I have been feeling once again like a B-grade version of Aeneas, stumbling into a place of shadows, of sleep, of endless darkness. Falling ill again I plummeted into a black hole. A bacterial infection. To submit or not to submit to antibiotics yet again (when it might have been the last round I took in Marfa, for a different infection, that caused this one)? For a week I lay slumped on the couch with a hot water bottle, watching *Gilmore Girls*, episode after episode, day in and day out. I had never seen this series but knew it was created by and much of it written by Amy Sherman-Palladino, she who created one of the most bravura shows on TV this past year, *The Marvelous Mrs. Maisel*. I enjoyed the witty, fast-paced repartee of *GG* and the fantasy of a mother-daughter relationship that is also a friendship. But eventually the smart dialogue and the panacea of familiarity—the staple generic device of a small community of eccentric but basically lovable characters—became claustrophobic, too white, too relentlessly assertive of a cheery heterosexual world. It made me sick. More sick than the bacterial infection and the antibiotics.

I knew that this was part and parcel of the returning CLL symptoms and vulnerability. I knew that another treatment was looming on the horizon. And I simply couldn't face it; all my stoicism, all the accumulated wisdom of the past ten years, all my Buddhist letting go, all of it went out the window in a flash. You would have thought that by now I would have become accustomed to the ups and downs of CLL, learned to take things in my stride, not to succumb to despair and sink into the black hole. I suppose that immersion in *GG* is better than cowering in a corner, indulging in self-flagellation and weeping buckets of remorse for a life lived wantonly. I've done enough of that in my time. Better, perhaps, but not much better. Can I say I learned something from this zoning out into another sphere, taking an unexpected detour? Not really. Except that I came out of it, having taken the antibiotics after much research and a long talk with the GI doctor and after embarking on a diet that cut out almost everything except meat but led to creative cooking, including a deliciously aromatic ginger and honey almond cake. I came out of it. I emerged from the thick black slurry.

I was apprehensive that Dr. K would veto my planned horticultural trip to New Zealand (meeting up with J, who has been in Australia, and Virginia and Helen B), but on the contrary, he was shocked that, having lived in Australia for so long, I had never been there. You need to travel, he said, it's good for you. I hope you're going to hike the Milford Trail. He has given me the literature for a new trial opening up in January. It will involve a cocktail of two drugs—Ibrutinib (a kinase inhibitor, to be taken orally), which has already been approved for CLL, and a new experimental drug, not yet approved, Cirmtuzumab (a monoclonal antibody, to be taken by infusion). It will last a year.

Preparing for New Zealand, I've been watching the films of Taika Waititi. In the hilariously anarchic *What We Do in the Shadows*, the vampire says of his way-out outfit, "I go for a look that I call dead but delicious." Taiku Waititi has another film that is equally anarchic and hilarious, *Boy*, that touched me elsewhere and even more, perhaps because of the romance of the kids in a world without grown-ups, and when the grown-up does appear he turns out to be more of a kid than any of them. It brings vividly to life a broken family, constantly and inventively patched up. I imagine that the New Zealand we are to see will not be this New Zealand, much of it will be seen through binoculars and botanical microscopes. But for me the spirit of these films will infuse the experience.

. . .

Holly is still alive. Faded, scruffy, but energized by deep reserves of venom mobilized against the young interlopers. During the day she scuffles and scratches around the yard with Eliza and Gigi, they appear to be a companionable trio. But when the evening shadows come, if she remembers to get to the coop where they sleep before they do, she will take up position in the doorway, rise up on her old scaly legs, puff out her feathers and peck furiously at them as they try to enter. She is like Cerberus guarding the gates to the underworld. Clearly I was wildly skew-whiff in my estimation of Holly's grief, and my attempt to project empathy, in the form of a gift and a solution, backfired. My grief was not like her grief. Empathy, sympathy, similes—tricky to enact. I hope that there are people out there with CLL and other afflictions who might recognize some of the experiences of this book and be able to say: Yes it's like that. But every simile also has its limit point. When well-meaning friends say, Oh I know how you feel; it's just like how I feel most of the time these days, tired, doesn't old age suck? I want to kick them in the teeth. This is like that, comparable but not the same. And sometimes you just have to say: There's no comparison.

Holly is a mystery, not least because she keeps on going, staying alive. A bit like me. Yet not like me. Still, I feel more like her than you might imagine.

As it has gradually dawned on me that I'm surviving, there is something unexpected that I have had to face. A cow in a slaughterhouse, that's what I felt like when I received the CLL diagnosis, a cow hit by a bullet, at close range, between the eyes. But unlike that putative cow I did not drop dead and, instead, received a curious kind of immunity. I was inoculated against a particular affliction or mode of suffering: able, on some level, to imagine that all my loved ones would outlive me, that being the one to go first I would not have to deal with the pain of separation and aloneness. Death itself, or the specter of one's own death, I have found, is not so frightening as facing up to the death of those who sustain one's own life. Elvis has gone, the chickens are going, and one day it is quite probable that I will have to witness and endure the passing of J, of being alone, without him. As I begin to apprehend this my breath stops, my heart speeds up, it's impossible to apprehend. I suppose I have gradually had to relinquish this fantasy of passing away first, of letting others, at least in my mind, cope with irreparable absence. Slowly, as I have survived and as others around me have not—others whom I love or have loved, others who have been friends for many years or fellow travelers—some who seemed when I was first ill to be in the prime of health, I have been deflected from this guiltless journey toward death and paradoxically had to inch slowly into living, into the question of how to live and how to rejig my understanding of the word *chronic*: How to nudge the notion of a chronic illness off from center stage and how to accommodate, somewhat grudgingly, to the idea of being chronically alive.

. . .

Remember Socrates's last words to his followers, after he had drunk the pharmakon or poison: "We owe a cock to Asclepius. Please, don't forget to pay the debt."

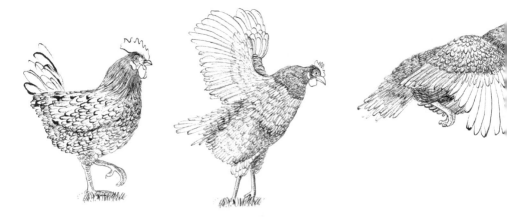

These words are often dismissed as the babble of a confused, dying man. But some commentators have intriguing interpretations. Nietzsche's proposition was that Socrates meant *life is a disease.* Asclepius was the Greek god of healing, and offering a cock in sacrifice was a way of thanking him for healing Socrates with the hemlock. A contemporary classicist, Emily Wilson, offers a different explanation: that Socrates is comparing death to childbirth and thus wishes to thank Asclepius for helping with the birth of his soul into the afterlife. Let's remember also that Asclepius not only had powers of healing but also the power to bring the dead back to life.

Perhaps we practice dying by finding out how to live. Hungry ghosts have haunted this diary but, also, spirits who have breathed inspiration. The experience of a Buddhist death, participating in Ryoko's passage from this world, being in the hospital with others for a week, before and during and after her passing, brought home to me the proximity of the dead and the living. Before and during and after: not so easily distinguished temporalities. Dead and alive: not such water-tight categories. The dead can sustain the living, the sociality of those remaining and the rituals associated with mourning and grief are also rituals of daily life, rituals of living and of celebration.

. . .

Between habit and ritual a thin line: between therapeutic and spiritual practices, between the gracious and orderly lighting of candles and the compulsive repetition of obsessive desire, between routine and observance. Many ritualistic practices— from the quotidian and idiosyncratic to those more formally prescribed—serve to preserve the way things are, to protect us against change, transformation, difference, grief. And yet, and yet . . . there is always the possibility of something mysterious happening.

. . .

But now this book is over. Perhaps we will meet in the afterlife, you and me and the foxes and Socrates. Or perhaps it is enough to meet here, to get on with living while we can. . . .

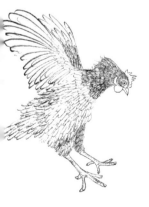 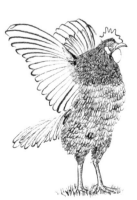 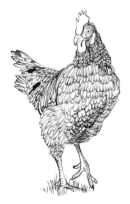

Notes

CHAPTER 2. THE TIME IT TAKES (BY WAY OF AN INTRODUCTION)

5   *Plato defined the human being*   Page Smith and Charles Daniel, *The Chicken Book* (Athens: University of Georgia Press, 2000), 16.

CHAPTER 5. EVENTS UNFOLD IN THE SNOW

13   *the book Miriam had finished*   Miriam Hansen, *Cinema and Experience: Siegfried Kracauer, Walter Benjamin, and Theodor W. Adorno*, ed. Edward Dimendberg (Los Angeles: University of California Press, 2011).

16   *"in a photograph a person's history is buried . . ."*   Siegfried Kracauer, *The Mass Ornament: Weimar Essays*, ed. Thomas Y. Levin (Cambridge, MA: Harvard University Press, 1995), 51.

CHAPTER 7. WHY CHICKENS, OR HOMAGE TO GLORIA

18   *"I remained loyal, as a man would to a bride . . ."*   E. B. White, "The Hen (An Appreciation)," in *The Second Tree from the Corner* (New York: Harper and Row, 1984), 235.

21   Backyard chickens dumped at shelters when hipsters can't cope, critics say   Jonel Aleccia, "Backyard Chickens Dumped at Shelters When Hipsters Can't Cope, Critics Say," NBC News, July 7, 2013, https://www.nbcnews.com/healthmain/backyard-chickens-dumped-shelters-when-hipsters-cant-cope-critics-say-6C10533508.

CHAPTER 8. BOOMERANG

22   *Akos's book is about plastic money*   Akos Rona-Tas and Alya Guseva, *Plastic Money: Constructing Markets for Credit Cards in Eight Postcommunist Countries* (Stanford, CA: Stanford University Press, 2014).

23 *You could give it a Žižekian spin*   Slavoj Žižek is a contemporary philosopher.

23 *Bryan Brown*   An Australian actor.

CHAPTER 9. A WAY OF MAKING ANOTHER EGG

27 *so vividly evoked by Kate Atkinson*   *Life after Life: A Novel* (Boston: Little, Brown, 2013), 228.

27 *reproduced in the magazine*   "Arzak Eggs," *Lucky Peach*, Summer 2011, 148–49.

CHAPTER 13. LIFE AFTER LIFE

40 *"He had trained in Vienna . . ."*   Atkinson, *Life after Life*, 155.

41 *"How sorry she felt for herself, as if she were someone else"*   Atkinson, *Life after Life*, 286.

CHAPTER 15. SOME MUSINGS ON METAPHOR

46 *Bittersweet like the Jane Campion movie*   *Sweetie*, directed by Jane Campion (Australia, 1989).

CHAPTER 16. TRICKING THE BODY

52 *With a group of graduate students*   After several years the group would crystallize to Kate Clark, Sara Solamaini, Matt Savitsky, Dominic Miller, and Emily Sevier. But the group was initially larger and included Alex Kershaw, Ilaria Tabusso-Marcyan, Samara Kaplan, and Nichole Speciale.

52 *a canyon in Tijuana*   See my article "A Garden or a Grave? The Canyonic Landscape of the Tijuana–San Diego Region," in *Arts of Living on a Damaged Planet: Ghosts and Monsters of the Anthropocene*, ed. Anna Lowenhaupt Tsing, Heather Anne Swanson, Elaine Gan, and Nils Bubandt (Minneapolis: University of Minnesota Press, 2016), 17–29.

CHAPTER 17. CHICKEN JOKE

53 *This joke is told by Alenka Zupančič*   *The Odd One In: On Comedy* (Cambridge, MA: MIT Press, 2008), 15.

55 *"In short, it is not simply that in analysis . . ."*   Zupančič, *The Odd One In*, 16.

CHAPTER 19. FRENZIED CALM

63 *Woman of the Dunes*   Title of a film directed by Hiroshi Teshigahara (Japan, 1964).

65 *Mary Douglas speaks to me*   Douglas, an anthropologist and cultural theorist, wrote the highly influential *Purity and Danger: An Analysis of Concepts of Pollution and Taboo* (London: Routledge, 1966).

67   *"The Florida criminal justice system has sent two clear messages today . . ."*   Corrine Brown, quoted in Mary Anne Franks, "Injury Inequality," in *Injury and Injustice: The Cultural Politics of Harm and Redress*, ed. Anne Bloom, David M. Engel, and Michael McCann (New York: Cambridge University Press, 2018), 235.

67   *During the Haiti crisis in 2004*   Corrine Brown, quoted in Teri Schultz and the Associated Press, "Bonilla: Muted Reaction to Brown Shows Double Standard," *Fox News*, February 27, 2004, https://www.foxnews.com/story/bonilla-muted -reaction-to-brown-shows-double-standard.

68   "Through time, in this country, what I like to call bleeding-heart . . ."   Josh Horwitz, "Arming Zimmerman," *huffpost.com*, March 20, 2012, https://www.huffpost .com/entry/arming-zimmerman_b_1367648.

CHAPTER 22. WHY ME, LORD?

75   *Joan Didion once wrote*   "Doris Lessing (1971)," in *The White Album* (New York: Simon and Schuster, 1979), 119.

79   *the question of how to live*   This perspective on Montaigne is indebted to Sarah Bakewell, *How to Live, or A Life of Montaigne in One Question and Twenty Attempts at an Answer* (New York: Other Press, 2010).

CHAPTER 24. THE WARRIOR SONG OF KING GESAR

82   The Warrior Song of King Gesar   Douglas J. Penick, *The Warrior Song of King Gesar* (Boulder, CO: Mountain Treasury Press, 2013).

83   *but most wonderfully to my mind in the film*   *The Forgotten Space*, directed by Noël Burch and Allan Sekula (United States, 2012).

83   *ranging from shamanistic declamation to rhythmic patter to song*   Mark Swed, "Review: Long Beach Opera's 'King Gesar' Channels a Legend," *Los Angeles Times*, September 9, 2013, http://articles.latimes.com/2013/sep/09/entertainment/la -et-cm-long-beach-opera-review-20130909.

CHAPTER 25. EUPHORIA

86   *I wrote a short book*   Lesley Stern, *Dead and Alive: The Body as Cinematic Thing* (Montreal: Caboose, 2012).

CHAPTER 29. BLUE / SHIMMER

94   *"Windsor and Newton Deep Ultramarine oil colour . . ."*   Sandra McGrath, *Brett Whiteley* (Sydney: Bay Books, 1979), 214.

94   *"The colours," she said "should not be put on subtly . . ."*   Quoted in the marvelous catalog J brought me from Australia: Deborah Edwards, Rose Peel, and Denise Mimmocchi, eds., *Margaret Preston*, exhibition catalog (Sydney: Thames and Hudson Australia, 2010), 260.

94   Norman Lindsay accused her of "violent crudities of pure colour"   Edwards, Peel, and Mimmocchi, *Margaret Preston*, 83.

95   *"It's like speaking in a French accent . . ."*   Alexa Moses, "Shadow Cast over a Painter's Legacy," *Sydney Morning Herald*, July 25, 2005, http://www.smh.com.au/news /arts/shadow-cast-over-a-painters-legacy/2005/07/24/1122143723289.html.

96   *"If you can understand the paintings . . ."*   Baluka Maymuru, son of Nänyin' Maymuru, interviewed by Andrew Blake, in Cara Pinchbeck, ed., *Yirrkala Drawings*, exhibition catalog (Sydney: Art Gallery of New South Wales, 2013), 106.

96   *I hear Deborah Bird Rose at a conference*   "Shimmer: When All You Love Is Being Trashed," lecture presented as part of the conference "Anthropocene: Arts of Living on a Damaged Planet," University of California Santa Cruz, May 8–10, 2014. See also Anna Lowenhaupt Tsing, Heather Anne Swanson, Elaine Gan, and Nils Bubandt, eds., *Arts of Living on a Damaged Planet: Ghosts and Monsters of the Anthropocene* (Minneapolis: University of Minnesota Press, 2017).

97   Bir'yun *refers to intense sources and refractions of light*   Howard Morphy, "From Dull to Brilliant: The Aesthetics of Spiritual Power among the Yolngu," *Man* 24, no. 1 (March 1989): 28. Morphy here is drawing on the field notes of the anthropologist Donald Thompson. Morphy has dealt with this concept of shimmer in a variety of writings; see, for instance (here I draw on), "Shimmering Light," in *Jörg Schmeisser: Bilder Der Reise; A Man Who Likes to Draw*, ed. Roger Butler (Lyneham, ACT: SFA Press in association with Macmillan Art Publishing, 2013); *Aboriginal Art* (London: Phaidon, 1998), 185–90; and "The Art of the Yirrkala Crayon Drawings: Innovation, Creativity and Tradition," in Pinchbeck, *Yirrkala Drawings*, 27–33.

97   *As Waka Mununggurr writes in the preface to the catalog*   Pinchbeck, *Yirrkala Drawings*, 13.

98   *It is estimated that as many as one thousand trepangers arrived each year*   Charles Campbell MacKnight, *The Voyage to Marege': Macassan Trepangers in Northern Australia* (Carlton, AU: Melbourne University Press, 1976), 29.

98   *"Their story is still alive today . . ."*   The video interview with Laklak Ganambarr is transcribed in Pinchbeck, *Yirrkala Drawings*, 146–47.

98   *Macassan culture was incorporated into Aboriginal Dreamtime*   Howard Morphy, "Engaging the Other: Art and the Survival of Aboriginal Society," in *Aboriginal Art*, 221–60.

98   *(Bununggu Yunupingu, whose* Ceremony with Macassan Influence *is densely imagistic)*   The crayon drawings were not given titles at the time they were made; the titles used in the exhibition and catalog were either in use from previous exhibitions or arrived at after extensive consultation with current clan leaders. Pinchbeck, *Yirrkala Drawings*, 6.

98   *"These beings had the power to travel over deep waters of the ocean"*   Pinchbeck, *Yirrkala Drawings*, 139.

99   *"We are all connected through the mixing of waters . . ."*   Maymuru interview in Pinchbeck, *Yirrkala Drawings*, 107.

100   *"So, two different styles to our sacred paintings . . ."*   Yalpi Yunupingu, interviewed by Andrew Blake, in Pinchbeck, *Yirrkala Drawings*, 139.

100　*"differing colors signify the differing states of water . . ."*　Andrew Blake, "Yirrkala: A Brief History," in Pinchbeck, *Yirrkala Drawings*, 37.

100　*"a sense of movement, that has references to the interwoven structure of the dam and the water . . ."*　Morphy, "Art of the Yirrkala Crayon Drawings," 31.

100　*In the Yirrkala drawings land and sea are connected*　Jens Korff, "Blue Mud Bay High Court Decision," Creative Spirits, last updated February 7, 2019, http://www .creativespirits.info/aboriginalculture/land/blue-mud-bay-high-court-decision. This article discusses the high court decision that accorded sea rights to the Yolngu.

100　*The Saltwater Collection consists of eighty bark paintings*　The Living Knowledge Project, "About the Saltwater Collection," Living Knowledge, Australian National University, 2008, http://livingknowledge.anu.edu.au/learningsites/seacountry/17 _collection.htm.

100　*After this desecration of Bäru*　This material is drawn from the Australian National Maritime Museum, where some of the barks were exhibited from May 2013 to February 2014.

102　*"the image remained that of a large imposing red hulk . . ."*　Lone Bertelsen and Andrew Murphie, "An Ethics of Everyday Infinities and Powers: Félix Guattari on Affect and the Refrain," in *The Affect Theory Reader*, ed. Melissa Gregg and Gregory J. Seigworth (Durham, NC: Duke University Press, 2010), 143.

103　*"asylum seekers who come here by boat . . ."*　Bianca Hall and Jonathan Swan, "Kevin Rudd to Send Asylum Seekers Who Arrive by Boat to Papua New Guinea," *Sydney Morning Herald*, July 19, 2013, https://www.smh.com.au/politics/federal/kevin -rudd-to-send-asylum-seekers-who-arrive-by-boat-to-papua-new-guinea-20130719 -2q9fa.html.

104　*As I write this . . . Australia has returned its seventh boatload of asylum seekers*　Michael Bachelard, "Another Turned Back Boat Lands in Indonesia," *Sydney Morning Herald*, February 25, 2014, https://www.smh.com.au/politics/federal/another -turned-back-boat-lands-in-indonesia-20140225-33dn7.html.

104　*Maritime law experts have voiced concern about the legality of Operation Sovereign Borders*　Jane McAdam, Kate Purcell, and Joyce Chia, "Inquiry into the Breach of Indonesian Territorial Waters: Submission to the Senate Standing Committee on Foreign Affairs, Defence and Trade," Andrew and Renata Kaldor Centre for International Refugee Law, March 19, 2014, https://www.kaldorcentre.unsw.edu.au /sites/default/files/kaldor_centre_submission_inquiry_into_breach_of_territorial _waters_final.pdf.

104　*"Here the word future is not a word"*　Suvendrini Perera and Joseph Pugliese, "'Here the Word Future Is Not a Word': Life as a Refugee on Nauru," *The Conversation*, August 4, 2014, http://theconversation.com/here-the-word-future -is-not-a-word-life-as-a-refugee-on-nauru-30079.

105　*Although Tony Abbott presents the current situation in terms of war*　"We are in a fierce contest with these people smugglers," Abbott has said. "And if we were at war, we wouldn't be giving out information that is of use to the enemy just because we might have an idle curiosity about it ourselves." Abbott is quoted in "Prime Minister Tony Abbott Likens Campaign against People Smugglers to 'War,'" *ABC*

News (Australian Broadcasting Corp.), February 3, 2014, http://www.abc.net
.au/news/2014-01-10/abbott-likens-campaign-against-people-smugglers-to-war
/5193546.

105   *Up to two million people were massacred*   For two reputable sources, see Robert
Cribb, "Introduction: Problems in the Historiography of the Killings in Indonesia,"
in *The Indonesian Killings of 1965–1966: Studies from Java and Bali*, ed. Robert Cribb
(Melbourne: Monash Asia Institute at Monash University, 1990), 1–43; and "Final
Report of the IPT 1965: Findings and Documents of the International People's Tri-
bunal on Crimes against Humanity Indonesia 1965," accessed November 15, 2019,
www.tribunal1965.org/en/final-report-of-the-ipt-1965.

105   *in fact, it was passed off as a civil war*   Thomas Reuter, "Australian Espionage and
the History of Foreign Intervention in Indonesia," *The Conversation*, November 25,
2013, https://theconversation.com/australian-espionage-and-the-history-of-foreign
-intervention-in-indonesia-20648.

105   *those Western powers that had knowledge*   Communiqués from U.S. and Australian
ambassadors reveal that the "politicide" was conducted with the full knowledge
and active complicity of those countries.

105   *A small boat in an ocean of impunity*   Galuh Wandita, "PREMAN NATION:
Watching *The Act of Killing* in Indonesia," *Critical Asian Studies* 46, no. 1 (March
2014): 167–70.

105   *the Coalition for Justice and Truth*   KKPK.org, https://asia-ajar.org/the-year-of-truth
-campaign-in-indonesia.

106   *"no country is more important to Australia than Indonesia"*   Bilveer Singh, *Defense
Relations between Australia and Indonesia in the Post–Cold War Era* (Westport, CT:
Greenwood, 2002), 89–93.

106   *This is a refrain that structures Joris Ivens's 1947 film*   *Indonesia Calling*, directed by
Joris Ivens (Australia, 1947).

107   *"They showed it preceding* Gone with the Wind . . ."   Hardjadibrata is quoted in
John Hughes, "Indonesia Calling: Joris Ivens in Australia," *Senses of Cinema*, MIFF
Premiere Fund/Post-Punk Dossier, no. 51 (July 2009): n.p., http://sensesofcinema
.com/2009/miff-premiere-fund-post-punk-dossier/indonesia-calling.

CHAPTER 31. BLOWN THROUGH THE AIR

111   *Feralization looks, on its surface, like domestication*   Ewen Callaway, "When Chickens Go Wild," *Nature* 529, no. 7586 (January 20, 2016): 270–73, https://www
.nature.com/news/when-chickens-go-wild-1.19195.

113   *"Like Michael said . . ."*   Pamela Brown, "Windows Wound Down," in *Home by
Dark* (Bristol, U.K.: Shearsman Books, 2013), 12.

CHAPTER 33. SPHERES OF GLASS

117   *"I was sitting alone in my wagon-lit compartment . . ."*   Sigmund Freud, "The Uncanny (1919)," in *Art and Literature*, ed. Angela Richards, trans. James Strachey

(London: Penguin, 1985), 339. Freud situates his essay as an investigation into aesthetics: "understood to mean not merely the theory of beauty but the theory of the qualities of feeling."

119 *"They look real enough . . ."* Jamaica Kincaid, "Splendor in the Glass," *Architectural Digest*, June 1, 2002, http://www.architecturaldigest.com/ad/archive/artnotebook _article_062002.

119 *Think of Ian Hamilton Finlay's glass poem* There are several iterations of this installation. The one I know was completed in 1987 as part of the Stuart Collection at the University of California, San Diego.

120 *"mental shift in scale (from individual item to larger combination)"* Leslie Dick, "Hyperbolic Crochet Coral Reefs," *X-tra* 11, no. 4 (Summer 2009): n.p., https:// www.x-traonline.org/article/the-institute-for-figuring-and-companions -hyperbolic-crochet-coral-reefs.

121 *"the potential for a large catastrophic failure"* Timothy Egan, "A Mudslide, Foretold," *New York Times*, March 29, 2014, https://www.nytimes.com/2014/03/30 /opinion/sunday/egan-at-home-when-the-earth-moves.html.

121 *"The 'taming' of this continent . . ."* Egan, "Mudslide, Foretold."

CHAPTER 36. DEAD AND ALIVE: A TENUOUS CONTINUUM

129 sadza A staple food in Zimbabwe, sadza is a thick porridge made from boiling maize meal.

130 *"a certain quantity of human perspiration . . ."* Katrin sends me this quote from Karl Marx, referring to a report on the baking trade by a Royal Commission of Enquiry in 1863. *Capital*, vol. 1 (New York: Penguin, 1976), 359.

132 *"correlative to life and to the organization of globules . . ."* Louis Pasteur, quoted in Bruno Latour, "From Fabrication to Reality: Pasteur and His Lactic Acid Ferment," in *Pandora's Hope: Essays on the Reality of Science Studies* (Cambridge, MA: Harvard University Press, 1999), 129.

132 *later writers, such as Michael Pollan* Pollan modifies the relationship between human and nonhuman in *Cooked: A Natural History of Transformation* (New York: Penguin, 2013).

133 *"converts a nonentity [yeast], the Cinderella of chemical theory, into a glorious and heroic character"* Latour, *Pandora's Hope*, 116–17.

133 *In the process yeast and lactic acid . . . mute world* Latour, *Pandora's Hope*, 140.

133 "we are allowed to speak interestingly by what we allow to speak interestingly" Vinciane Despret, quoted in Latour, *Pandora's Hope*, 144.

133 *That canonic Buddhist text* The Tassajara Bread Book Edward Espe Brown, *The Tassajara Bread Book* (Boulder, CO: Shambhala, 1970), http://www.xedizioni.it /Numeri-due/Tassajara-bread-book-p.pdf.

135 *"What has been the staff of life . . ."* Stephen Jones, quoted in Tom Philpott, "Could This Baker Solve the Gluten Mystery?," *Mother Jones*, February 12, 2014, https:// www.motherjones.com/food/2014/02/toms-kitchen-100-whole-wheat-bread -doesnt-suck-and-pretty-easy.

CHAPTER 38. LANDSCAPE

140   *he liked to listen to opera*   Marilyn Ann Moss, *Giant: George Stevens, a Life on Film*
(Madison: University of Wisconsin Press, 2004), 220.

CHAPTER 39. TOOTIN POOTIN

144   *there is the issue of how many courses of Flagyl she has taken*   Celiac disease is massively on the rise. About 40 percent of patients taking Flagyl are more likely to
have had antibiotics recently. For those who are prescribed more courses of Flagyl, the risk of celiac disease is greater. Per Martin Blaser, Flagyl had "the greatest association with celiac disease. People who were prescribed it ran more than
twice the risk of getting celiac disease compared to those who were not recently
prescribed any antibiotics." Blaser admits it's only an association between antibiotic use and celiac disease. No causal connection. See Martin J. Blaser, *Missing
Microbes: How the Overuse of Antibiotics Is Fueling Our Modern Plagues* (New York:
Henry Holt and Co., 2014), 175.

144   *"El Niagara en Bicicleta"*   Juan Luis Guerra, "Juan Luis Guerra—El niagara en
bicicleta," YouTube video, 4:02, January 10, 2007, https://www.youtube.com
/watch?v=b4i7tbqkWp4. A translation into English of the Spanish lyrics can be
found at Miley Lovato, ed., "El Niagara en Bicicleta (English translation)," April 27,
2016, https://lyricstranslate.com/en/el-niagara-en-bicicleta-niagara-falls-bicycle.
html.

145   *Albutt Einstein, Dumpledore, Vladimir Pootin, and Winnie the Poo*   Emily Eakin,
"The Excrement Experiment: Treating Disease with Fecal Transplants," *New
Yorker*, December 1, 2014, http://www.newyorker.com/magazine/2014/12/01
/excrement-experiment.

146   *A 2013 Dutch study*   Blaser, *Missing Microbes*, 212–13. See also Rob Knight with
Brendan Buhler, *Follow Your Gut: The Enormous Impact of Tiny Microbes* (New York:
Simon and Schuster, 2015), 69. Knight also reports on a study he did with others at
the University of Minnesota that showed that within a few days after fecal transfer, symptoms vanished.

146   *"It's the closest thing to a miracle I've seen in medicine"*   Zain Kassam, cited in Eakin, "Excrement Experiment."

147   *"Like a lion escaped from the zoo"*   Blaser, *Missing Microbes*, 188.

147   *The inspired figures (at the time grad students at MIT)*   See the OpenBiome web
page, a fine example of lucidity and transparency: http://www.openbiome.org.

148   *a kind of Red Cross for poop*   Eakin, "Excrement Experiment."

148   *"we don't yet know if this altered behavior is caused by the body's immune
response . . ."*   Knight and Buhler, *Follow Your Gut*, 40.

CHAPTER 42. A LION'S ROAR

157   "How to move from whining . . ."   Gretel C. Kovach, "Pastor Exhorts Married Cou-
ples to Have More Sex," New York Times, October 24, 2008, https://www.nytimes
.com/2008/11/24/world/americas/24iht-24sex.18094364.html.

CHAPTER 43. THE ECOLOGY OF CANCER, AND WHAT DO ANTS
HAVE TO DO WITH IT?

158   When I heard Deborah Gordon   In her talk "The Evolution of Collective Behavior
in Ant Colonies," presented as part of "Anthropocene: Arts of Living on a
Damaged Planet," University of California, Santa Cruz, May 8–10, 2014. Now
published as "Without Planning: The Evolution of Collective Behavior in Ant
Colonies," in Arts of Living on a Damaged Planet: Ghosts and Monsters of the Anthropocene, ed. Anna Lowenhaupt Tsing, Heather Anne Swanson, Elaine Gan,
and Nils Bubandt (Minneapolis: University of Minnesota Press, 2017), M125–31.
This paper also draws on her TED talks: "The Emergent Genius of Ant Colonies,"
TED Talks video, 20:22, February 2013, https://www.ted.com/talks/deborah
_gordon_digs_ants?language=en; and "What Ants Teach Us about the Brain,
Cancer and the Internet," TED Talks video, 14:06, March 2014, https://www
.ted.com/talks/deborah_gordon_what_ants_teach_us_about_the_brain
_cancer_and_the_internet?language=en. See also "Deborah Gordon: Why Don't
Ants Need a Leader?," NPR TED Radio Hour video, April 24, 2015, https://www
.npr.org/2015/04/24/401735715/why-don-t-ants-need-a-leader.

160   this is how the great and pioneering ant scholar E. O. Wilson described ant society
"The Social Biology of Ants," Annual Review of Entomology 8 (January 1963):
345–68, https://doi.org/10.1146/annurev.en.08.010163.002021.

161   the researcher group called them "nurse-like cells"   Jan A. Burger, Nobuhiro
Tsukada, Meike Burger, Nathan J. Zvaifler, Marie Dell'Aquila, and Thomas J.
Kipps, "Blood-Derived Nurse-Like Cells Protect Chronic Lymphocytic Leukemia
B Cells from Spontaneous Apoptosis through Stromal Cell–Derived Factor-1,"
Blood 96, no. 8 (October 15, 2000): 2655–63, http://bloodjournal.org/content
/96/8/2655?variant=long.

162   chickens (with whom we share about 60 percent DNA)   National Human Genome
Research Institute, "Researchers Compare Chicken, Human Genomes," NIH News
Release, December 8, 2004, http://www.genome.gov/12514316.

CHAPTER 47. TOUCHED BY A WHALE

175   "mobilizes in him a tenderness akin to vulnerability . . ."   James Hamilton-Paterson,
Seven Tenths: The Sea and Its Thresholds (New York: Europa Editions, 2009), 279.

176   so bitingly satirized by the Australian writer Murray Bail   Homesickness (New York:
Farrar, Straus and Giroux, 1980).

178   *except on two recent occasions*   Carl Zimmer, "Whales on the Wrong Side of the World," *National Geographic*, March 10, 2015, http://phenomena.national geographic.com/2015/03/10/whales-on-the-wrong-side-of-the-world.

178   *Gray whales may be about to move back into the Atlantic*   Amy Wilson, "Whales Behaving Weirdly: Gray Whales Have Wandered into the Atlantic for the First Time in Nearly 300 Years. How Did They Get There?," *Orange County Register*, February 10, 2014, http://www.ocregister.com/articles/whales-600918-gray-whale.html.

179   *"If a Lion could talk we could not understand him"*   Ludwig Wittgenstein, *Philosophical Investigations*, trans. G. E. M. Anscombe (Oxford: Basil Blackwell, 1986), 223.

CHAPTER 49. THE ANSWER IS NOT COMING

182   *"The answer is not coming"*   Rachel Kushner, *The Flamethrowers* (New York: Scribner, 2013), 383.

CHAPTER 50. NIGHTCLUB BOUNCERS

185   *Fine Gardening*   Jeff Gillman, "Setting the Record Straight on Glyphosate," *Fine Gardening*, November/December 2013, 56–59.

185   *between 1987 and 2012, according to* National Geographic   Elizabeth Grossman, "What Do We Really Know about Roundup Weed Killer?," *National Geographic*, April 23, 2015, http://news.nationalgeographic.com/2015/04/150422-glyphosate -roundup-herbicide-weeds.

186   *a simple video . . . of how herbicides like Roundup work*   Amro Hamdoun, "How Do Our Bodies Fight Off Dangerous Chemicals?," MSN video, 2:22, February 24, 2015, http://www.msn.com/en-us/video/watch/how-do-our-bodies-fight-off -dangerous-chemicals/vp-BBi4p07.

CHAPTER 51. ALL NATURAL

187   *Each person in this country*   These statistics are taken from the website of the National Chicken Council, the trade association for the companies that raise broiler chickens and make and market chicken products. These companies provide about 95 percent of the chicken, as they say, "on America's table." See "Broiler Chicken Industry Key Facts 2019," National Chicken Council, accessed November 19, 2019, http://www.nationalchickencouncil.org/about-the-industry/statistics /broiler-chicken-industry-key-facts.

188   Chicken, *by Annie Potts*   (London: Reaktion Books, 2012).

188   *Val Plumwood, the Australian ecophilosopher*   "Meeting the Predator," in *The Eye of the Crocodile*, ed. Lorraine Shannon (Canberra: Australian National University, 2012), 9–21.

188   *antibiotics, arsenic, caffeine, and the active ingredients in Benadryl*   "Whole Chickens," *Cooks Illustrated*, September 2012, http://www.cooksillustrated.com /tastetests/overview.asp?docid=38414&extcode=L3HN4AA00.

188   The broiler industry produces billions of pounds of feathers   Potts, *Chicken*, 170.

188   *Cannibals, wrote Montaigne*   "On the Cannibals," in *The Complete Essays*, trans. M. A. Screech (London: Penguin, 2004), 482.

188   *America's Test Kitchen has an excellent report*   See "Whole Chickens."

CHAPTER 52. ANZA BORREGO

191   *"Certain desert areas have a distinctive and subtle charm . . ."*   Frederick Law Olmsted Jr., "Report of State Park Survey of California," *San Diego Union*, October 12, 1938, B1; cited in Diana Lindsay, "History in the California Desert," *San Diego Historical Society Quarterly* 19, no. 4 (Fall 1973): n.p., https://sandiegohistory.org/journal/1973/october/anza.

195   *In 1998 the U.S. Fish and Wildlife Service (USFWS) listed this population segment as an endangered species*   Janene Colby and Randy Botta, "Peninsular Bighorn Sheep Annual Report 2014," California Department of Fish and Wildlife, accessed November 19, 2019, https://nrm.dfg.ca.gov/FileHandler.ashx?DocumentID =97891&inline.

195   *"attentive shepherds"*   Ellen Meloy, *Eating Stone: Imagination and the Loss of the Wild* (New York: Pantheon, 2005), 9.

195   *Helen Macdonald writes*   "Flight Paths," *New York Times Magazine*, May 15, 2015, http://www.nytimes.com/2015/05/17/magazine/flight-paths.html?_r=0.

CHAPTER 55. STINGING NETTLES

205   *"the low level of research that continued on thalidomide . . ."*   "Lenalidomide," Wikipedia, accessed November 20, 2019, https://en.wikipedia.org/wiki/Lenalidomide.

208   *"E. E. Evans-Pritchard, in his study of the magic practices . . ."*   Page Smith and Charles Daniel, *The Chicken Book* (Athens: University of Georgia Press, 2000), 32.

209   *"antibiotics are essentially poisons . . ."*   Rob Knight with Brendan Buhler, *Follow Your Gut: The Enormous Impact of Tiny Microbes* (New York: Simon and Schuster, 2015), 75.

209   *"Alternatively, you could say the microbes . . ."*   Ed Yong, *I Contain Multitudes: The Microbes within Us and a Grander View of Life* (New York: HarperCollins, 2016), 91.

210   *"They are harmless if they stay in the gut . . ."*   Yong, *I Contain Multitudes*, 80–81, based on research by Nichole Broderick.

211   *"They live to infect and reproduce . . ."*   Siddhartha Mukherjee, *The Gene: An Intimate History* (New York: Scribner, 2016), 204.

CHAPTER 56. A TALENT FOR CANCER

212   *"My relative examined you"*   Octavia Butler, *Dawn* (New York: Warner Books, 1987), 22.

212   *cancer is as old as time*   Paul Davies says, "Scientists have identified genes implicated in cancer that are thought to be hundreds of millions of years old. Clearly,

we will fully understand cancer only in the context of biological history." He and Charles Lineweaver have proposed a theory of cancer based on its ancient evolutionary roots. See Davies, "Cancer Can Teach Us about Our Own Evolution," *Guardian*, November 18, 2012, http://www.theguardian.com/commentisfree/2012/nov/18/cancer-evolution-bygone-biological-age.

213   *but as Donna Haraway has written*   "Sowing Worlds: A Seed Bag for Terraforming with Earth Others," epilogue to *Beyond the Cyborg: Adventures with Donna Haraway*, ed. Margret Grebowicz and Helen Merrick (New York: Columbia University Press, 2013), 138.

CHAPTER 57. PHOBIA: THE CHICKENS COME HOME TO ROOST

214   *"Now take your average brain tumor"*   I quote myself here. This is from an earlier book where it is a joke. Lesley Stern, *The Smoking Book* (Chicago: University of Chicago Press, 1999).

216   *She even wrote a book*   Lesley Stern, *The Scorsese Connection* (London: British Film Institute; Bloomington: Indiana University Press, 1995).

CHAPTER 58. WALKING MEDITATION

219   *"When I walk alone . . ."*   Michel de Montaigne, "When I Walk Alone," in *Essays: Montaigne, The Complete Works*, vol. 3, ed. and trans. Donald Frame (London: Everyman, 2005), 1036, quoted in Sarah Bakewell, *How to Live, or A Life of Montaigne in One Question and Twenty Attempts at an Answer* (New York: Other Press, 2010), 38.

CHAPTER 60. REACHING YIRRKALA

230   *"The care of returned materials . . ."*   Australian Government, Parks Australia, "Sorry Rocks: Fact Sheet, Uluru–Kata Tjuta National Park," accessed November 21, 2019, http://www.environment.gov.au/system/files/resources/a44a0273-2b69-4c90-8067-87c8ecf80139/files/uktnp-a4factsheet-sorryrocks-small.pdf.

235   *generated out of a key ancestral story embedded in the site*   My thanks to Will Stubbs, via Ruark Lewis, for this description. See also the biographical note by Will Stubbs, "Yarrinya: Barayuwa Mununggurr," Art Gallery of New South Wales, accessed November 22, 2019, https://www.artgallery.nsw.gov.au/collection/works/248.2015. Later iterations of this installation exist, for instance, in the MCA, Sydney.

236   *The linear design of Ruark's drawings resonate*   Jane O'Sullivan, "Undiscovered: Barayuwa Mununggurr," *Art Collector*, no. 68 (April–June 2014): n.p., https://janeosullivan.com.au/2014/07/08/undiscovered-barayuwa-mununggurr. See also Noelene Cole and Alice Buhrich, "Endangered Rock Art: Forty Years of Cultural Heritage Management in the Quinkan Region, Cape York Peninsula," *Australian Archeology*, no. 75 (December 2012): 66–77, https://researchonline.jcu.edu.au

/24268/1/cole%26buhrich_2012.pdf; and Julie Marcus, "Pink, Olive Muriel (1884–1975)," *Australian Dictionary of Biography*, vol. 16 (Melbourne: Melbourne University Press, 2002), http://adb.anu.edu.au/biography/pink-olive-muriel-11428.

239 *"What's important is that they should be in the same space"* Sylvia Lawson, *How Simone de Beauvoir Died in Australia* (Kensington, AU: UNSW Press, 2002), 31.

239 *leveled at the museum for building the show around stolen objects* Particularly by Zoe Pilger, John Pilger's daughter.

240 Quinkan Country P. J. Trezise, *Quinkan Country: Adventures in Search of Aboriginal Cave Paintings in Cape York* (Sydney: Reed, 1969). See also P. J. Trezise, *Rock Art of South-East Cape York*, Australian Aboriginal Studies, no. 24 (Canberra: Australian Institute of International Affairs, 1971).

244 *"What we learn..."* Writing in the "Guide to the Olive Pink Botanic Garden," 5, Alice Springs Town Council, http://www.alicesprings.nt.gov.au/events/2014-11-05 /guide-olive-pink-botanic-garden-launch.

244 *The ghost of Lévi-Strauss* Claude Lévi-Strauss, *Tristes Tropiques*, trans. John and Doreen Weightman (Harmondsworth, U.K.: Penguin, 1992).

CHAPTER 62. CHICKEN SHIT

246 *There is a Shambhala saying* Chögyam Trungpa Rinpoche, *Training the Mind and Cultivating Loving Kindness* (Boston: Shambhala, 1993), 150. Slogan: "Work with the greatest defilements first."

246 *"Habit is the ballast..."* Samuel Beckett, *Proust* (New York: New Directions, 1931), 7–8.

248 *"...his certitudes perched like fat chickens"* J. G. Farrell, *The Siege of Krishnapur* (New York: New York Review Books, 1973), 211.

CHAPTER 63. MIMETIC PAIN

253 *The Essays falls open on a passage about the power of speech* Michel de Montaigne, "An Apology for Raymond Sebond," in *The Complete Essays*, trans. M. A. Screech (London: Penguin, 2004), 512.

253 *That reminds me of a film, El Circo* Directed by Miguel M. Delgado (Mexico, 1943). My thanks to Patricia Montoya for drawing my attention to this film and indeed to so many Mexican films.

CHAPTER 64. YOU ARE MOSTLY NOT YOU

254 *the human genome has about twenty-three thousand genes* Martin J. Blaser, *Missing Microbes: How the Overuse of Antibiotics Is Fueling Our Modern Plagues* (New York: Henry Holt and Co., 2014), 35.

255 *If you take a group of people* Curtis Huttenhower from the Harvard School of Public Health, commenting on the findings of the Human Microbiome Project when they were released in June 2012. See Ed Yong, "Microbial Menagerie," *The Scien-*

tist, June 13, 2012, http://www.the-scientist.com/?articles.view/articleNo/32215
/title/Microbial-Menagerie.

255 "*Animals and plants are far more similar . . .*" Lynn Margulis, *Symbiotic Planet: A New Look at Evolution* (New York: Basic Books, 1998), 56.

255 "*You do not of course you do not . . .*" Gertrude Stein, *Everybody's Autobiography* (London: Virago, 1985), 85.

256 "*The human body isn't just what you see in the mirror . . .*" Lita Proctor, director of the National Institute of Health's Human Microbiome Project, cited in Rebecca Jacobson, "Can We Save Our Body's Ecosystem from Extinction?," *Science*, April 23, 2014, http://www.pbs.org/newshour/updates/theres-extinction -happening-stomach.

256 "*microbes don't just 'rule' the world . . .*" Margaret McFall-Ngai, "Noticing Microbial Worlds: The Postmodern Synthesis in Biology," in *Arts of Living on a Damaged Planet: Ghosts and Monsters of the Anthropocene*, ed. Anna Lowenhaupt Tsing, Heather Anne Swanson, Elaine Gan, and Nils Bubandt (Minneapolis: University of Minnesota Press, 2017), M59.

256 "*They sentenced me to twenty years of boredom . . .*" Leonard Cohen, "First We Take Manhattan," track 1 on *I'm Your Man* (Columbia, 1988).

256 "*a symbiotic, interactive view of the history of life on Earth*" Lynn Margulis and Dorion Sagan, *Microcosmos: Four Billion Years of Microbial Evolution* (Los Angeles: University of California Press, 1997), 16.

257 "*There are no 'higher' beings . . .*" Margulis, *Symbiotic Planet*, 3.

257 *In the past scientists focused their attention* Michael Pollan, *Cooked: A Natural History of Transformation* (New York: Penguin, 2013), 323.

257 "*not a marginal or rare phenomenon . . .*" Margulis, *Symbiotic Planet*, 9.

257 *the imagined autonomy of the individual* "Beyond Individuals," in Tsing et al., *Arts of Living*, M71.

257 *A major engine of accelerated adaptation* Stewart Brand, "Rethinking Extinction," ed. Ross Andersen, *Aeon*, April 21, 2015, http://aeon.co/magazine/science/why -extinction-is-not-the-problem.

257 "*Genes are jumping around*" Chris Thomas, a conservation biologist at York University, U.K., cited in Brand, "Rethinking Extinction."

257 *During the birth process* Scott F. Gilbert, "Holobiont by Birth: Multilineage Individuals as the Concretion of Cooperative Processes," in Tsing et al., *Arts of Living*, M73–89.

258 "*In reality the tree of life . . .*" Margulis, *Symbiotic Planet*, 52.

258 "*So while mothers nourish this microbe . . .*" Ed Yong, *I Contain Multitudes: The Microbes within Us and a Grander View of Life* (New York: HarperCollins, 2016), 95.

258 *Sea otters, by eating sea urchins* James A. Estes and John F. Palmisano, "Sea Otters: Their Role in Structuring Nearshore Communities," *Science* 185 (1974): 1058–60; cited in Ingrid M. Parker, "Remembering in Our Amnesia, Seeing in Our Blindness," in Tsing et al., *Arts of Living*, M164.

258 *As Gregory Bateson famously said* in "Form, Substance, and Difference," in *Steps to an Ecology of Mind: Collected Essays in Anthropology, Psychiatry, Evolution, and Epistemology* (Chicago: University of Chicago Press, 1972).

259 *"And now, both poets and scientists . . ."* Ursula K. Le Guin, "Deep in Admiration," in Tsing et al., *Arts of Living*, M15.

CHAPTER 65. RIP ELVIS, THE KING OF THE CATS

260 Michel de Montaigne "On Cruelty (1595)," in *The Complete Essays*, trans. M. A. Screech (London: Penguin, 2004), 487.

CHAPTER 66. AFTERLIFE

265 *"When I play with my cat . . ."* Michel de Montaigne, "An Apology for Raymond Sebond," in *The Complete Essays*, trans. M. A. Screech (London: Penguin, 2004), 505.

265 *"Drizzled with sadness"* Manohla Dargis, "Review: 'Heart of a Dog,' Laurie Anderson's Meditation on Loss," *New York Times*, October 20, 2015, https://www.nytimes.com/2015/10/21/movies/review-heart-of-a-dog-laurie-andersons-meditation-on-loss.html.

266 *As Chögyam Trungpa Rinpoche points out* See Rinpoche, *Training the Mind and Cultivating Loving Kindness* (Boston: Shambhala, 1993).

267 *"Florence, which I visited after New York . . ."* Lévi-Strauss, *Tristes Tropiques*, trans. John and Doreen Weightman (Harmondsworth, U.K.: Penguin, 1992), 408–15.

CHAPTER 68. BODIES IN PIECES

273 *Tershia's book* Tershia d'Elgin, *The Man Who Thought He Owned Water: On the Brink with American Farms, Cities, and Food* (Boulder: University Press of Colorado, 2016).

274 *"when that revolution was over, France would never be dominated by an absolutist monarchy again . . ."* Rebecca Solnit, *A Paradise Built in Hell: The Extraordinary Communities That Arise in Disaster* (New York: Penguin, 2009), 19.

CHAPTER 70. FIG FUTURE

279 *"But I have dug fifty-six large holes . . ."* Samuel Beckett to Barney Rosset, *The Letters of Samuel Beckett*, vol. 1: *1929–1940*, ed. Martha Dow Fehsenfeld and Lois More Overbeck (New York: Cambridge University Press, 2009), 608.

CHAPTER 71. BETWEEN FRESH AND ROTTEN

280 *"Between fresh and rotten there is a creative space . . ."* Sandor Ellix Katz, *The Art of Fermentation: An In-Depth Exploration of Essential Concepts and Processes from around the World* (White River Junction, VT: Chelsea Green, 2012), 35.

283 *He was, as Harold McGee says, "prescient"* On Food and Cooking: The Science and Lore of the Kitchen (New York: Scribner, 2004), 47.

283 *"Particular strains of these bacteria . . ."* McGee, *On Food and Cooking*, 47.

283 *a series of articles, later condensed in* I Contain Multitudes Ed Yong, *I Contain Multitudes: The Microbes within Us and a Grander View of Life* (New York: Harper-Collins, 2016), 221.

283 *And other doubting voices were raised* For instance, Martin J. Blaser, *Missing Microbes: How the Overuse of Antibiotics Is Fueling Our Modern Plagues* (New York: Henry Holt and Co., 2014), 210–12.

285 *when I see a film that sets sparks flying* *Pastori di Orgosolo*, directed by Vittorio De Seta (Italy, 1958).

285 *Every pastoral since* Gilgamesh Brad Kessler, *Goat Song: A Seasonal Life, a Short History of Herding, and the Art of Making Cheese* (New York: Scribner, 2009), 198.

287 *Enzymes extracted from the flowers of two plants* Paul S. Kindstedt, "The Basics of Cheesemaking," in *Cheese and Microbes*, ed. Catherine W. Donnelly (Burlington: Vermont Institute of Artisan Cheese and the University of Vermont, 2014).

288 *The company characterizes it as a "dramatically provocative . . ."* Michelle Nijhuis, "The Book That Colored Charles Darwin's World," *New Yorker*, January 27, 2018, https://www.newyorker.com/tech/elements/the-book-that-colored -charles-darwins-world.

288 *A much more ingenious method of recycling whey* Noella Marcellino and David R. Benson, "The Good, the Bad, and the Ugly: Tales of Mold-Ripened Cheese," in Donnelly, *Cheese and Microbes*.

289 *Michael Pollan would say* *Cooked: A Natural History of Transformation* (New York: Penguin, 2013), 360; see also "Earth," episode 4 of the Netflix documentary series *Cooked*, created by Alex Gibney and Michael Pollan, which aired February 19, 2016, https://michaelpollan.com/uncategorized/netflix-documentary-series -cooked.

290 *home to a fast-growing community of immunotechnology drug developers* Esther and Andrew Schorr have already started working with some of these pharmaceutical companies to bring together researchers and patients with the goal of speeding up clinical trials. See Pam Kragen, "Carlsbad Couple Shedding Light on Rare Cancers," *San Diego Union Tribune*, January 13, 2017, https://www.sandiegounion tribune.com/communities/north-county/sd-no-patient-power-20170105-story.html.

290 *Rob Knight, cofounder of the Human Gut Project* American Gut Project, University of California San Diego, accessed November 26, 2019, http://americangut.org /about.

290 *"The reason I'm so interested in food microbes"* Rachel Dutton, "72 Ways Food Can Change the World," *Eater*, accessed November 26, 2019, https://www.eater.com /a/72-ways-food-can-change-the-world/rachel-dutton, 41.

291 *Articles about her have appeared in the* New York Times Peter Andrey Smith, "For Gastronomists, a Go-To Microbiologist," *New York Times*, September 17, 2012, https://www.nytimes.com/2012/09/19/dining/for-gastronomists-a-go-to -microbiologist.html.

291 *Dutton and Wolfe had shown that the environment* Larissa Zimberoff, "Small Cheese Makers Invest in a Stinky Science," *New York Times*, February 6, 2017,

https://www.nytimes.com/2017/02/06/dining/jasper-hill-farm-cheese-science .html?_r=o.

292 *As a post-pastoralist*   Heather Paxson, *The Life of Cheese: Crafting Food and Value in America* (Los Angeles: University of California Press, 2013). Paxson calls Kehler and other contemporary U.S. artisanal cheesemakers, who combine traditional dairying with scientific acumen and resources, post-Pasteurian and post-pastoral.

292 *"Tamie thus is a cheese . . ."*   Marcellino and Benson, "The Good, the Bad, and the Ugly," 121.

292 *Using the cheese rind microbiome as a model system*   Kevin S. Bonham, Benjamin E. Wolfe, and Rachel J. Dutton, "Extensive Horizontal Gene Transfer in Cheese-Associated Bacteria," *eLife*, June 23, 2017, https://elifesciences.org/articles/22144.

293 *wooden vats, a reservoir of microbial biodiversity*   For this argument, see Sylvie Lortal, Giuseppe Licitra, and Florence Valence, "Wooden Tools: Reservoirs of Microbial Biodiversity in Traditional Cheesemaking," *Microbiology Spectrum* 2, no. 1 (January 2014): 1–8, doi:10.1128/microbiolspec.CM-0008-2012. See also Bronwen Percival and Francis Percival, *Reinventing the Wheel: Milk, Microbes, and the Fight for Real Cheese* (Oakland: University of California Press, 2017).

293 *Sister Noella says*   Gibney and Pollan, "Earth."

CHAPTER 77. THE STRUCTURE THAT A LIFE HAS

310 *"it seems to me that the state of this country . . ."*   David Antin, *john cage uncaged is still cagey* (San Diego: Singing Horse Press, 2005), 56.

310 *"how do I build something . . ."*   Antin, *john cage uncaged is still cagey*, 71.

CHAPTER 79. THE MALVOLIO GENE

315 *Where do the chickens we know today come from?*   Jonas Eriksson, Greger Larson, Ulrika Gunnarsson, Bertrand Bed'hom, Michele Tixier-Boichard, Lina Strömstedt, Dominic Wright, et al., "Identification of the Yellow Skin Gene Reveals a Hybrid Origin of the Domestic Chicken," *Public Library of Science (PLOS) Genetics* 4, no. 2 (February 29, 2008): n.p., https://journals.plos.org/plosgenetics/article?id=10.1371 /journal.pgen.1000010.

315 *complicating the debate that began with Darwin and Dixon*   Darwin kept chickens in his backyard and was intrigued by the question of inheritance they posed. He brought together his own experience of domestic relations with a theoretically elaborated account of the origin of the species. The Rev. Edmund Saul Dixon, author of *Ornamental and Domestic Poultry: Their History and Management*, challenged Darwin's proposal that species can be traced to a single origin, specifically that domestic chickens are descended from a wild bird, because this suggests that species are mutable, that they might change. The Christian view of evolution was that God created each species as distinct and immutable. See Dixon, *Ornamental and Domestic Poultry: Their History and Management*, cited in Andrew Lawler, *Why*

Did the Chicken Cross the World? The Epic Saga of the Bird That Powers Civilizations (New York: Atria Books, 2014), 136.

316　"*Tyrannosaurus rex Basically a Big Chicken*"　Cited in Lawler, *Why Did the Chicken*, 158–59.

316　*Either way, African multiregionalism*　Ed Yong, "The New Story of Humanity's Origins in Africa," *Atlantic*, July 11, 2018, https://www.theatlantic.com/science /archive/2018/07/the-new-story-of-humanitys-origins/564779.

CHAPTER 81. CHIMERA

320　"*The invincible . . .*"　Homer, *The Iliad*, trans. Peter Green (Los Angeles: University of California Press, 2015), 124, lines 179–82.

320　"*Let's make America the country that cures cancer, once and for all*"　Barack Obama, "Obama: 'Let's Make America the Country That Cures Cancer,'" PBS News Hour, YouTube video, 1:17, January 12, 2016, https://www.youtube.com/watch?v =EJDyBBGncQc.

320　*In December of that year a full-page advertisement*　Siddhartha Mukherjee, *The Emperor of All Maladies: A Biography of Cancer* (New York: Scribner, 2010), 180–81.

322　*Some, like Paul Davies, have even proposed*　Davies, "Cancer Can Teach Us about Our Own Evolution," *Guardian*, November 18, 2012, http://www.theguardian.com /commentisfree/2012/nov/18/cancer-evolution-bygone-biological-age.

322　*He and Charles Lineweaver propose an understanding of cancer*　Paul Charles William Davies and Charles H. Lineweaver, "Cancer Tumors as Metazoa 1.0: Tapping Genes of Ancient Ancestors," *Physical Biology* 8, no. 1 (February 7, 2011): n.p., http://iopscience.iop.org/article/10.1088/1478-3975/8/1/015001.

323　*In the early 1890s a bone sarcoma surgeon*　I'm grateful to Dr. Castro for alerting me to this historical dimension in his talks to our patient education group at UCSD.

324　*One way the immune system attacks foreign substances*　See American Cancer Society, "Monoclonal Antibodies and Their Side Effects," accessed November 27, 2019, https://www.cancer.org/treatment/treatments-and-side-effects/treatment-types /immunotherapy/monoclonal-antibodies.html.

325　*Researchers identified a mouse antibody*　Emma Stokes, "From Mouse to Monkey to Humans: The Story of Rituximab," *Speaking of Research*, accessed November 27, 2019, https://speakingofresearch.com/2009/07/13/from-mouse-to-monkey-to -humans-the-story-of-rituximab.

326　*the "darling" of current research*　CLL Society, "E.R.I.C. Barcelona European Research Initiative on CLL October 2018: Dr. Cameron Turtle on CAR-T Therapy," November 6, 2018, https://cllsociety.org/2018/11/e-r-i-c-barcelona-european -research-initiative-on-cll-october-2018-dr-cameron-turtle-on-car-t-therapy.

326　"*turning the wrath of the immune system against cancer . . .*"　Denise Grady, "Harnessing the Immune System to Fight Cancer," *New York Times*, July 30, 2016, https://www.nytimes.com/2016/07/31/health/harnessing-the-immune-system-to -fight-cancer.html.

327 *"No bells rang . . ."* Brian Koffman, "DAY ZERO: CAR-T cells are aboard and getting ready to seek out and destroy all my CLL (chronic lymphocytic leukemia) cells," CAR-T blog, March 22, 2018, https://cllsociety.org/2018/03/day-zero-car-t -cells-aboard-getting-ready-seek-destroy-cll-chronic-lymphocytic-leukemia-cells/.

327 *"We've been in touch . . ."* Heather Koffman, "DAY +7 Post CAR-T," CAR-T blog, March 29, 2018, https://cllsociety.org/2018/03/day-7.

328 *groups like the CLL Society* See the CLL Society and Patient Power websites, cllsociety.org and https://www.patientpower.info.

329 *By 1976, Steingraber says, sixty-two thousand synthetic chemicals* Sandra Steingraber, *Living Downstream: An Ecologist's Personal Investigation of Cancer and the Environment* (Philadelphia: Da Capo, 2010), 101.

329 *New research projects* For example, the Halifax project. See Ronald Piana, "The Halifax Project: A New Approach to Combination Therapy," September 25, 2016, accessed January 20, 2020, https://www.ascopost.com/issues/september-25-2016 /the-halifax-project-a-new-approach-to-combination-therapy/.

330 *"Some tinker with our hormones . . ."* Steingraber, *Living Downstream*, 94.

331 *Scott Pruitt, has reversed or indefinitely postponed* Scott Faber, "Scott Pruitt Has Literally Made Washington—and America—More Toxic," Environmental Working Group, April 4, 2018, https://www.ewg.org/news-and-analysis/2018/04/scott-pruitt -has-literally-made-washington-and-america-more-toxic#.WslEvC-ZNvc.

332 *"Most Americans," he writes, "don't like to think . . ."* Paul Stoller, *Stranger in the Village of the Sick: A Memoir of Cancer, Sorcery, and Healing* (Boston: Beacon, 2004), 39.

334 *Every "I" is also a "we"* Margaret McFall-Ngai, "Noticing Microbial Worlds: The Postmodern Synthesis in Biology," in *Arts of Living on a Damaged Planet: Ghosts and Monsters of the Anthropocene*, ed. Anna Lowenhaupt Tsing, Heather Anne Swanson, Elaine Gan, and Nils Bubandt (Minneapolis: University of Minnesota Press, 2017), M52.

CHAPTER 83. ARRIVEDERCI

338 *"Arrivederci, come le volpi in pellicceria"* Charles Nicholl, "Unliterary, Unpolished, Unromantic," *London Review of Books* 40, no. 3 (February 2018): 7–10, https:// www.lrb.co.uk/v40/n03/charles-nicholl/unliterary-unpolished-unromantic.

341 *Nietzsche's proposition* Friedrich Nietzsche, *The Gay Science*, trans. Walter Kaufmann (New York: Vintage, 1974).

341 *A contemporary classicist, Emily Wilson* *The Death of Socrates* (Cambridge, MA: Harvard University Press, 2007).

CPSIA information can be obtained
at www.ICGtesting.com
Printed in the USA
FSHW020856060221
78408FS